THE NEUROBEHAVIORAL TREATMENT OF EPILEPSY

THE NEUROBEHAVIORAL TREATMENT OF EPILEPSY

Edited by

David I. Mostofsky
Boston University

Yngve Løyning
The National Center for Epilepsy, Norway

LEA LAWRENCE ERLBAUM ASSOCIATES, PUBLISHERS
1993 Hillsdale, New Jersey Hove and London

Lawrence Erlbaum Associates, Inc., Publishers
365 Broadway
Hillsdale, New Jersey 07642

Library of Congress Cataloging-in-Publication Data

The Neurobehavioral treatment of epilepsy / edited by David I. Mostofsky, Yngve Løyning.
p. cm.
Includes bibliographical references and index.
ISBN 0-8058-1106-0
1. Epilepsy—Psychological aspects. 2. Behavior therapy.
I. Mostofsky, David I. II. Løyning, Yngve.
[DNLM: 1. Behavior Therapy. 2. Epilepsy—therapy. WL 385 N49335]
RC372.N38 1993
616.8′5306—dc20
DNLM/DLC
for Library of Congress 92-48966
CIP

Books published by Lawrence Erlbaum Associates are printed on acid-free paper, and their bindings are chosen for strength and durability.

Printed in the United States of America

10 9 8 7 6 5 4 3 2 1

Contents

Preface

Traditionally, a volume concerned with the treatment of epilepsy restricts itself to alternatives and options that fall within the confines of pharmacological or surgical protocols. Indeed, the literature on the medical management of the epilepsies is vast, and such works often include reviews of basic neurophysiology and neurochemistry, technical issues of electroencephalography and related recording methodologies, and even animal models. Yet almost without exception, they fail to report the range of behavioral or psychological interventions and therapeutic programs that have been validated scientifically and that are available to contribute to the comprehensive management of epileptic disorders. Such techniques, properly applied, may well lead to significant reductions in the frequency and severity of clinical seizures, perhaps even with concurrent reduction or elimination of abnormal electrical discharges.

The evidence strongly suggests that the inclusion of behavioral methods in a comprehensive treatment program may offer much to the clinical neurologist. At the very least, they foster increased compliance with medication regimens and stem emotional and interpersonal crises that have been shown frequently to exacerbate seizure disorders. Conventionally separated from medical management, the psychological considerations have been relegated to what has become a minor role for clinical neurologists (i.e., enhancing quality of life, teaching a restrictive lifestyle, and monitoring sequelae of the patient's condition on his or her family).

Contemporary neurology had its roots in anecdotal and clinical lore, which made frequent reference to the interplay of body and mind. Yet, paradoxically, many medical practitioners now express a seemingly hostile attitude toward theories and techniques that appear to them to stray from the path. Remarkably, it is forgotten that Gowers (1901), a giant in epileptology, had no such compunctions when he advocated *limb ligation* to arrest seizures, for which there was empirical evidence dating back to the 17th century, but no scientific support.[1] The academic training of most neurologists fosters a rigid dualism and a curious reluctance to examine controversial findings. This has resulted in few collaborations with other behavioral sciences—to the detriment of all, especially the seizure sufferer.

Nevertheless, an increasing number of these patients, on their own initiative, are seeking professional assistance from unconventional quarters. Increasing numbers of physicians are now joining the ranks of psychologists and other health-care workers who are scrutinizing the claims, promises, and limitations of these options. It is to their great credit, as well as to that of the many agencies, foundations, and hospitals, that such research has been pursued for some years, now resulting in a growing number of cases and a change of attitude among even the most hard-core nonbelievers. To be sure, there have been notable exceptions when illustrious neurologists and clinics have embraced and fought for the inclusion of behavioral strategies in their epilepsy clinical services, but their numbers are small.

The efforts of nontraditionalists are beginning to gain acceptance by the weight of their demonstrated successes, achieved most often in the face of patients intractable to surgery and/or conventional medication. Furthermore, the rapidly expanding neurosciences databases confirm the interactions between the *milieu internal* and the *milieu external*. Such factors as environment, conditioning, and personality, and such functions as thinking, imagining, and even breathing may have a rightful place in the therapeutic armamentarium of clinical epileptology.

This volume is the first of its kind, addressed principally to the professional reader. Although it is not intended to be exhaustive or comprehensive, its aim is to sketch a broad picture of some of the nondrug and nonsurgical treatment strategies with a demonstrated basis in conventional scientific method. Likewise, although it does not include all those who have contributed to the emergence of this exciting new field, it assembles those authors whose seminal work has earned them international reputations.

Our purpose in producing this volume is to provide a state-of-the-art guide to methods and techniques used in the behavioral treatment of epilepsy, and to their basis in theory. We hope that it will catalyze the evolution of their acceptance as standard elements, where appropriate, in the clinical activities of independent practitioners, clinics, and agencies that service those with convulsive disorders.

This book draws on a rich scientific and clinical history, including the bio-

[1]Gowers, W. R. (1901). *Epilepsy and other chronic convulsive diseases*. Philadelphia, PA: P. Blakiston's Sons.

psychological links to epilepsy described by such early pioneers as Hughlings Jackson and William Lennox. Giants in this field, they fueled the courage of those who later conducted clinical investigative programs, such as those of the Seizure Unit at Boston Children's Hospital and the Norwegian National Center for Epilepsy, whose programs are notable for their humane and insightful concepts. All those who trained at such institutions were imbued with a special sensitivity to multidisciplinary treatment options.

The last 20 years, especially, have witnessed a dramatic increase in interest in biobehavioral approaches to the management of convulsive disorders, and a number of influential scientific journals have published comprehensive reviews of ongoing research and clinical applications. The creation of an international *interest group,* whose name was adopted as the title of this book, attests to the vitality of this new discipline. We, the editors of this volume, wish to express our warmest thanks to our many colleagues from all disciplines. We are particularly grateful to Peter Fenwick and Joanne Dahl for their encouragement of this project, and for their vigorous promotion of this topic area at international meetings. To them, and to the many others whose encouragement and advice made this book a valuable and appreciated addition to the epilepsy literature, we are most grateful.

—David I. Mostofsky
—Yngve Løyning

1 Sensorimotor EEG Feedback Training in the Study and Treatment of Epilepsy

M. B. Sterman
Veterans Administration Medical Center, Sepulveda, and UCLA School of Medicine

BACKGROUND

For the past three decades, my laboratory has investigated the nature, origin, and functional significance of both normal and pathological electroencephalographic (EEG) patterns in sensorimotor cortex. EEG studies in behaving animals supported the fact that well-defined rhythmic patterns, which appear in this area of cortex during immobility or after experimental interruption of afferent somatosensory pathways, are generated by gated ventrobasal thalamocortical volleys (Bowersox & Sterman, 1981; Harper & Sterman, 1972; Howe & Sterman, 1972; Shouse & Sterman, 1979; Sterman & Wyrwicka, 1967). This work with behaving animals was consistent with earlier findings based primarily on acute preparations and summarized comprehensively by the important conceptual treatise of Andersen and Andersson (1968). The dominant intrinsic thalamocortical 12–15 c/sec frequency was exclusive to alert but motionless waking states. Both the frequency and general distribution of this activity was similar to the well-known "spindle burst" seen during non-REM sleep. In deference to function, we labeled this band the *Sensorimotor Rhythm,* or SMR.

In a novel series of behavioral studies, we found that cats and monkeys could be trained to facilitate this 12–15 c/sec activity through the application of operant conditioning techniques (Sterman, Goodman, & Kovalesky, 1978; Wyrwicka & Sterman, 1968). Perhaps the most interesting aspect of this work was the serendipitous discovery that both cats and monkeys trained behaviorally to enhance the SMR were subsequently resistant to seizures induced by the injection of convulsant hydrazine compounds (Sterman, 1973; Sterman, LoPresti, & Fairchild, 1969; Sterman, Goodman, & Kovalesky, 1978).

A series of studies focusing on the neurophysiological basis for this effect showed that specific changes in somatosensory and motor excitability accompanied trained SMR activity. In particular, attenuation of somatic afferent discharge, related thalamic sensory relay transmission, and efferent motor and striate muscle activity were all seen in strict relationship to the appearance of this pattern in the sensorimotor EEG (see review by Sterman & Bowersox, 1981). Additionally, EEG dynamics indicated that physiological and pharmacological manipulations that facilitated SMR activity were associated with a corresponding decrease in slower 4–7 c/sec rhythmic patterns (Bowersox & Sterman, 1981; Sterman & Kovalesky, 1983). The opposite effects had been reported in epileptogenic conditions, where experimentally produced increases in cortical excitability replaced normal rhythmic EEG patterns with such slower frequencies and, ultimately, with spike-and-wave discharge (Gloor, Pellegrini, & Kostopoulos, 1979).

Collectively, these and other findings led us to propose that epileptogenic pathology involving motor manifestations is generically associated with a disturbance of normal sensorimotor regulation, with a consequent disturbance of conductive patterns and associated EEG manifestations. Under these circumstances, influences that further increase intracortical excitability and/or alter thalamocortical interactions (i.e., drowsiness, slow-wave sleep, metabolic changes, etc.) facilitate abnormal patterns as well as ictal and interictal discharge. Conversely, influences that decrease intracortical excitability and/or stabilize normal thalamocortical interactions attenuate abnormal discharge. Thus, EEG feedback training directed to an enhancement of normal thalamocortical regulation could potentially support the latter effect and increase seizure threshold.

In extending these investigations to man, we observed the so-called "wicket" or "mu" rhythm in the sensorimotor EEG during motor quiescence, as described earlier by Gastaut (1952) and Chatrian, Petersen, & Lazarte, (1959), among others. However, our analyses were dominated by quantitative rather than visual methods. Bandpass and spectral analysis techniques disclosed frequency components not clearly seen with visual scrutiny and confirmed the presence of sensorimotor patterns similar to those seen in our animal work (Sterman, 1977; Sterman, Macdonald, & Stone, 1974). However, the limitations of scalp rather than direct cortical recording and voltage differences in the human EEG made this higher frequency pattern difficult to observe visually. Operant conditioning could be used selectively to enhance 12–15 c/sec activity but sleep studies were the most effective means of characterizing changes in this frequency band due to the clear expression of a related pattern during Stage 2 sleep, the sleep spindle. When normal and poorly controlled epileptic subjects were compared in this regard, SMR and sleep-spindle patterns were found to be significantly attenuated and 4–7 c/sec activity increased in the epileptics, particularly when anticonvulsant medication influences were decreased or absent (Sterman, 1977, 1981).

In 1972, we reported our first attempt at EEG feedback-based enhancement of the SMR pattern in a human epileptic patient (Sterman & Friar). Response acquisition was demonstrated over a 3-month period and was accompanied by a dramatic decline in reported seizures. This work was followed by expanded studies in 1974 (Sterman, Macdonald, & Stone), 1978 (Sterman & Macdonald), 1980 (Sterman & Shouse), and 1984 (Sterman). After the 1974 report, we began controlling for nonspecific effects and included noncontingent "placebo" training conditions as well as the suppression of abnormal EEG frequencies, together with enhancement of the SMR in contingent training conditions. Normalization of the EEG and significant seizure reductions were associated exclusively with contingent feedback training and response acquisition in all of these studies (see, for example, Fig. 1.1).

Neuropsychological assessment was included in a study of 24 patients with poorly controlled complex-partial seizure disorders (Lantz & Sterman, 1988). This study confirmed previously reported deficits in psychosocial and cognitive functioning in this population. Additionally, however, specific psychomotor disturbances were documented as well, and these were found to predict success with EEG feedback training. Further, patients who successfully normalized central cortical EEG patterns showed significant improvements in both cognitive and motor functioning. These improvements, unlike psychosocial changes, were specific to successful contingent training in this controlled, crossover design study.

Starting in 1975, many other laboratories began to explore EEG feedback training in relation to epileptic pathology. Numerous reports have appeared in the EEG and neurological literature from other laboratories, all of which documented significant seizure reductions with this approach (Cott, Pavloski, & Black, 1979; Ellertsen & Kløve, 1976; Finley, Smith, & Etherton, 1975; Kaplan, 1975; Kuhlman, 1978; Lubar & Bahler, 1976; Lubar et al., 1981; Quy, Hutt, & Forrest, 1979; Tozzo, Elfner, & May, 1988; Wyler, Lockard, Ward, & Finch, 1976; Wyler, Robbins, & Dodrill, 1979). Controversy arose, of course, over the "active ingredient" in this methodology. Despite the evidence already reviewed and the development of other theoretical explanations for this therapeutic effect (Kuhlman & Kaplan, 1979; Wyler, 1984), profound differences between the clinical epilepsies and animal models, together with the complexities of human epilepsy, have precluded a definitive resolution of this question.

Some clues as to mechanism were provided by a preliminary study of complex-partial seizure patients who were candidates for neurosurgical treatment involving resection of anterior temporal lobe tissues (Sterman & Bloomfield, 1987). During Phase 2 of the neurosurgical protocol, these patients had fine-wire microelectrodes implanted bilaterally into deep anterior temporal lobe sites. Unit recordings, indicating cellular discharge behavior at these sites, were obtained from 3 patients during several EEG feedback training sessions for the enhancement of SMR activity. A comparison of cortical and subcortical EEG patterns showed a general and significant reciprocity, in that the presence of SMR trains

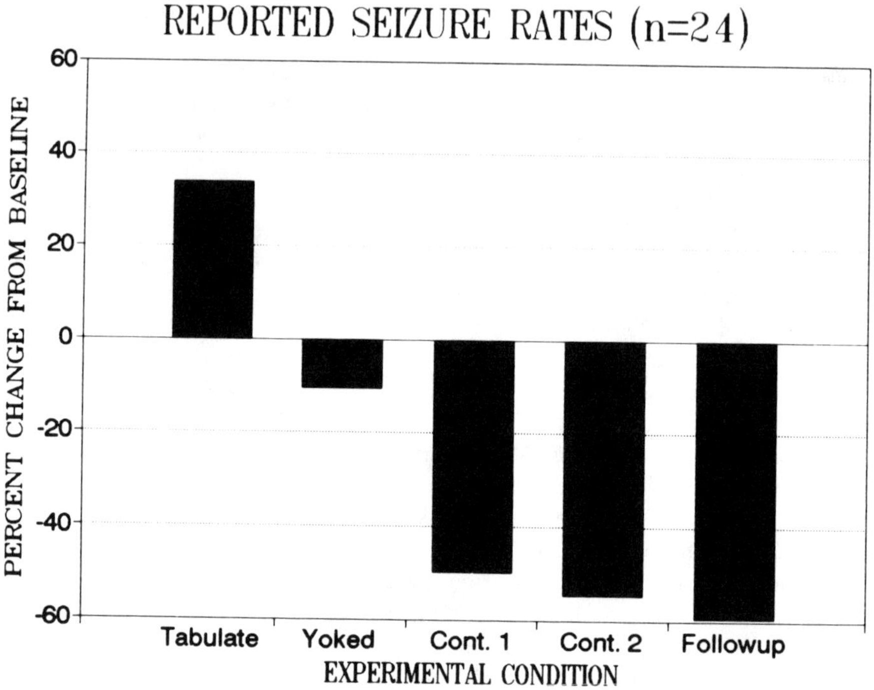

FIG. 1.1. Comparison of mean percent change from baseline seizure rates during the last month of four sequential experimental treatment conditions, as reported by 24 poorly controlled partial-complex seizure subjects. Three-month treatment periods included: (a) seizure tabulation with special seizure logs, (b) noncontingent, yoked control EEG feedback training, (c) contingent feedback training for EEG normalization (Cont. 1), and (d) gradual withdrawal from contingent training (Cont. 2). Data reported after a 6-month follow-up period are also shown. Rates registered during the Tabulation period were significantly elevated ($p = <0.05$). Rates reported following contingent training were significantly depressed ($p = <0.05$). Data reported during the final phase of contingent training and with follow-up were also significantly reduced ($p = <0.01$). No significant change was reported with noncontingent, yoked training (data from Sterman, 1984).

in the sensorimotor EEG was accompanied by normal electrical activity at deep sites. Conversely, subcortical paroxysmal discharge occurred almost exclusively in association with activated or slow-frequency EEG patterns. Feedback training sessions that produced an enhancement of the SMR across trials were accompanied by a sustained suppression of unit firing at many hippocampal recording sites (Fig. 1.2). These findings demonstrated a surprisingly consistent relationship between the sensorimotor cortical EEG and subcortical focal pathology.

Abnormal subcortical EEG patterns and related unit discharge were suppressed when normal sensorimotor rhythmic EEG activity was present or behaviorally enhanced through feedback training. This implies that cortical and/or thalamocortical regulatory mechanisms can have a significant effect upon limbic neuronal excitability.

In summary, several decades of animal and human research have established a relationship between thalamocortical EEG mechanisms and seizure pathology. These studies clearly showed that animals can be trained to produce discrete,

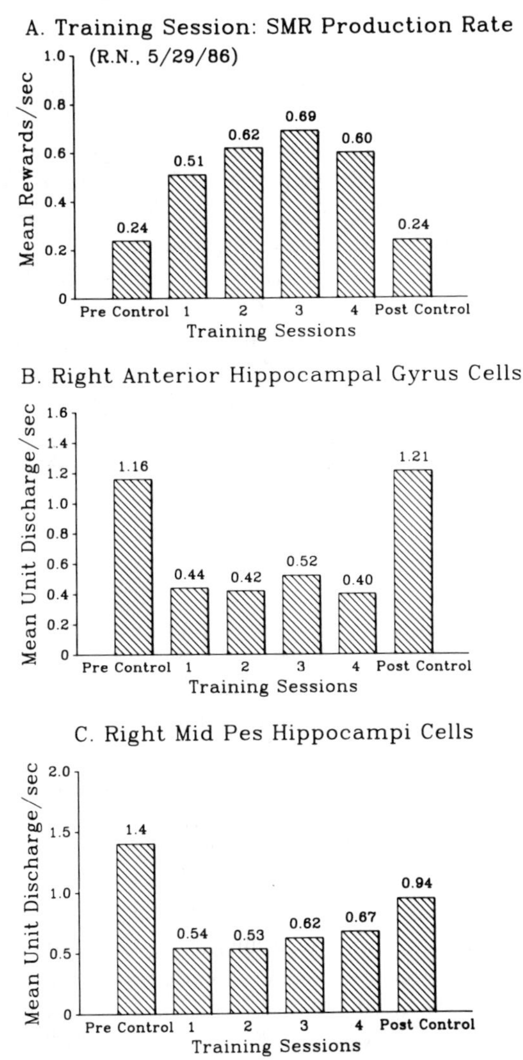

FIG. 1.2. Mean incidence of automatically detected cortical (C3) SMR activity is compared here with corresponding mean integrated extracellular unit discharge rates at limbic sites in a presurgical patient with partial-complex seizures. Data were collected before, during, and after four sequential 7-minute EEG feedback training trials. A clear enhancement of SMR activity across feedback trials was associated with a significant and sustained decrease in unit discharge rates at these sites.

voluntary changes in sensorimotor EEG patterns that are not directly mediated by behavioral events and that can alter susceptibility to experimental seizures. Numerous controlled studies evaluating the effects of sensorimotor EEG feedback training in epileptics documented a significant therapeutic effect and ruled out nonspecific factors. Neurophysiological evidence suggests that this methodology can produce significant changes in underlying neuronal regulation that can also alter seizure susceptibility.

RECENT DEVELOPMENTS

In recent years, work in this area has been greatly facilitated by the emergence of highly sophisticated computer-based quantitative EEG analysis systems. These systems provide a comprehensive analysis of background EEG abnormalities in epileptics, with the resulting advantage of objective and quantitative data for the development of appropriate EEG feedback training strategies. Our efforts with this new technology were initially directed to the development of an appropriate methodology for the application of the greatly expanded capability it provided.

We worked exclusively with the Lexicor NRS-24 topographical mapping system (Boulder, CO). This system performs a digital conversion of the analog EEG signal and calculates real-time spectral magnitudes, using the Fast Fourier Transform, for selected EEG frequency bands from 19 cortical recording sites. These quantified frequency magnitudes can then be displayed sequentially over time as compressed spectral arrays, trends, or topographic maps.

Despite the complex and attractive visual displays that this system provides, it was necessary to develop software for the organization of data within analytic spreadsheet programs that provide for appropriate quantitative comparisons and statistical analysis. It was necessary, also, to standardize procedures for system settings, data collection, and artifact removal. Most importantly, however, it was essential to collect a comprehensive body of EEG data with this system from a sufficiently large group of confirmed neurologically normal subjects. These normative data would provide the critical reference needed for the evaluation of epileptic pathology in the background EEG.

This was accomplished over an extended period during which 30 data sets were obtained from normal, right-handed male subjects participating in a standardized EEG study protocol (Sterman, Mann, Kaiser, & Suyenobu, 1993). Quantitative EEG data were tabulated for three standard test conditions, each lasting 2 min. These included: (a) eyes closed, (b) eyes open, and (c) numerical calculations. Standardized recordings were obtained from a fitted electrode cap, with leads placed according to the International 10/20 System at 19 cortical sites. A monopolar montage was used with reference to linked earlobes. Electrode impedances of less than 10 Kohms were required at all sites prior to recording. EEG signals were fed directly to the analysis system where they were digitized at a rate of 512 samples per second. Input characteristics provided common mode rejection, Hanning window smoothing, and bandpass filtering between 2 and 16 Hertz. Data were acquired in 4 sec epochs to a hard disc for subsequent quantitative analysis.

For the past 2 years, we have entered a series of poorly controlled epileptic subjects into an identical assessment protocol, with the addition of a respiratory hyperventilation test. This assessment was used to confirm and characterize background EEG abnormalities in these subjects. The data obtained were used as the basis for selection of subjects for a new EEG feedback-training study and for determination of appropriate EEG training sites and strategies.

In addition to the hyperventilation test, which often activates EEG pathology in epileptics, we found that the eyes-closed, resting condition also provides valuable information for the assessment of background EEG abnormalities. Further, our normative database does not include a hyperventilation test, thus precluding quantitative comparisons. For these reasons, we focus here on assessment data obtained from the eyes-closed test condition. Further, we examine EEG spectral findings in the 4–8 Hz frequency band; as already mentioned, this activity has been most closely associated with epileptic pathology in the background EEG.

Figure 1.3 compares mean log magnitude values at 4–8 Hz with the eyes-closed condition from sites across the central coronal cortical plane in 6 epileptic subjects with the mean and mean plus one standard deviation for each of these sites from our database. The normative means are seen at the bottom of this figure as a solid curve with filled boxes, and the means plus standard deviations just above this as a solid curve with empty boxes. The values for epileptic subjects are arrayed primarily above these with various other curve and symbol formats. It is immediately apparent that each subject showed unique background EEG abnormalities but that all displayed significantly abnormal 4–8 Hz values at one or another of these sites. Not surprisingly, this reflects the variable pathologies underlying the seizure disorders manifested in these patients. Thus, 2 of these patients had partial-motor (Jacksonian) seizures secondary to focal cortical lesions, the sites of which were identified by unusually elevated 4–8 Hz activity. One other had partial-complex seizures with clearly lateralized enhancement of 4–8 Hz activity on the right. Finally, 3 had partial-complex seizures with generally increased 4–8 Hz activity.

These findings demonstrate the value of the background EEG in characterizing epileptic pathology and the utility of this approach in localizing (and verifying) that pathology. The potential accuracy of this localization is demonstrated in Fig. 1.4, which compares CT scan findings with topographic EEG findings in one of the patients with Jacksonian seizures. These seizures persisted despite the removal of a right, parasaggital central-parietal hamartoma, shown as the bright region in the CT study of the cerebral hemispheres (horizontal perspective). On the right is a comparable EEG topographic map based on a 2-min average of

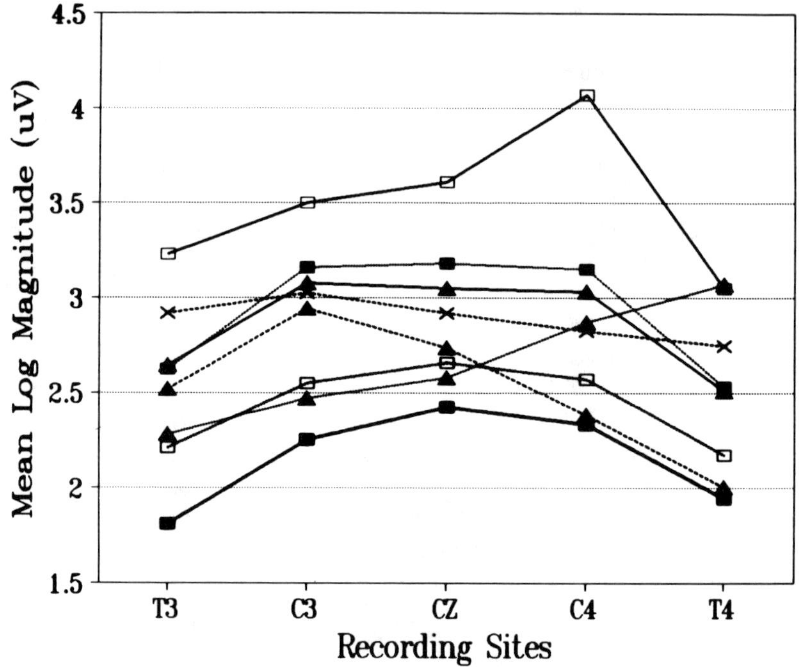

FIG. 1.3. Mean log spectral magnitudes at 4–8 Hz are shown here for a standardized 2-min eyes-closed period at recording sites across the central cortical coronal plane. Data from 6 subjects with varying seizure disorders are compared with mean and mean plus one standard deviation values from a normal database population. Normative data are represented by the two parallel solid line curves at bottom of graph, showing means (filled boxes) and means plus standard deviation (empty boxes). Values greater than two standard deviations from normal were considered to reflect epileptic pathology.

sequential 4-sec spectral-magnitude estimates at 4–8 Hz, with eyes closed. The topographic EEG image was originally in color and showed a single region of incrementing 4–8 Hz density in the right central-parietal area. This is shown in this black-and-white rendition as the large bright region with a dark center on the right. Given the slightly different horizontal planes of the head in these two images, the topographic EEG findings were in very close agreement with the CT study in localizing this pathology. Additionally, however, the EEG findings disclosed more than just morphology by also indicating an expanded extent of functional abnormality.

These considerations demonstrate again the importance of a quantitative frequency assessment of the topographic EEG in selecting appropriate sites for the application of a frequency-based EEG feedback procedure in what is always a diverse population of epileptic patients. In earlier studies, we did not have the advantage of the rapid and relatively inexpensive collection of such comprehensive data. Instead, we standardized training to left central cortex, using a bipolar lead from C1–C5. Further, feedback was based on bandpass filter analysis of this signal, with electronic relays activated when both positively and negatively rewarded frequencies reached criterion levels. The new topographic equipment allows for feedback to be applied selectively to previously determined sensorimotor sites of maximal abnormal background activity. This localization is made possible through the use of monopolar (referential) recording methods and bases feedback on real-time spectral-magnitude values calculated in frequency bands matched to patient pathology. High- and low-pass filters and adjustable band frequencies provide for attenuation and continuous monitoring of signal artifacts. Session data can be stored digitally for further analysis. Additionally, feedback modalities can be varied with ease and adapted for different patient groups. As a result of these advances, such important factors as localization, feedback accuracy, and data retrieval are all greatly facilitated.

This new capacity for "customized" training makes the rigid experimental protocols used previously both difficult and inappropriate, particularly if the

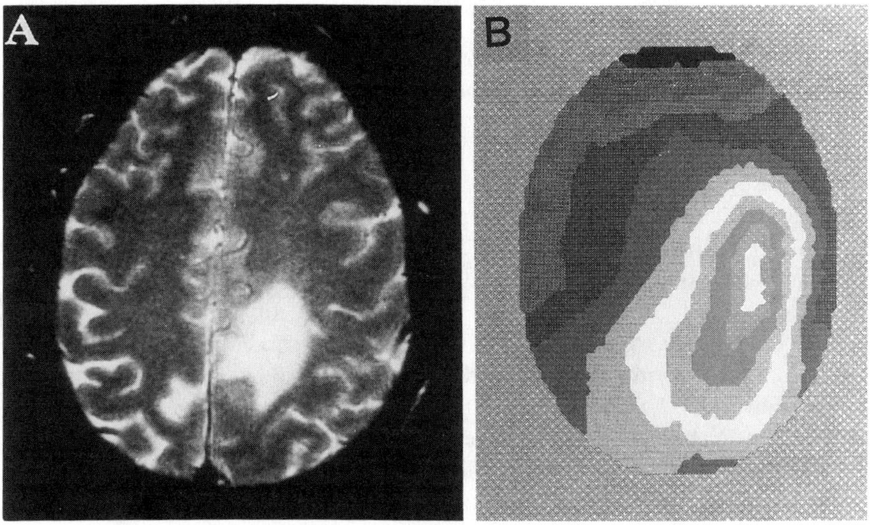

FIG. 1.4. Comparison of computer tomography (CT) image and topographic spectral analysis of 4–8 Hz EEG activity in a subject with severe focal-motor seizures secondary to a right central-parietal, parasaggital hamartoma. Tumor location is indicated by the bright area on the right in both studies. EEG study also discloses expanded region of functional disturbance.

patient's welfare is considered. The objective of training remains the same, namely normalization of the disturbed epileptic EEG. Confirmation of EEG abnormalities in sensorimotor cortex is still essential to our approach because it is based on animal and human research focused on sensorimotor mechanisms and pathological manifestations. However, this objective can now be addressed in a more individualized manner. The cortical site or sites primarily implicated can be identified objectively, the abnormal frequencies specified, and the optimal format of feedback for response acquisition determined. Further, flexibility with regard to frequency bandwidth and complexity of displays facilitates the shaping of desired responses.

Some discussion of the new and rather remarkable feedback modality capabilities is in order. All formats achieve essentially the same objective, that of portraying both desired and undesired frequency components in a manner that best facilitates their learned enhancement or suppression, respectively. This can be done separately or together, from one or several sites, and with a number of different displays. For example, it may be beneficial initially to focus on the suppression of abnormally elevated, and often dominant, slow activity in the 4–8 Hz range. Sequential mean spectral magnitudes for samples ranging from 0.5 to 2 sec can be represented by modulated bars, circles, or real-time trends. These can be displayed in any color the subject desires. Maintenance of the signal below predetermined magnitude threshold levels can be rewarded by auditory or numerical reinforcement. Subsequently, attention can be directed to the enhancement of the desirable higher frequencies. A different, perhaps more soothing, color and tone is used for shaping frequencies within the 12–16 Hz range component in this phase. One can then alternate between low-frequency suppression and high-frequency enhancement. Finally, the two can be displayed together in any of these formats and the subject rewarded for their differentiation. Experience has indicated that subjects respond best to the more recently achieved capacity for real-time frequency trend displays.

Quantitative spectral magnitude data for each trial can be stored for later evaluation and are also used to summarize the trial for the subject. Two trial summary sets (approximately 1 min in duration) are shown in Fig. 1.5 and Fig. 1.6, which present smoothed, trended outputs in 12–16 Hz (upper curve in each graph) and 5–7 Hz (bottom curve) bands for 2 different subjects. Figure 1.5 presents data from a normal subject recorded at C3 and taken from an early (top) and late (bottom) trial in a single training session. These data demonstrate the frequency differentiation that can sometimes be achieved fairly quickly with nonepileptic subjects.

Figure 1.6, on the other hand, presents data from two different sites (C4 top and C3 bottom) at approximately the same point in a training session but in an epileptic subject. Note that these two frequency bands show variable but significant reciprocity at each site. They also show very different magnitudes at each site and in comparison to Fig. 1.5. Finally, it is clear that at the point in training

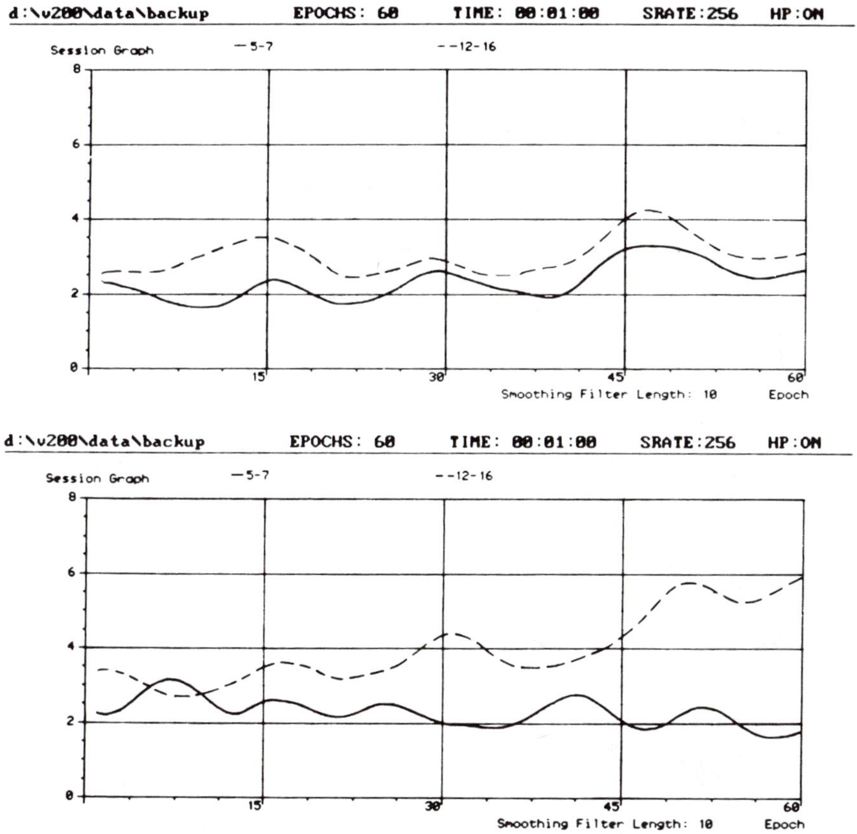

FIG. 1.5. Summary trends of 12–16 (dashed) and 5–7 Hz (solid) EEG spectral data from two 1-min EEG feedback trials at the beginning (top) and end (bottom) of the same training session. Subject in this case was a 27-year-old nonepileptic male. Ordinate is spectral magnitude and abscissa time in seconds. Reinforcement was for increasing 12–16 Hz and decreasing corresponding 5–7 Hz activity. Early trials were characterized by lack of differentiation and parallel modulation. With repeated trials, these frequency bands became differentiated and showed increased reciprocity.

depicted here, the subject was able to follow reward contingencies more effectively at the more normal C3 site.

Subjects were provided with two 1-hour training sessions per week, and re-evaluated at approximately 3-month intervals. The objective of training in all cases was the normalization of sensorimotor EEG frequencies, focused on a structured suppression of abnormal components within the 4–8 Hz range and a corresponding enhancement or stabilization of higher frequencies within the 12–

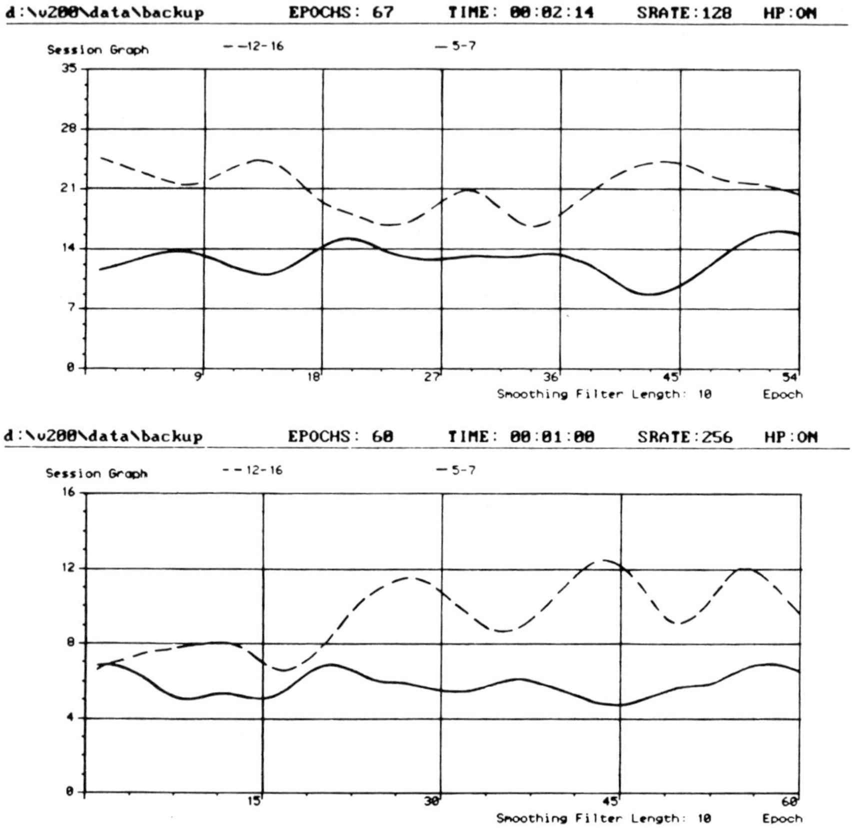

FIG. 1.6. Summary EEG spectral magnitude trends as in Fig. 1.5 but showing, instead, data from two different sites studied during the same session in epileptic subject. At this point in training, this subject had significantly higher spectral magnitude values at C4 (top) and was able to follow reward contingencies better at C3 (bottom). Note some degree of frequency band reciprocity at both sites.

16 Hz range. Because this review is based on cumulative data from a recent outpatient series, quantitative findings concerning EEG and seizure effects are limited. In fact, only 2 of these patients have had sufficient training for review at this time. Both were high functioning females in their late 50s.

As in previous studies, seizure logs have documented significant attenuation in the intensity and frequency of seizures. Further, these clinical improvements have been registered despite meaningful reductions in anticonvulsant medications. Details from each case will be reviewed separately.

Figure 1.7 compares baseline, eyes-closed sensorimotor EEG data from these 2 patients with comparable normative data from laboratory studies, both prior to

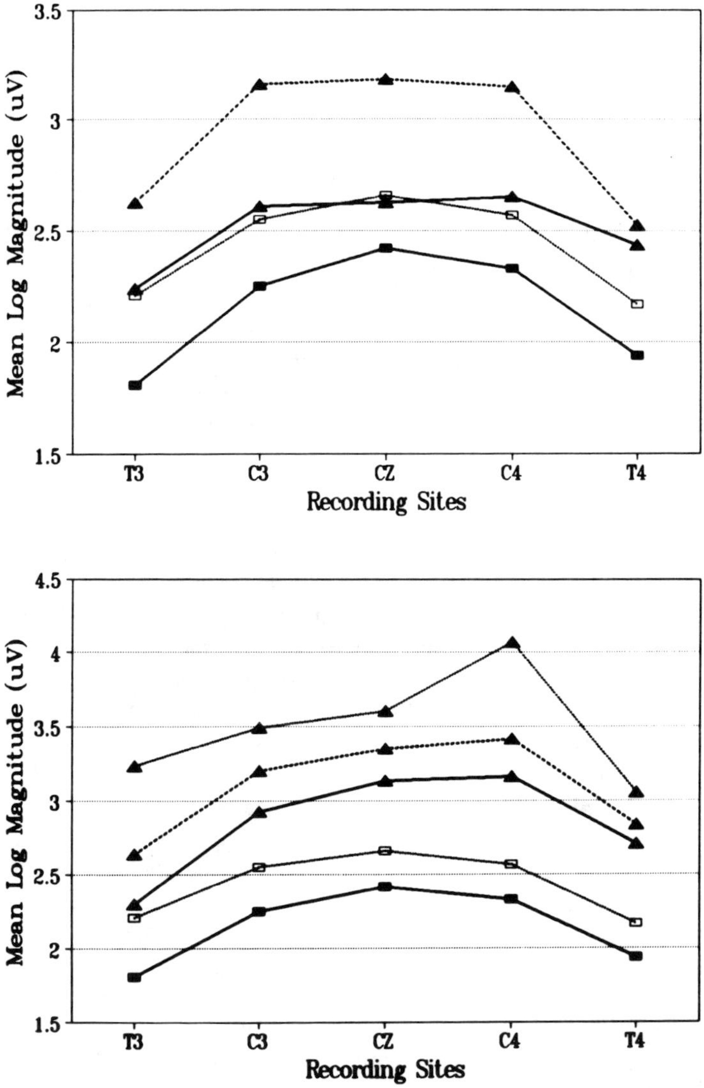

FIG. 1.7. Repeated baseline assessments (eyes closed) showing central cortical EEG spectral magnitudes at 4–8 Hz are compared here with normative data in 2 epileptic subjects at different stages of EEG feedback training. Database means (filled box) plus one standard deviation (empty box) at bottom can be contrasted to epileptic subject values (triangles). For subject in top graph, initial assessment (dashed curve) is compared with identical data acquired 6 months into EEG feedback training for normalization (solid curve) and shows decline of 4–8 Hz activity at most sites to within normal range. Data for subject in bottom graph reflect initial (dotted) and two sequential 6-month follow-up assessments (dashed and solid curves). This subject has shown a progressive attenuation of 4–8 activity, particularly at the site of epileptogenic tumor focus (C4).

training and at regular assessment intervals after training began. The patient in the top graph suffers from relatively frequent partial-complex seizures and showed a significant, general increase in 4–8 Hz background activity across the central cortical plane in pretraining, eyes-closed data. Training was alternated between C3, CZ, and C4 in this subject. After approximately 6 months of training, this subject demonstrated a significant attenuation of central 4–8 Hz activity during a retest eyes-closed assessment. Because normative data are very stable over time, this change is best explained as a result of the EEG feedback training. Seizure rate decreased and became stable at a significantly lower level in this patient, which encouraged the responsible neurologist to allow a subsequent withdrawal from Tegretol anticonvulsant therapy. The patient has sustained these gains and is currently on monotherapy, having continued with a relatively low dosage of Mysoline only.

The second patient (bottom graph, Fig. 1.7) experienced frequent Jacksonian focal-motor seizures secondary to right central cortical-tumor pathology (see Fig. 1.4). The initial pretreatment, eyes-closed assessment EEG data for this patient showed a remarkable and highly significant elevation of background 4–8 Hz activity, with a specifically elevated secondary peak at C4. After approximately 6 months of training focused on the primary C4 site, these levels declined across the central strip, most dramatically at C4. An additional 6 months of training resulted in a further reduction, bringing some sites within two standard deviations of normal mean values. Training emphasis during this period alternated between C4, C3, and T4. Although 4–8 Hz magnitudes on the right remained elevated compared to the left, the specific discrepancy at C4 was abolished.

This patient maintained comprehensive seizure logs before and since the initiation of EEG feedback training. These logs have documented an irregular but progressive decline in the rate and intensity of focal motor seizures during the course of training. She now experiences unique seizure-free periods and can abort many seizures in their earliest phase. During this same period, and as a result of these gains, she has been permitted to reduce her Phenobarbital and Tegretol medications by 30 and 40%, respectively.

Although proper application of this new computer technology is still in its infancy, initial findings are very encouraging. The ability to achieve a facile quantification of background EEG abnormalities and changes associated with training fortifies documentation significantly. Later reports will expand on these initial findings.

GENERAL CONCLUSIONS

It has been difficult to summarize 20 years of research on the voluntary control of sensorimotor EEG patterns, not to mention the complications added with its application to the clinical morass of epilepsy. We take some pleasure in the fact that our animal findings were rather straightforward. Healthy cats and primates showed a distinct, behaviorally significant EEG rhythmic pattern recorded from implanted electrodes placed directly on sensorimotor cortex. Well-controlled studies showed that cats and monkeys could, indeed, learn to regulate the incidence of this EEG pattern and, in so doing, provide a basis for the disclosure of relevant underlying neuronal dynamics. Changes in cell-firing patterns, sensory conduction, and motor excitability were all objectively demonstrated. So, too, was the fact that seizure thresholds could be raised.

In applying this methodology to human seizure disorders, the circumstances were very different. The EEG was recorded from surface electrodes in subjects whose signals were often characterized by an inherent deficiency in the EEG patterns of interest. Additionally, the influence of medications and the variety of epileptic pathologies further complicated matters. Finally, and of equal importance, was the impact of such factors as history, expectations, and, for lack of a better term, personal styles, on the effectiveness of behavioral intervention. Certainly, none of these issues burdened our animal work.

Despite these problems, we and others have demonstrated that EEG feedback training for normalization can have a lasting effect on brain electrical activity and on the clinical manifestation of seizure pathology. Achieving these outcomes, however, is no easy matter. Because effective EEG feedback training probably depends on the gradual alteration of underlying neural substrates achieved through voluntary learning, it is not surprising that success requires a serious and sustained effort. The cost in terms of time and resources for such an effort is not trivial. Neither, however, are the alternatives.

Our experience indicates that this therapy modality is not for everyone. Studies have shown that outcomes vary as a function of seizure type, intelligence, and social adjustment. Generalized motor, focal motor, and partial-complex seizures with motor manifestations respond best. As with medications, good mental and social competence are associated with better results. Perhaps most important, however, is the personal variable previously mentioned. Successful patients are those who are best able to immerse themselves effectively in the task and to achieve awareness and control of their subjective state. This is difficult territory to chart objectively but clearly deserves more systematic attention. It must, in reality, be a simple skill, because cats seem quite competent in this regard.

REFERENCES

Andersen, P., & Andersson, S. A. (1968). *Physiological basis of the alpha rhythm.* New York: Appleton-Century-Crofts.

Bowersox, S. S., & Sterman, M. B. (1981). Changes in sensorimotor sleep spindle activity and seizure susceptibility following somatosensory deafferentation. *Experimental Neurology, 74,* 814–828.

Chatrian, G. E., Petersen, M. C., & Lazarte, J. A. (1959). The blocking of the rolandic wicket rhythm and some central changes related to movement. *Electroencephalography and Clinical Neurophysiology, 11,* 497–510.

Cott, A., Pavloski, R. P., & Black, A. H. (1979). Reducing epileptic seizures through operant conditioning of central nervous system activity: Procedural variables. *Science, 203,* 73–75.

Ellertsen, B., & Kløve, H. (1976). Clinical application of biofeedback training in epilepsy. *Scandinavian Journal of Behavior Therapy, 5,* 133–144.

Finley, W. W., Smith, H. A., & Etherton, M. D. (1975). Reduction of seizures and normalization of the EEG in a severe epileptic following sensorimotor biofeedback training: Preliminary study. *Biological Psychology, 2,* 189–203.

Gastaut, H. (1952). Etude electrocortique de la reactivite des rhythmes rolandiques [Electrocortical study of rolandic rhythm dynamics]. *Reveux Neurologique, 87,* 176–182.

Gloor, P., Pellegrini, A., & Kostopoulos, G. K. (1979). Effects of changes in cortical excitability upon the epileptic bursts in generalized penicillin epilepsy of the cat. *Electroencephalography and Clinical Neurophysiology, 46,* 274–289.

Harper, R. M., & Sterman, M. B. (1972). Subcortical unit activity during a conditioned 12–14 Hz sensorimotor EEG rhythm in the cat. *Federation Proceedings, 31,* 404.

Howe, R. C., & Sterman, M. B. (1972). Cortical–subcortical EEG correlates of suppressed motor behavior during sleep and waking in the cat. *Electroencephalography and Clinical Neurophysiology, 32,* 681–695.

Kaplan, B. J. (1975). Biofeedback in epileptics: Equivocal relationship of reinforced EEG frequency to seizure reduction. *Epilepsia, 16,* 477–485.

Kuhlman, W. N. (1978). EEG feedback training of epileptic patients: Clinical and electroencephalographic analysis. *Electroencephalography and Clinical Neurophysiology, 45,* 699–710.

Kuhlman, W. N., & Kaplan, B. J. (1979). Clinical applications of EEG feedback training. In R. J. Gatchel & K. P. Price (Eds.), *Clinical applications of biofeedback: Appraisal and status.* New York: Pergamon.

Lantz, D., & Sterman, M. B. (1988). Neuropsychological assessment of subjects with uncontrolled epilepsy: Effects of EEG feedback training. *Epilepsia, 29*(2), 163–171.

Lubar J. F., & Bahler, W. W. (1976). Behavioral management of epileptic seizures following biofeedback training of the sensorimotor rhythm. *Biofeedback and Self-Regulation, 1,* 77–104.

Lubar, J. F., Shabsin, H. S., Natelson, S. E., Holder, G. S., Whitsett, S. F., Pamplin, W. E., & Krulikowski, D. I. (1981). EEG operant conditioning in intractable epileptics. *Archives of Neurology, 38,* 700–704.

Quy, R. J., Hutt, S. J., & Forrest, S. (1979). Sensorimotor rhythm feedback training and epilepsy: Some methodological and conceptual issues. *Biological Psychology, 9,* 129–149.

Shouse, M. N., & Sterman, M. B. (1979). Changes in seizure susceptibility, sleep time, and sleep spindles following thalamic and cerebellar lesions. *Electroencephalography and Clinical Neurophysiology, 46,* 1–12.

Sterman, M. B. (1973). Neurophysiologic and clinical studies of sensorimotor EEG biofeedback training: Some effects on epilepsy. *Seminars in psychiatry, 5,* 507–525.

Sterman, M. B. (1977). Clinical implications of EEG biofeedback training: A critical appraisal. In G. E. Schwartz & J. Beatty (Eds.), *Biofeedback theory and research* (pp. 389–411). New York: Academic Press.

Sterman, M. B. (1981). Power-spectral analysis of EEG characteristics during sleep in epileptics. *Epilepsia, 22,* 95–106.

Sterman, M. B. (1984). The role of sensorimotor rhythmic EEG activity in the etiology and treatment of generalized motor seizures. In T. Elbert, B. Rockstroh, W. Lutzenberger, & N. Birbaumer (Eds.), *Self-regulation of the brain and behavior* (pp. 95–106). Berlin: Springer-Verlag.

Sterman, M. B., & Bloomfield, S. (1987). Limbic neuronal discharge correlates of sensorimotor

EEG feedback training in presurgical patients with intractable epilepsy. *Proceedings of the 18th Annual Meeting of the Biofeedback Society of America,* 102.

Sterman, M. B., & Bowersox, S. S. (1981). Sensorimotor EEG rhythmic activity: A functional gate mechanism. *Sleep, 4,* 408–422.

Sterman, M. B., & Friar, L. R. (1972). Suppression of seizures in an epileptic following sensorimotor EEG feedback training. *Electroencephalography and Clinical Neurophysiology, 33,* 89–95.

Sterman, M. B., Goodman, S. J., & Kovalesky, R. A. (1978). Effects of sensorimotor EEG feedback training on seizure susceptibility in the rhesus monkey. *Experimental Neurology, 62*(3), 735–747.

Sterman, M. B., & Kovalesky, R. A. (1983). Baseline studies and anticonvulsant drug effects on the sleep EEG power spectral profile. *Electroencephalography and Clinical Neurophysiology, 5,* 212–222.

Sterman, M. B., LoPresti, R. W., & Fairchild, M. D. (1969). *Electroencephalographic and behavioral studies of monomethylhydrazine toxicity in the cat* (Technical Report No. AMRL-TR-69-3). Wright-Patterson Air Force Base, OH: Air Force Systems Command.

Sterman, M. B., & Macdonald, L. R. (1978). Effects of central cortical EEG feedback training on incidence of poorly controlled seizures. *Epilepsia, 19,* 207–222.

Sterman, M. B., Macdonald, L. R., & Stone, R. K. (1974). Biofeedback training of the sensorimotor EEG rhythm in man: Effects on epilepsy. *Epilepsia, 15,* 395–416.

Sterman, M. B., Mann, C. A., Kaiser, D. A., & Suyenobu, B. Y. (in preparation). Topographic patterns of state and task-specific EEG desynchronization.

Sterman, M. B., & Shouse, M. N. (1980). Quantitative analysis of training, sleep EEG and clinical response to EEG operant conditioning in epileptics. *Electroencephalography and Clinical Neurophysiology, 49,* 558–576.

Sterman, M. B., & Wyrwicka, W. (1967). EEG correlates of sleep: Evidence for separate forebrain substrates. *Brain Research, 6,* 143–163.

Tozzo, C. A., Elfner, L. F., & May, J. G., Jr. (1988). EEG biofeedback and relaxation training in the control of epileptic seizures. *International Journal of Psychophysiology, 6,* 185–194.

Wyler, A. R. (1984). Operant conditioning of single neurons in monkeys and its theoretical application to EEG operant conditioning in human epilepsy. In T. Elbert, B. Rockstroh, W. Lutzenberger, & N. Birbaumer (Eds.), *Self-regulation of the brain and behavior* (pp. 85–94). Berlin: Springer-Verlag.

Wyler, A. R., Lockard, J. S., Ward, A. A., & Finch, C. A. (1976). Conditioned EEG desynchronization and seizure occurrence in patients. *Electroencephalography and Clinical Neurophysiology, 41,* 501–512.

Wyler, A. R., Robbins, C. A., & Dodrill, C. B. (1979). EEG operant conditioning for control of epilepsy. *Epilepsia, 20,* 279–286.

Wyrwicka, W., & Sterman, M. B. (1968). Instrumental conditioning of sensorimotor cortex EEG spindles in the waking cat. *Physiology and Behavior, 3,* 703–707.

2 Breathing Training for the Self-Regulation of Alveolar CO_2 in the Behavioral Control of Idiopathic Epileptic Seizures

Robert Fried
Hunter College of the City University of New York,
and *Institute for Rational Emotive Therapy*

In the United States, *idiopathic* seizure sufferers are estimated to constitute about 75%–80% of the total population of individuals said to have epilepsy—about 16 million or more persons, and growing by about 100,000 cases annually. In this subpopulation, seizures typically first emerge in the late teens, or about the time that most of them enter the labor market. A genetic predisposition to idiopathic seizures has been postulated, but no convincing scientific evidence suggests that it is strong. But there may be a cluster of related inherited disorders such as migraine, Raynaud's, and angina, principally involving the vascular and oxygen transport systems, that they and their family seem to share (Deutsch, Ehrentheil, & Pierson, 1941; Fried, 1990, in press; Hauptmann & Meyerson, 1948).

Seizures are classified by etiology, manifestations, and physiological correlates; those of readily determinable origin are said to be "symptomatic." They may take various forms (i.e., petit mal, grand mal, psychomotor, etc.) and may be accompanied by premonitory sensations (auras) that may take different forms, such as auditory, visual, abdominal, and so forth (Gastaut, 1970).

WHAT IS EPILEPSY?

In antiquity, seizure sufferers were variously admired or reviled, praised, or persecuted. The "falling disease," the "sacred illness," was often said to be demonic possession—hence the word *seizure*—or caused by winds (*aura*). It was described in considerable detail by Hippocrates (460–357 B.C.) and Galen (130–200 A.D.) and references to it may be found in the New Testament (Mark 9.17). With time, the treatment of epilepsy came to be the concern of neurology.

The theory of seizure etiology currently in vogue in neurology stipulates spontaneous individual brain neuron dysfunction, with subsequent recruiting of an aggregate whose critical mass results in total brain involvement in electrical seizure discharge. This theory is based on the electroencephalographic (EEG) observations during the seizure. But, in fact, it satisfactorily explains neither why the seizure starts nor why it stops. Wolfe and Elliott (1962) were typical:

> Convulsive activity may now be conceived, not as an enhancement of the normal excitation of neurons, but as the partial or complete block of normal inhibition. A biochemical abnormality of some neurons is thought by many investigators to underlie the initiation of gradually increasing depolarization in their dendritic fields so that minimal stimuli may initiate a seizure discharge. The spread to adjacent neurons and the propagation axonally to other areas of the nervous system of the discharge results in the striking manifestation of the convulsion. (p. 694)

This elaborate definition raises more questions than it answers. Which biochemical neuronal abnormality? In well over 5,000 books and research articles available on the subject, there is little more than speculation. Ginter (1955) cited "inherent metabolic defects carried on transmissible genes;" birth defects, or birth injury traceable to "definite pathologic evidence [of] microgyri or glial scars;" disturbance in prenatal or neonatal oxygen (O_2) or foodstuffs supply; "poisoned" enzyme or hormone disturbance; and last, although by no means least, latent viruses that "may cause a decrease in the rate of glycolysis and inhibit glucose phosphorylation, or later the formation of amino acids from protein." Himwich (1951) also cited hypoglycemia, but Maccario, Messis, & Vastola (1965) proposed hyperglycemia. Cogan, Schulman, Porter, & Mudd (1980) suggested methylmalonic acidurea and homocystinurea. There are suggestions that inhibitory mechanisms, such as those involving gamma-aminobutyric acid (GABA; Tower, 1968) and more recently taurine (Rozen, Goodyer, & Scriver, 1982), may play a role. They are diverse and cover a broad spectrum of metabolic processes.

The study of seizures as brain events dates from about the middle 19th century. Wilks (1859, cited in Penfield & Jasper, 1954) introduced the therapeutic use of *bromide*—the term later came to mean a universal palliative—and distinguished between functional (idiopathic) and focal seizures. But Merritt & Putnam (1938), who pioneered the use of dilantin, brought to our attention that:

> Good results in the treatment of patients with convulsive seizures have been obtained by a variety of methods, such as medical treatment with bromides or barbituric acid compounds, the ketogenic diet, restriction of fluids, and the surgical excision of scars or irritable cortical foci. (p. 1068)

This would lead one to believe that uncontrolled seizures are, excepting extremes, a thing of the past. They continued, "In spite of these various therapeutic means, there are a great number of patients who are not relieved of their attacks or are helped only temporarily by treatment" (p. 1068). In 1952, Yahr, Sciarra, Carter, & Merritt, reporting on the effectiveness of dilantin, concluded that it was about "87% effective" in the 319 patients they studied, but that 87% included only 48% whose seizures were controlled, whereas 37% showed varying degrees of improvement. Technically, this is "87% effective."

Hughlings Jackson (1870, cited in Taylor, 1931) rejected the possibility of seizures in the absence of histopathology. Gowers (1881, 1901), supporting Wilks, disagreed:

> The naked eye appearance of the nerve-centers in idiopathic epilepsy is for the most part that of healthy organs. . . . Great as is the aid which the microscope has afforded in the investigation of the structural changes in many diseases of the nervous system, it cannot be said to have thrown much light on the nature of idiopathic epilepsy. Of the minute histological changes which have been described, most, if not all, of those which are not common to many other diseases, are simply secondary. . . . (Gowers, 1901, p. 213)

Disciples of Hughlings Jackson were left to hope that histopathological evidence would emerge as technology advanced. It is not surprising that the EEG discoveries of Berger (1929) and Bremer (1938) resurrected the faithful; for here, finally, was the evidence for histopathology, (i.e., the biochemical lesion). But, they might have done well to heed Gower's (1901) warning:

> [T]he subject of the pathology of epilepsy resolves itself, in the main, into four questions: What is the seat of the discharge which thus produces the symptoms of the fit? Is the seat of the discharge the seat of the disease? How far does such discharge explain all the symptoms of the attack? What is the nature of the morbid change which causes the discharge? (p. 215)

According to tradition, neurology, like the youngest son, did not seem to know that there were questions to be asked. Berger (1929) and Bremer (1938) were, parenthetically, entirely at odds. The first held the EEG to be due to the electrophysiology of the vascular bed of the brain; the latter assigned it to neurons. No one else seemed to have paid much attention to this critical distinction, and thus it faded from view.

In fact, for some time it seemed not to matter much what the etiology of seizures actually was. As late as 1965, the renowned British neurologist, Lord Brain, stated, in what is considered by many the classic textbook of neurology, that we do not yet understand the physiological relationship between cortical dysrhythmia and the epileptic attack. Elsewhere, such an assertion would have been taken as parochial, if not curious agnosia, for the publications of countless scientists, especially in the United States, which promulgated quite creditable specifics (Gibbs, Lennox, & Gibbs, 1940; Gibbs, Williams, & Gibbs, 1949;

Himwich, 1951; Lennox, Gibbs, & Gibbs, 1938; Madsen, 1943; Meyer & Waltz, 1961; Millichap & Ulrich, 1962; Penfield & Jasper, 1954; Schwab, Grunwald, & Sargant, 1941; Swanson, Stavney, & Plum, 1958; Tower, 1960; Wolfe & Elliott, 1962). Brain (1965) continued:

> There seems no doubt, however, that whatever its immediate or remote cause, an epileptic attack is that manifestation of a paroxysmal discharge of abnormal electrical rhythms in some part of the brain. If one adds that such discharges are likely to be repetitive, one has defined the cardinal features of epilepsy. (p. 129)

Epilepsy . . . "whatever its immediate or remote cause!" (p. 129). He might have cited Penfield (1933): "The vasomotor spasms and changes seen so characteristically in the cerebral cortex of epileptics are due to vasomotor reflexes . . ." (p. 310), right or wrong. Barolin (1966) was as vague as Brain and postulated an initial "pathological activity in the nervous cells" (p. 56). So was Merritt (1979), codeveloper of dilantin, who explained that seizures are due to ". . . excessive repetitive firing of [a] single or small group of neurons in the brain . . . [with] recruitment of adjacent neurons spreading to the entire system until it is out of control." So if a few brain neurons seize and enough of them do it at the same time, a seizure results. If recruitment is how they get each other to join in the act, what limits recruitment to a lesion, or focus, that can be excised surgically?

Metabolic etiology of seizures, most notably where the body's CO_2 economy plays a central role, has been proposed by numerous investigators (Brill & Seidmann, 1942; Caspers & Speckmann, 1972; Gotoh, Meyer, & Takagi, 1965; Meyer & Gotoh, 1960; Meyer & Waltz, 1961; Morrice, 1965; Raichle & Plum, 1972). But its division from electroclinical seizure etiology is demarcated so sharply that Gastaut & Tassinari (1966), proponents of the electroclinical view, assigned just one paragraph to "hyperpnea" and six short paragraphs to metabolic factors, limited to hypocalcemia in infants. All other research was dismissed with: "[Epileptogenic metabolic disorders] . . . are not only particularly interesting from the physiopathogenic point of view, but very important from the clinical point of view and must always be considered and studied in each subject. . . ." (p. 96). So why not tell us what they are? Even the paragraph on hyperpnea mentions nothing about CO_2, dismissing hundreds of respected investigations into its link to seizures.

Most metabolic theories of seizure etiology implicate hypoxia, relating it to the body's CO_2 economy and the way that economy affects the O_2 transport system. They stem from observations of brain blood flow and metabolism, EEG, and seizures, following hyperventilation (HV) (Caspers & Speckmann, 1972; Gibbs, Williams, & Gibbs, 1949; Kerr, Dalton, & Gliebe, 1937; Penfield & Jasper, 1954; Raichle & Plum, 1972; Withrow, 1972). Brody and Dusser de Barenne (1932) may have been the first of many investigators to have reported inducing seizures with HV, and it has been verified repeatedly (Darrow & Graf, 1945). Gibbs, Lennox, and Gibbs (1940), stated unequivocally that:

> Considering all those links between carbon-dioxide and epilepsy, namely that (1) the influence of carbon dioxide on the EEG, (2) the abnormal values of carbon dioxide in arterial and jugular blood of patients with petit mal and grand mal, and (3) the abnormal variation of carbon dioxide preceding grand mal seizures in such a way as to indicate a causal relationship, we may conclude that carbon dioxide plays a significant role in the etiology of epileptic convulsions. (p. 109)

Himwich (1951) supported this position: "In addition to exerting physiological effects, carbon dioxide may also be involved in pathological conditions, for instance, epilepsy" (p. 103). Holmberg (1953) asserted that "hypocapnia is probably the essential factor which produces slow waves in the EEG" (p. 374). Penfield and Jasper (1954) also allowed the possibility that etiological variables might include a spectrum of events broader than just "vasomotor reflexes," or the prevailing theories of neuronal hyperexcitability: "The possibility that there may be intermediary metabolic defects, or abnormal reactivity of certain cerebral vessels . . . must also be considered. . . . It might be related to migraine . . . or to some obscure metabolic defect" (p. 495). With hypocapnia, they also saw brain arterial vessels "blanching," but they did not cite Darrow and Graf (1945), who previously had produced it experimentally by HV in cats. The latter must have been astonished at the sight, because they reported, "A striking effect of hyperventilation was the occasional appearance of waves of constriction passing along the vessels, giving them the appearance of sausage links" (p. 456). Penfield and Jasper (1954) actually witnessed what Lennox et al. (1938) had hypothesized (i.e., paroxysms of cerebral arterioles *during* seizures in the brain exposed to view) and likened it to a small thread tied around the artery. But, they ultimately more or less dismissed vascular and metabolic variables:

> The mechanism whereby hyperventilation elicits changes in the EEG and seizures in epileptic patients is still unknown; it may act by causing a partial ischemia due to cerebral vasoconstriction, and there may be some increase in excitability accompanying the lowered CO_2 concentration. (p. 230)

The links between low alveolar CO_2 (hypocapnia), alkalosis, brain arterial paroxysmal vasonconstriction, ictal EEG patterns, and seizures did not turn most investigators toward a metabolic dysfunction theory of the seizure etiology. Even today, neurophysiological theory of the etiology of idiopathic seizures involves the hypothetical destabilization of one or more hyperexcitable brain neurons, which, in concert, recruit surrounding such neurons until a critical mass has been achieved. Such a critical mass of destabilized neurons is thought to result in the local paroxysmal discharge called a focus, though in some cases it may involve the brain as a whole. The destabilization of the neurons is attributed by some to indeterminate chemical factors, which alter cell membrane characteristics. The seizure terminates when the activity is exhausted:

> Review of the literature reveals that most experimental studies are concerned with the problem of initiation. . . . It is well known that seizure activity is accompanied

> by a considerable increase in energy metabolism of the brain. . . . [I]t has been suspected that each convulsive discharge outlasting a certain period ceases automatically when the supply of energy is exhausted. . . . [P]articular attention has been directed to changes in gas tension in blood and tissue. (Caspers & Speckmann, 1972, p. 699)

This *hybrid* tells us that seizures end because they are self-terminating; but, in case they do not, they run out of steam—steam lost because of blood gas levels. In such theories, seizure activity is likened, by analogy, to the action potential of individual neurons, but on a grand scale.

The search for metabolic etiology has led many to compare biochemical factors in seizure sufferers and nonsufferers, reporting detectable differences (Batt et al., 1975; Davis & Wallace, 1941, 1942; Faurbye, 1943; Glaser, 1979; Groen, 1975; Himwich, 1951; Ikonomoff, 1970; Laidlaw & Richens, 1976; Latham, 1975; Lowenthal, 1965; Lubin & Price, 1942; Madsen, 1943; Meyer & Waltz, 1961; Millichap & Ulrich, 1962; Shinozaki & Furutani, 1968). It would not add immeasurably to this report to detail each finding. But, the most consistent is that concerning the body's CO_2 economy and the acid–base balance of the blood.

THE EFFECT OF CO_2 ON THE EEG AND SEIZURE THRESHOLD

It has been known for over 50 years that arterial blood CO_2 concentration ($PaCO_2$) is the most powerful intrinsic influence on cerebral blood flow and metabolism (Gibbs et al., 1940; Himwich, 1951; Holmberg, 1953; Lennox et al., 1938; Meyer & Waltz, 1961). Some maintained that the autonomic nervous system (ANS) plays little role in cerebral vasotonus, and that CO_2, therefore, is the only such factor (Heistad, Marcus, & Abboud, 1978).

Figure 2.1 shows the relationship between cerebral blood flow (CBF) and $PaCO_2$. At normal $PaCO_2$—38 torr (about 5%)—CBF is about 45 cc/100g/min. When $PaCO_2$ decreases to 30 torr, a value commonly observed in chronic HV (Fried, 1987a, 1992), CBF drops to about 35 cc/100g/min—a decrease of over 20%.

Figure 2.2 shows the relationship between pulmonary (alveolar) ventilation and alveolar and blood CO_2, O_2, and blood pH levels. *Alveolar ventilation* (i.e., respiration volume) is conventionally expressed as minute volume (Vmin), and is given here in liters/minute. When ventilation increases above the reference norms line at a little below 5.4 1/min, alveolar CO_2 (PCO_2), (A), and arterial blood CO_2 ($PaCO_2$), (B), decrease; oxihemoglobin (OHb) saturation (SaO_2), (C), remains constant, although alveolar O_2 concentration (PO_2), (D), rises; and pH rises (alkalosis), (E). With increased Mv, PCO_2 and $PaCO_2$ decrease; SaO_2 remains unchanged, whereas pH rises. Some investigators erroneously focus on

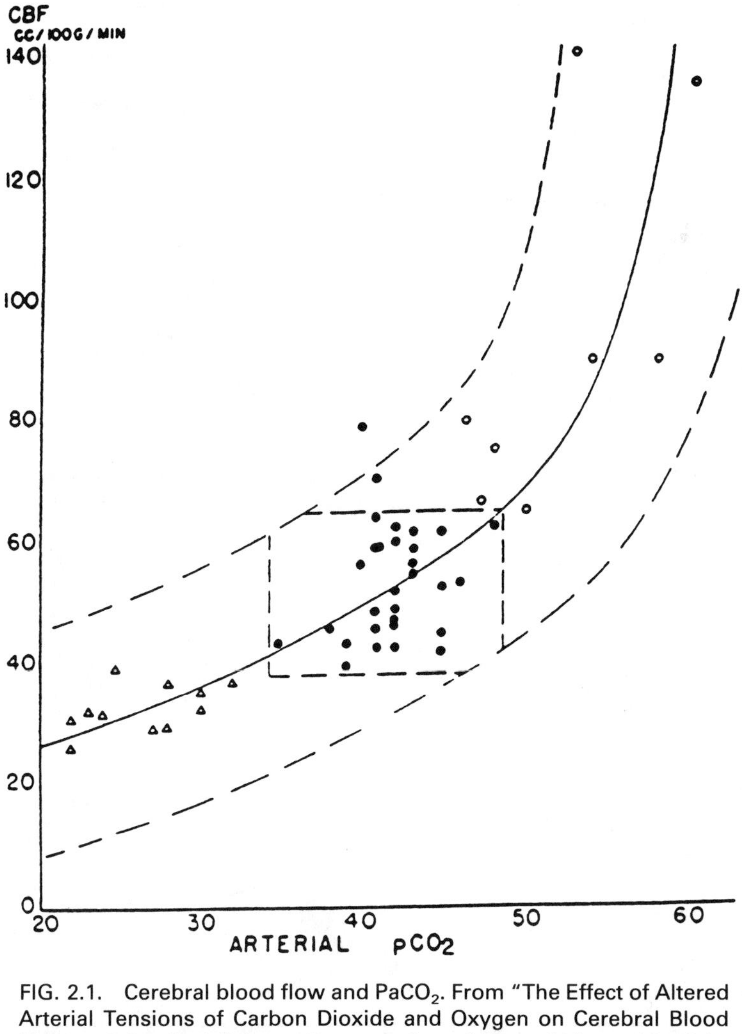

FIG. 2.1. Cerebral blood flow and $PaCO_2$. From "The Effect of Altered Arterial Tensions of Carbon Dioxide and Oxygen on Cerebral Blood Flow and Cerebral Oxygen Consumption of Normal Young Men" by S. S. Kety and C. F. Schmidt, 1948, *Journal of Clinical Investigation, 27,* pp. 484–492. Copyright 1948 by *Journal of Clinical Investigation.* Reprinted by permission.

breathing rate (RR) as the measure of HV. Although logically related to pulmonary ventilation, varying activity level makes it an unreliable measure of CO_2 loss. For instance, an individual who is running and breathing rapidly to reduce excess CO_2, or one with metabolism accelerated by cocaine, is not hyperventilating simply because he or she may be breathing rapidly (hyperpnea).

Cerebral blood flow is affected directly by alkalosis. Figure 2.3 shows the

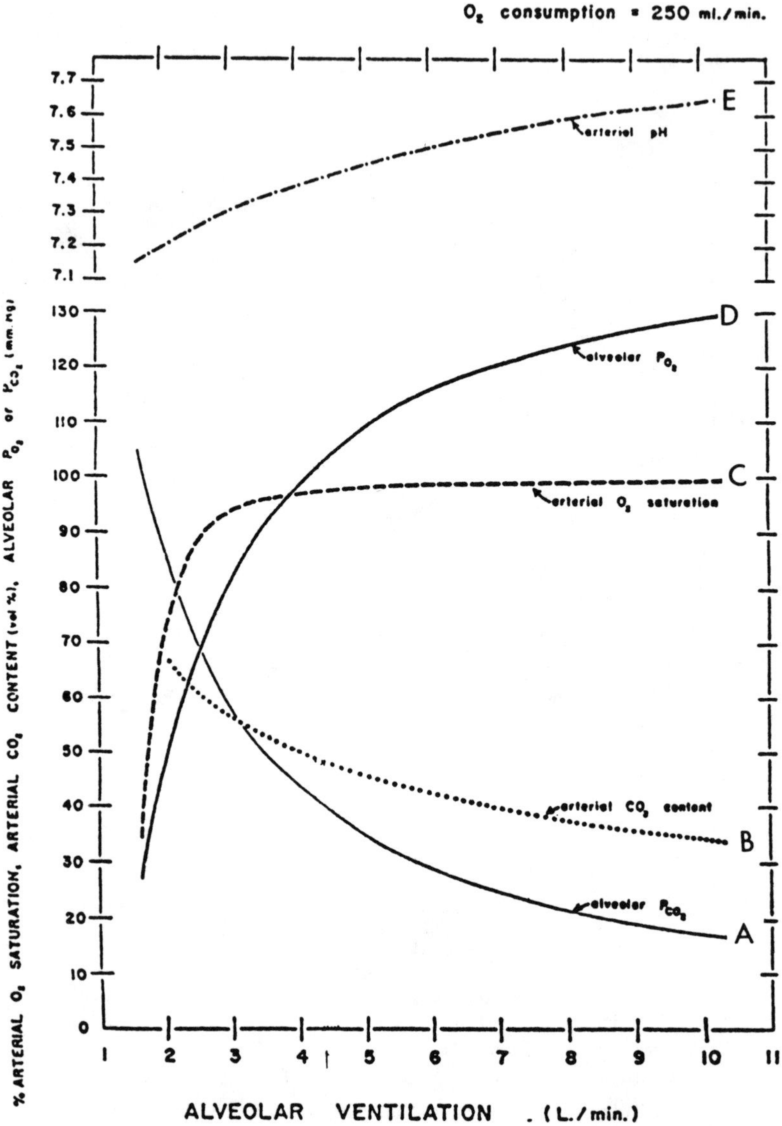

FIG. 2.2. The effect of changing alveolar ventilation on alveolar gas and arterial blood O_2, CO_2, and pH. From *The Lung: Clinical Physiology and Pulmonary Function Tests* (2nd ed., p. 47), by J. H. Comroe, R. E. Forster, H. Dubois, A. B. Briscoe, & E. Carlsen, 1962, Chicago: Year Book Medical Publishers. Copyright 1962 by Year Book Medical Publishers. Reprinted by permission.

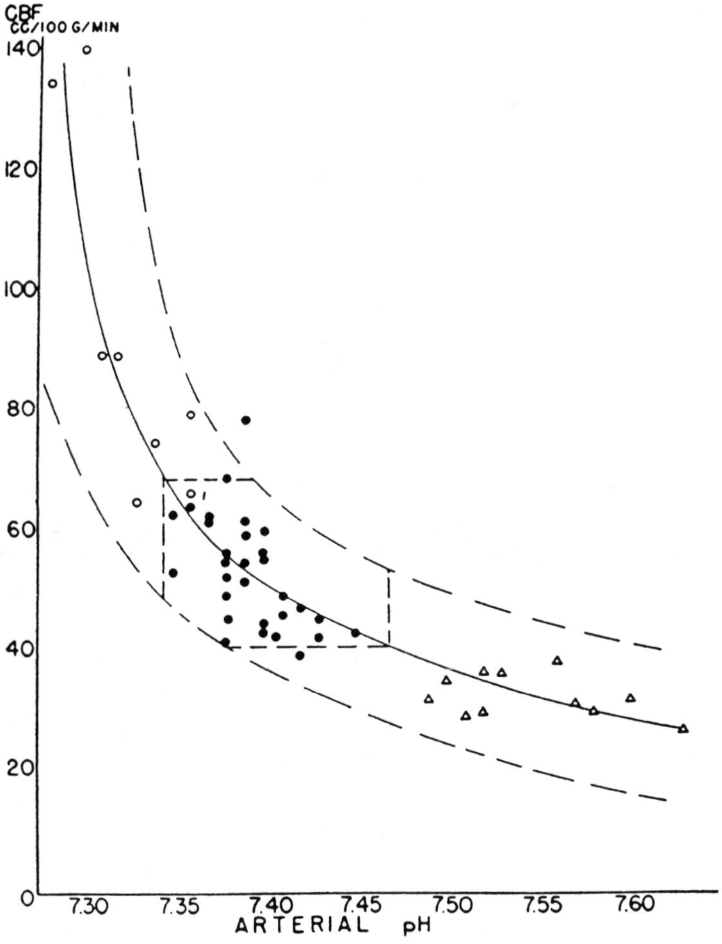

FIG. 2.3. The relationship between cerebral blood flow and arterial pH. From "The Effect of Altered Arterial Tension of Carbon Dioxide and Oxygen on Cerebral Blood Flow and Cerebral Oxygen Consumption in Normal Young Men" by S. S. Kety & C. F. Schmidt, 1948, *Journal of Clinical Investigation, 27,* pp. 484–492. Copyright 1948 by *Journal of Clinical Investigation.* Reprinted by permission.

relationship between CBF and pH: At normal alveolar ventilation, arterial blood pH is about 7.38, and CBF is about 45 cc/100g/min. If alveolar ventilation doubles—which is not uncommon in chronic HV—arterial blood pH rises to 7.6 (see Fig. 2.2) and CBF drops to about 35 cc/100g/min—a little over 20%.There is a parallel relationship between alveolar HV and arterial blood CO_2 in their adverse effect on CBF. This adversity is aggravated further by the effect of alkalosis on the OHb-dissociation curve (Bohr-effect).

In 1904, Bohr, Hasselbach, and Krogh noted the effect of blood CO_2 concentration on the affinity of hemoglobin (Hb) for O_2. CO_2, contributing to the acidification of blood by biochemically affecting its concentration of hydrogen ion (H+), and therefore its acid–base balance, is critical in Hb function. Figure 2.4 shows the OHb-dissociation curve (ODC) at three values for pH. When pH rises, the curve shifts to the left; when it drops, the curve shifts to the right. A left-shifted ODC means higher affinity, which is detrimental to metabolism because O_2 and Hb are more tightly bound and therefore less is released to tissues. A right-shifted ODC favors O_2 release. According to Woodson (1979), one of the reasons for an acute increase in in vivo oxygen affinity in man is respiratory alkalosis due to inadvertent HV. He added, "Hyperventilation may likewise be hazardous, because, in addition to increasing oxygen affinity, it appreciably reduces cerebral and coronary blood flow" (p. 372).

Other pH-dependent factors further jeopardize the O_2 transport system. Alkalosis promotes decreased red blood cell calcium efflux, making them rigid and less able to traverse capillaries; and increased production of organic phosphates, including 2,3-diphosphoglycerate (DPG), which competes with O_2 for binding on

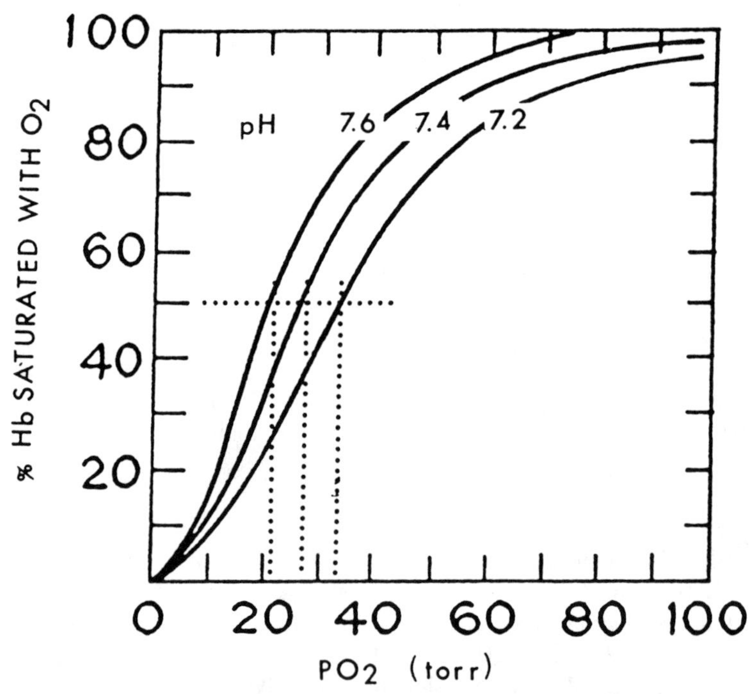

FIG. 2.4. Oxyhemoglobin (OHb) dissociation curve (ODC).

Hb (Altura, 1982; Brewer, 1974; Bunn & Jandi, 1970; Chanutin & Curnish, 1967; George et al., 1964; Levine & Coburn, 1984; Mairbaurl & Humpeler, 1981).

Loss of CO_2 by HV was reported by Lennox et al. (1936) as one of the conditions affecting the EEG and influencing seizure activity. Parenthetically, Lennox had noted, as early as 1928, that disordered breathing was a common feature in seizure sufferers. Inhaling O_2 had no influence on the EEG or seizures, so Lennox et al. (1938) hypothesized that inhaling CO_2 might wipe out the EEG slow waves preceding the seizures. That is precisely what happened. Then, in 1938, they reported the near-linear relationship between hypocapnia and the *fundamental frequency* of the EEG (Fig. 2.5). A decrease in CO_2 of 3% (volume) from normal control reduces the EEG frequency from 11 Hz, *alpha,* to 7.5 Hz, *theta,* right where ictal EEG waves appear.

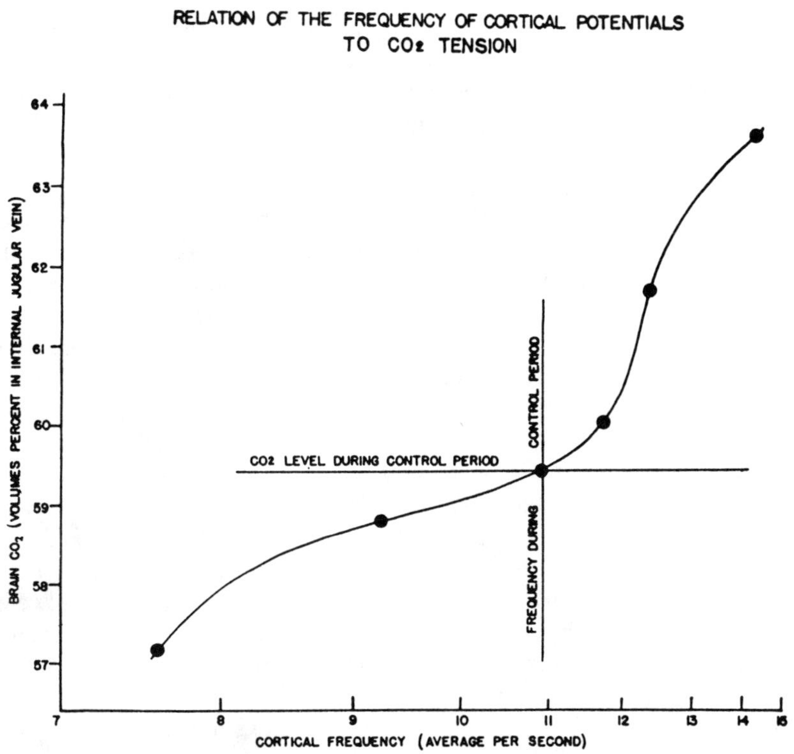

FIG. 2.5. The relation of cortical potentials to the CO_2 content of internal blood. From "The Relationship in Man of Cerebral Activity to Blood Flow and Blood Constituents" by W. G. Lennox, F. A. Gibbs, and E. L. Gibbs, 1938, *Journal of Neurology & Psychiatry, 1,* pp. 222–225. Copyright 1938 by *Journal of Neurology & Psychiatry.* Reprinted by permission.

Engel, Ferris, and Logan (1947) also showed that the EEG frequency dropped at a near constant rate from 10Hz, *alpha,* to about 3 Hz, *theta,* when hyperventilating in room air over a 3 min time span. Conscious awareness was negligible at 150 sec and most subjects did not recall losing it after the procedure (see Fig. 2.6).

These interrelated components form a mosaic: Hypocapnia is a vasoconstrictor, reducing cerebral blood flow and, consequently, the O_2 supply of the brain; hypocarbia leads to alkalosis that left-shifts the ODC increasing OHb affinity and also reduces CBF, compounding reduction of the brain O_2 supply. CO_2 loss is near-linearly related to decreased EEG frequency and the onset of seizures. One may reasonably conclude that the etiology of seizures (i.e., the cause of neuronal instability) is metabolic depression by hypoxia. But, hypocapnia is the more immediate causal factor, because hypocarbia is renal compensated in the long run.

EEG power spectral analysis led Gibbs et al. (1949) to conclude that there is a shift in energy toward the slow side of the spectrum as brain CO_2 concentration falls, although little change is noted with O_2 reduction until it reached the 40% saturation level. Since then, the technique has been refined considerably (Gersch & Goddard, 1970; Lubar & Bahler, 1976; Sterman, 1981; Tharp & Gersch, 1975; Walter, Rhodes, Brown, & Adey, 1966).

A number of theories attempt to explain HV in seizure sufferers. Mattson, Henniger, Gallagher, and Glaser (1970) proposed an anxiety mechanism that leads to HV lowering $PaCO_2$, thus triggering seizures. They based this theory on polygraphic studies of HV and the EEG. Their patients, who showed a marked tendency to unconscious HV when anxious, showed no obvious overbreathing; yet, end-tidal CO_2 ($ETCO_2$) fell nearly 50% and abnormal EEG and clinical seizure activity increased. In a more recent review of clinical research, Mathew and Wilson (1990) strongly supported the belief that the mechanism responsible for observed reduction in CBF during severe anxiety is most likely hypocapnia.

Swanson et al. (1958) noted that EEG follows change in PCO_2, not in arterial pH, when these are changed independently. They concluded that "carbon dioxide possesses unique properties that influence nerve cell function and cerebral electrical activity" (p. 792). Curiously, this conclusion overlooks the seemingly clear evidence of impaired neuronal function by reduced cerebral blood flow resulting from the vasoconstrictive effects of hypocapnia. Despite the weight of evidence, there is considerable controversy over the precise role of CO_2 in seizure etiology, but little doubt that it only compromises brain neurons already predisposed to destabilization in the presence of reduced CBF and hypoxia, where brain arteries tend to paroxysmal vasospasm or, sometimes, transient ischemia (TIA).

In this scenario, organic, or psychogenic, factors initiate chronic arousal with HV, and the consequent hypocapnia causes reduced CBF and brain hypoxia by cerebral arterial vasoconstriction, and pH related change of the O_2 transport system. When brain arterial blood CO_2 levels drop below a crucial set point,

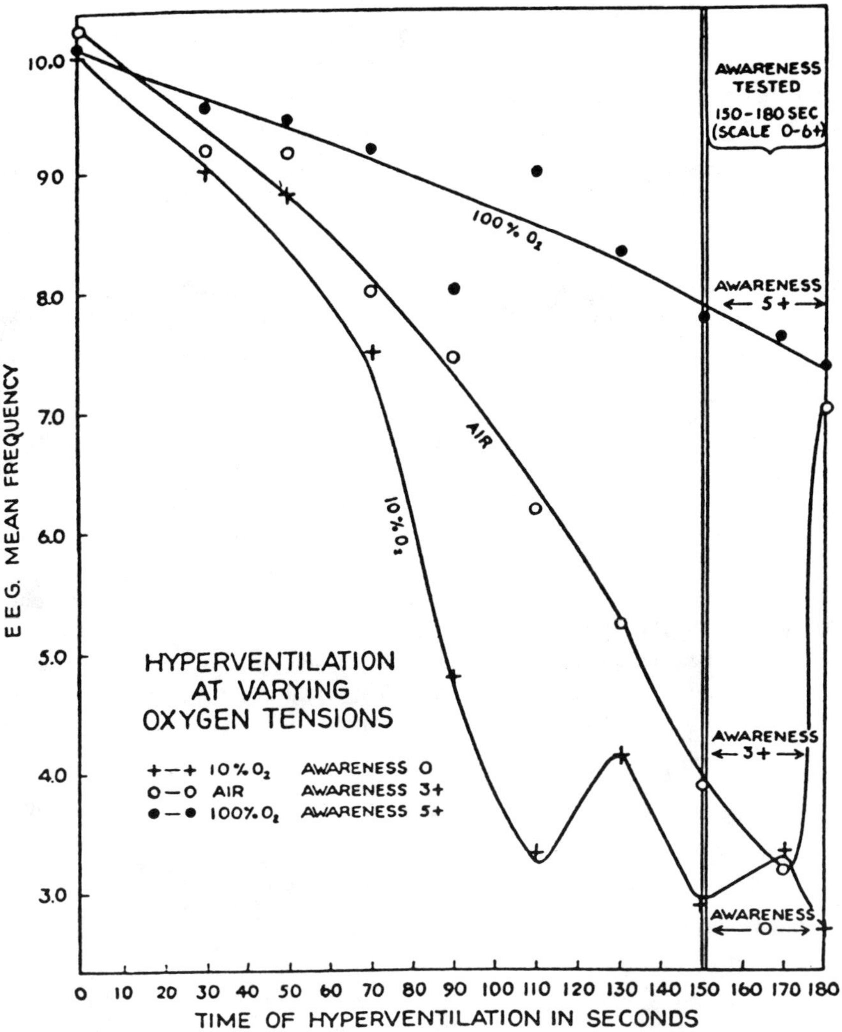

FIG. 2.6. EEG mean frequency changes during hyperventilation at different oxygen tension, and correlation with level of awareness. From "Hyperventilation: Analysis of clinical symptomatology" by G. L. Engel, E. B. Ferris, and M. Logan, 1947, *Annals of Internal Medicine, 5,* pp. 683–704. Copyright 1947 by *Annals of Internal Medicine.* Reprinted by permission.

some cerebral arteries, selected by local factors, respond with paroxysmal vasospasm, which induces further ischmic hypoxia causing regional shunting in CBF microcirculation. Consciousness is impaired as metabolism drops rapidly, and respiration ceases as hypocapnia depresses respiratory drive. But, in this anaerobic environment, brain levels of glutamate rise rapidly, metabolism surges, and brain CO_2 rises rapidly causing vasodilation and a surge in blood flow followed by return of consciousness as the hypoxia lifts. Each element in this scenario has been shown to take place, in the studies cited earlier, and its aggregate played a prominent role in my decision to pursue the behavioral control of seizures through the self-regulation of PCO_2. The elegance of this scenario is not hampered by the fact that it provides the only logical mechanism for the termination of the seizure. Because the seizure is initiated by hypoxia due to an ischemic attack, it ends when the vasoconstriction is lifted by restoration of normocapnia. I hold this to be somewhat superior to the "neurons-gone-bonkers are exhausted" theory.

THE BEHAVIORAL CONTROL OF SEIZURES

The 1970s witnessed the emergence of behavioral seizure control methods with varying degrees of success. Summarized in a comprehensive review by Mostofsky and Balaschak (1977), these methods fall into three major categories: (a) psychotherapy, (b) behavior modification, and (c) biofeedback. Excepting psychotherapy, they have two principal aims: (a) the control of specific behaviors that lead to seizures, or (b) the control of the internal, physiological milieu. These include:

- denial of reward
- punishment
- penalty program (time out)
- avoidance
- overt and covert reward
- relaxation
- desensitization
- hypnosis
- habituation/extinction
- biofeedback

These methods may be thought to be dependent on conditioning; and two seemingly unrelated methods are of particular relevance here, because they set the stage for behavioral control of EEG and seizures by PCO_2 biofeedback: (a) the nonspecific relaxation/desensitization, and (b) EEG biofeedback. The initial success of EEG biofeedback (Chase & Harper, 1971; Harper & Sterman, 1972; Lubar & Bahler, 1976; Lubar et al., 1981; Sterman, 1977; Sterman & Friar, 1972) was questioned (Gastaut, 1975; Kaplan, 1975) because seizures frequently are intractable even to medication.

The reduction of seizures by these methods was often attributed to either a temporary generalized attention effect, stress reduction, or placebo. There is little reason to believe that placebo played a major role in the reduction of seizure frequency and severity, but there is ample evidence for the role of stress reduction in seizure control.

Stress Reduction and Relaxation

Temkin and Davis (1984) examined the role played by major life events, daily hassles, uplifts, and daily stress levels in seizure risk. In adults with severe epilepsy, they devised a statistical risk ratio and reported that daily stressful events and perceived stress levels tend to increase the incidence of seizures. Comparing both positive events and hassles, they concluded that uplifting events seldom result in seizures.

Williams, Gold, Shrout, Shaffer, and Adams (1979) distinguished between neurogenic and hysterical seizures on the basis that the latter are triggered by emotional stress. They cited clinical reports suggesting that psychotherapy can play a useful role in treating uncontrolled seizures. Presumably, they viewed *psychiatric intervention* as a form of emotional stress reduction, bolstering their argument by pointing out that some seizures can be initiated and/or inhibited by specifiable external or internal events. Feldman and Paul (1976) previously reported that, although emotional factors played an important role in poor seizure control, psychotherapeutic efforts were without benefit, because retroactive ictal amnesia erased the memory for the stressful antecedents to the seizure. Using videotaped recordings of specific problematic social interactions, they taught their clients to avoid the events that previously had been sufficient to induce seizures.

Aird (1983) cited prolonged and intense emotional stress among seizure triggers. He also emphasized metabolic factors such as hypoxia, HV, acid–base imbalance, and hypoglycemia. He reported that daily activities may be epileptogenic; even those that vary from hour to hour may alter seizure incidence in as many as 17% of the drug refractory. Aird stated, "In epilepsy, as with other medical disorders, it is important to control all factors that significantly influence the underlying condition" (p. 581).

Some effort has gone into reducing stress by behavior modification techniques. Dahl, Melin, and Lund (1987) tested a form of desensitization, or counterconditioning (Wolpe, 1973), contingent-relaxation, in refractory epilepsy. Patients learned to identify and discriminate high- and low-risk preseizure warning signals by a behavioral analysis, using daily mapping of preseizure situations and signs. They also were taught to recognize safe, low-risk situations and signs incompatible with increased seizure risk. When they could identify these low-risk signs reliably, they were told to vividly imagine the high-risk situation and switch to a relaxed state with a low-risk scene. As is the common practice in behavior therapy, this was done first with visualization, then, finally, in vivo. Dahl et al. (1987) reported a statistically significant 66% reduction in seizures in their treatment group, as compared with no change and increased seizure frequency in the controls.

Standage (1972) reported a case in which he treated epilepsy by reciprocal inhibition of anxiety, aided by intravenous (IV) injection of diazepam (Valium) to induce relaxation (diazepam has anticonvulsant properties). This 29-year-old woman had a 7-year history of grand mal seizures, preceded by bilateral myoclonic jerking and occasional psychomotor attacks, at the rate of one to two per month, often triggered by tension and feelings of panic before they began. Since the onset of epilepsy, she often experienced anxiety attacks when left alone, or when faced with the prospect of going out, until she ceased to go out unaccompanied. A strong connection between seizure and panic disorder has been documented (Bear, Freeman, & Greenberg, 1985; Brodsky, Zuniga, & Casenas, 1983; Weilburg, Bear, & Sachs, 1987).

In the relaxed state, the patient was asked to imagine a situation from a previously established hierarchy involving being alone, and the onset of a seizure:

> At the bottom of the hierarchy was the scene of being alone for short periods indoors, after which the scenes progressed to longer periods by herself, shopping unaccompanied and eventually, the experience of prodromal jerking while alone indoors. Finally, she was asked to imagine the progression from jerking to loss of consciousness. (p. 218)

If anxiety was expressed during a particular scene presentation, the patient was instructed to relax and was taken back to a less threatening scene in the hierarchy. During the first 6 months of treatment, she experienced only one grand mal and one psychomotor seizure. Then, she also was taught "autogenous relaxation" (Stafford-Clark, 1964), in which a combination of therapist suggestions and concentration on muscle sensations induce relaxation. During the next 6 months, she experienced only one attack.

Similarly, Parrino (1971) used desensitization of several social-anxiety hierarchy triggers in a 36-year-old man with grand mal seizures and Jakob-Creutzfeld syndrome. Seizure activity declined from about 30 per week to about 10, on the 14th inpatient week; to just fewer than 5, over the next 5 outpatient weeks. Whitman, Dell, Legion, Eibhlyn, and Statsinger (1990) proposed to (a) abbreviate the 10-session protocol for progressive relaxation training of Bernstein and Borkovec (1973); (b) determine the degree of experience a therapist requires before being able to successfully teach progressive relaxation to clients; and (c) determine its long term-effect on seizures. Their subjects experienced six or more seizures during the baseline period (8 weeks). The abbreviation of the Bernstein and Borkovec (1973) protocol consisted of combining their Sessions 1 through 5 on Session 1; their Sessions 6 and 7 on Session 2; and incorporating their "recall," "recall and counting," and "counting," of their Sessions 8, 9, and 10 on Session 3: "Patients were asked to recall the feelings of the release of tension and to practice this recognition as they relaxed all muscle groups at once while the trainer counted from 1 to 10" (p. 19). They were instructed to practice the procedure twice per day and to keep an 8-week calendar on which to record seizure frequency daily; and were contacted by phone each month, for 4 months, to obtain seizure data. Of the 12 clients, 10 experienced a statistically significant seizure decrease. Group median seizure frequency decreased 21% from baseline to the first follow-up; then, 54% after 6 months. There seemed to be no appreciable untoward effect of the modification of the Bernstein and Borkovec (1973) protocol and, indeed, most studies they cited report fewer than 10 sessions, but at least 4 or more. Finally, despite lack of formal clinical psychology training, the lay therapists seemed to have obtained good results with their clients.

Because my main interest is the biobehavioral control of seizures by self-regulation of alveolar PCO_2, one may wonder why I give stress reduction by relaxation training—stress is only one of the many factors in the incidence of seizures—so seemingly detailed a description. It is because I believe that, by whatever technique relaxation obtains, it normalizes breathing and improves peripheral and cerebral circulation. I have detailed this elsewhere, in connection with different forms of mediation (Fried, 1987a, 1987b, 1990, 1993; Fried, Rubin, Carlton, & Fox, 1984); but, because there is no literature citing it in connection with seizure control, I am not doing so here. Relaxation training, deep-diaphragmatic breathing, and zen and yoga meditation (Kasamatsu & Hirai, 1969), including the well-documented "respiratory suspension" phenomenon (Badawi, Wallace, Orme-Johnson, & Rouzere, 1984; Kesterton & Clinch, 1985), all have been shown to produce a state in which EEG *alpha* dominates over *theta*—a signature of unimpeded CBF, a state inimical to seizures.

EEG Feedback Training of Seizure Inhibiting Brain Activity

In 1935, Gibbs, Davis, and Lennox reported the normal EEG of epileptic patients to consist of various dominant frequencies including *alpha* (Berger's rhythm, an 8–12 Hz waveform at 10–50 μv). When they became drowsy, EEG frequency decreased and amplitude rose somewhat to about 60 μv. Petit mal seizures accompanied a particular EEG waveform—a low frequency, sinusoidal, and sharp negative spike in the 3–4 Hz range, at about 100–300 μv, whereas grand mal was accompanied by dominant waves, 5–18 Hz, becoming larger and faster just before the patient's cry. Then, as the seizure subsided, slower rhythms appeared among the fast ones and the electrical activity decreased along with the muscle activity. After this phase, an abnormal flat EEG prevailed during stupor, returning to normal about 20 min later.

It is the control of the *alpha* rhythm that came to popular attention in the 1960s and 1970s, in connection with biofeedback and operant conditioning (Kamiya, 1969). These studies, erroneously thought to be the first, applied brain wave biofeedback to enhance a number of altered states of consciousness thought to benefit mood and reduce anxiety. As the technology used to produce these meditative states advanced, attempts to condition other cortical biopotentials were reported (Brown, 1975).

The first such study, as best I can determine, is that of Schwab et al. (1941) entitled "Regulation of Epilepsy by Synchronized Recording of Respiration and Brain Waves." It is astonishing that this study, published in *Archives of Neurology & Psychiatry,* a major medical journal, has never been cited in a single report on EEG biofeedback. Any doubt about what this publication reports is dispelled quickly by reading the opening paragraph:

> The technic of Cobb, Sargant, and Schwab [1939] in recording the synchronous respiration and electroencephalographic activity of epileptic patients at once suggested the possibility of using this method in controlling the treatment of such patients. In this paper the clinical application of the technic to the therapeutic management of 59 patients with epilepsy is described. (p. 1017)

This is not, of course, standard biofeedback fare, but it is a recognizable beginning, used to adjust medication. It yielded some interesting observations, all germane to the present concern. First, Schwab et al. (1941), not surprisingly, did not induce seizures with 3 min of deep hyperpnea at 20 to 30 breaths per sec despite increased *theta*. Why? Cobb et al. (1939) had done so previously. You may recall that in the previously cited study by Engel et al. (1947), *theta* appeared at about 90 sec, and significant loss of awareness did not occur until about 150 sec into the procedure (see Fig. 2.6), when EEG frequency had dropped sharply to about 5 Hz. In other words, Schwab et al. simply did not hyperventilate their clients long enough. Consequently, they arrived at the clearly contrary conclusion that "convulsions are rarely produced by hyperventilation." In fact, Robinson (1944) reported that it took 6 min to induce seizures. Second, Schwab et al. reported that, after taking anticonvulsants, phenobarbital, and dilantin in their study, epileptic patients tended to breathe more quietly: "[P]henobarbital and other anticonvulsant drugs act in a sedative manner, quieting the respiration so that spontaneous overbreathing is less likely" (p. 1030). Do anticonvulsants reduce chronic HV? Sedatives tranquilize, just like relaxation. Third, some epileptic patients did not show significant increase in *theta* until the 3rd min of HV. But, in the Engel et al. (1947) study, it appeared by 100 sec in nonepileptic subjects. This means that the precipitating factor in *theta* production in "respiratory alkalosis" is hypocapnia and not increased pH, because, in non-HV persons, there is no renal compensation for alkalosis: HV induces double whammy as CO_2 drops and blood pH rises before compensation can occur.

In 1967, Sterman & Wyrwicka reported a discrete EEG rhythm, consisting of 12–20 Hz bursts localized to the coronal gyrus of the cat, and called it the sensorimotor rhythm (SMR). They described it in the cat withholding somatomotor responses, and concluded that the SMR is observed in response to a "negative conditioned-stimulus" (CS). A negative CS is the occasion for response inhibition, in operant terms. In 1968, Wyrwika and Sterman followed with an elaboration of the SMR—production of the SMR by the cat was rewarded with milk for a number of sessions of 50 reinforcements each. Episodes of production of the SMR became more frequent; it was evidently conditionable. It became increasingly clear that the behavioral correlates of this rhythm were stereotyped posture, and more or less complete cessation of spontaneous activity. Apparently it seemed to them that they were observing the conditioning of "a central state related to inhibition of the phasic motor behavior."

In 1971, Chase and Harper, in a similar study, confirmed the conditionability of the SMR, now confined to the 12–14 Hz segment of the EEG. They also observed the accompanying cessation of movement and suppression of somatic activity. Their analysis of the respiratory correlates of the SMR led them to state, "Visual observation of the animals gave us the impression that they were regulating closely their pattern of respiration during epochs of conditioned EEG activity" (p. 87). Respiratory mechanisms are involved as well as the motor cortex. But, either the cats need to control their breathing to produce the SMR (in which case it is not operant conditioning of the SMR), or producing the SMR controls their breathing. Is breathing change primary or secondary?

In a subsequent study, Harper and Sterman (1972) also reported that conditioned SMR show a functional relationship to regulation of respiration. Chase and Harper (1971) had stated, in the previously cited study, that:

> Onset of each epoch [of SMR] was correlated positively with the termination phase. . . . Termination of 12 to 14 c/sec activity tended to occur during expiration in all cats (p 0.005). . . . Short bursts as well as long trains of 12 to 14 c/sec activity were time-locked to the respiration pattern described above. (p. 87)

Then, in 1972, Sterman and Friar reported the suppression of seizures in an epileptic, for the first time, by training her to increase her production of SMR. The procedure was relatively simple: Production of SMR triggered a visual biofeedback stimulus. Subsequent communications (Sterman, 1973) yielded these conclusions: (a) a 12–14 Hz rhythm can be recorded in humans over the Rolandic region; (b) its operant level and amplitude are low (3–4 μv); and (c) it shows an increase after about 2 weeks of training. Six seizure sufferers were studied over a period of 6–20 months, reportedly showing decreased spontaneous production of low frequency (*theta*) discharges and petit mal, grand mal seizures, and improvement of the quality of sleep.

However, Kaplan (1975), replicating Sterman and colleagues, concluded that the procedure had no effect on seizure reduction in her subjects, discounting previous findings and attributing whatever seizure reduction was observed to relaxation training or placebo. Her critique was supported immediately by Gastaut (1975), who essentially stated that reports of SMR conditioning are premature. In fact, the Kaplan (1975) study was not a replication, nor was that by Upton and Longmire (1975), who also failed to corroborate SMR findings. Differences in procedure may have considerable impact on outcome. The argument that no matter what you do, significant seizure reduction will be obtained because of generalized effects such as relaxation or placebo is patently untenable. Epileptic syndromes, in some, are notoriously intractable to any form of treatment; if placebo were a powerful control agent, it would have gained wider therapeutic acceptance.

Lubar and Bahler (1976) conducted their own study of SMR conditioning in 8 severely epileptic patients, following the same procedure. They confirmed previous findings, corroborated also by Finley (1977); Sterman, MacDonald, and Bernstein (1977); and Sterman (1977). It became evident that psychobiological control of seizures was feasible and that a number of different methods could be employed. Although Kuhlman (1980) essentially corroborated previous findings, he hedged about whether SMR conditioning was responsible for the observed change in seizure activity, contending that the procedure is nonspecific despite the fact that EEG power spectral composition in his subjects shifted to higher frequencies. Finally, he stated that normalization of the EEG is taking place, which was the same conclusion as that drawn by Lubar and Bahler (1976). No reference was made to the pioneering investigators who, from the 1920s to the 1940s, reported it in connection with their studies of CO_2 in abnormal EEG and epilepsy (Gellhorn, 1953; Meduna, 1958). Kuhlman's (1980) position was supported by Quy, Hutt, and Forrest (1979), who concluded that evidence for SMR conditioning is slender, but the procedure still works.

Sterman and Kovaleski (1979) reported that, in hydrazine seizures in monkeys, physical restraint raises seizure threshold comparably to pyridoxine (vitamin B6). Seemingly self-imposed physical restraint was observed in cats enhancing SMR. Vitamin B6 is a well-known anticonvulsant, especially in children with idiopathic seizures (Soulayrol, Mesdjian, Lob, Tassinari, & Rogers, 1965). Carlton and Fried (1983) have proposed that vitamin B6 (pyridoxal-5-phosphate) affects cell excitability thresholds and O_2 availability by its action on cellular magnesium transport and its opposition to excess cell calcium (Altura & Altura, 1982; Levine & Coburn, 1984). Both B6 and magnesium deficiency have been noted in epilepsy (Canelas, Marques de Assis, & Dejorge, 1965; Durlach, Verdeaux, & Henrotte, 1973).

Coupled with DeLorenzo's (1980) report that dilantin is a calcium antagonist, the effect of vitamin B6 should have prompted a look at its role in respiratory alkalosis. It did not. Sterman and Kovaleski (1979) replicated the study by showing that chair-restraint immobilization is accompanied by an increase in SMR observed at the lateral and mid-Rolandic region (Holcombe, Sterman, Goodman, & Fairchild, 1979), and by surmising that SMR corresponds to the operation of a motor inhibitory center. This conclusion was supported in Bowersox and Sterman (1981). They observed that dorsal column transsection decreases hydrazine seizure susceptibility. Such findings were reported in seizure sufferers with traumatic spine severation (Sterman, personal communication, 1982).

Alteration of the power spectrum by SMR conditioning was reported by Lubar et al. (1981) in a double-blind, crossover study of 8 persons with seizures refractory to medical control. When seizures decreased, power rose in the frequency band 16–23 Hz, and decreased in the low frequency band, 0–7 Hz. The latter encompasses the 4–7 Hz component typically associated with seizures. No neuropsychological changes were noted.

I am inclined to interpret the SMR studies this way: The brain may emit a detectable rhythm (13–15 Hz) at very low amplitude, in phase with breathing and associated with motion inhibition. Biofeedback training may enhance the covert behavior that raises its amplitude. In the process, the EEG normalizes (i.e., *alpha* increases and *theta* decreases), and there is a decreased incidence of seizure activity.

These studies typically have been carried out on those intractable to medication control. They have not, in all instances, yielded uniform results, or results that lend themselves to interpretation within a unified model of behavioral control. In the search for something to unify a core of conclusions into a synthesis of these research findings, it seemed that the covert behavior that results in the appearance of the SMR, or the SMR itself, is functionally related to respiration; or, possibly, that cerebral events are controlled by a breathing-related mechanism that both inhibits motor behavior and enhances the SMR. The law of parsimony was not of much help here. But early studies of arterial CO_2 tension, the EEG, and epilepsy suggested that the SMR and inhibition of motor activity was the consequent condition, whereas breathing was the antecedent.

In the first phase of the behavioral control program at ICD, SMR conditioning was tried simultaneously with end-tidal CO_2 monitoring. However, it quickly became evident that in a procedure like Lubar and Bahler's (1976), in which epileptic patients learned to increase high frequency (12–15 Hz), EEG was locked entirely to end-tidal CO_2, as predicted by Lennox et al. (1938). Because it is easier to control breathing than to enhance a cortical rhythm, I dropped EEG training and focused on producing the optimum breathing pattern—the one that would produce the normalized EEG that we observed during breathing training.

REDUCING EEG ABNORMALITY AND SEIZURE FREQUENCY BY THE SELF-REGULATION OF PERCENTAGE OF END-TIDAL CO_2 ($PETCO_2$)

In 1980, the behavioral seizures control program of the *Rehabilitation Research Institute,* ICD-International Center for the Disabled, NY, undertook the procedures reported to enhance SMR. We simultaneously monitored $PETCO_2$, because we were aware of its relationship to EEG and seizures. My colleagues and I observed a continuous and exact inverse relationship, breath by breath, between the video monitor analog bars of $PETCO_2$ and EEG *theta*. As one rose, the other fell, both in seizure and in nonseizure subjects. *Alpha* was related directly to $PETCO_2$. As the literature predicted, no irrelevant connection between breathing, EEG, and seizures can exist—a vast literature attests to that fact. At first, we wondered why it never came up in the SMR studies; the knowledge of the effects of CO_2 on the motor cortex goes back at least to Brody and Dusser de Barenne, who, in 1932, were the first to use the term *hyperventilation*. It seemed then, and still seems now, a curious omission.

Findings were used to convince the ICD directors that controlling seizures by self-regulation of alveolar PCO_2 was not an indication that we had taken leave of our senses. These studies included Brick (1958), who observed over 50% seizure reduction with CO_2 inhalation; Caspers and Speckmann (1972); and others (Caspers & Simmich, 1966; Pollock, 1949; Wang & Sonnenschein, 1955; Woodbury & Kemp, 1970). Holmberg (1953) found an eightfold increase in spike-and-wave activity with room-air HV; and Robinson (1944) found an inverse relationship between daily arterial CO_2 blood content and incidence of petit mal in epileptics. Raichle and Plum (1972) reported a 2% decline in cerebral blood flow (CBF) for every 1 torr decline in alveolar PCO_2, but Morrice (1956) cautioned, "The first appearance of slow wave activity in the EEG occur[s] over a wide range of tensions [$PaCO_2$]. In other words . . . individual constitution overshadows the effect of respiratory effort and change in blood chemistry" (p. 67).

PHASE I: THE PILOT STUDY

Before undertaking a full-scale investigation, preliminary answers to basic hypotheses were obtained:

- Seizure sufferers hyperventilate prior to seizure onset, resulting in profound hypocapnia.
- Individuals can learn to regulate their breathing and reduce hypocapnia.
- Normocapnia normalizes the EEG and reduces the likelihood of seizure.

The physiological mechanisms that link HV and seizures, and the studies that affirm two of these three hypotheses are detailed elsewhere (Fried, 1987a,

1987b, 1990, 1993; Fried, Fox, & Carlton, 1990; Fried et al., 1984). The evidence that idiopathic seizures are preceded by hyperventilatory breathing changes goes back at least to Lennox (1928); and Rosett (1924) showed that they may be induced by HV. The second hypothesis, bolstered by the report of Ingvar, Siesjo, and Hertz (1959), is that PCO_2 can be self-regulated by controlled breathing. The third hypothesis is tenable because normocapnia by CO_2 inhalation has shown the desired effect on the EEG and seizure incidence (Brick, 1958).

Method

Subject. There were 3 men and 2 women ranging in age between 22 and 43 years in this preliminary study; there were a variety of seizures, including partial, partial complex, and generalized seizures, despite therapeutic range levels of anticonvulsants. Data are summarized in Table 2.1. Seizure type, severity, and frequency were established on the basis of medical records and corroborative testimony from friends, relatives, and physicians. Seizure logs were issued with detailed instructions in their use. A project physician examined each subject and his or her medical record before admission to the study. No organic basis for seizures was noted in any of the subjects in this study.

Apparatus. A slender tube, one end inserted about $\frac{1}{4}$in. into the subject's right nostril, was taped to the upper lip to sample end-tidal air for CO_2 analysis by a P.K. Morgan infrared gas analyzer. The analog output of the gas analyzer was transmitted to an ASI Matrix 9400, which transformed the percentage of CO_2 concentration ($PETCO_2$) in end-tidal air to a blue trace on a video monitor in front of the subject. Simultaneously, it was transmitted to an analog-to-digital (A/D) converter so that it could be analyzed by an Apple II+ computer, which determined mean and peak percent CO_2 for any preselected number of 15 sec epochs (3–5, usually).

EEG Power Spectral Analysis. Grass gold-plated electrodes were attached to the scalp of the subject, midway between F3–C3 and C3–P3 (International 10/20 System). The signal was transmitted to two WPI (DAM) preamplifiers, simultaneously recorded on a Vetter (Model A) FM tape recorder for subsequent fast-Fourier analysis by the computer, and also monitored online by a Hewlett-Packard spectrum analyzer (Model 3582A). Power values were based on ten 3-sec samples, 27 sec apart. The computer was programmed to do power/frequency distribution for 25 discrete ordinates, from 1 to 25 Hz units in bar-graph, or curve form. Figure 2.7 illustrates this in a control subject, for the range of 1–21 Hz.

Diaphragmatic Breathing Training with $PETCO_2$ Biofeedback. With the $PETCO_2$ video monitor trace as a biofeedback cue, deep-diaphragmatic respiration was taught by a biofeedback trainer who instructed the subjects in the proper

TABLE 2.1
Description of Patient Sample in Pilot Study

Subject No.	*Sex*	*Age*	*Age of Onset*	*Seisure Type*	*Entered Program*	*Disposition*	*Medication*
107	M	39	21	GM, PM, Pm, blackouts	Jul. 82	Withdrew: Jan. 83	Dilantin, 600 mg; Phenobarb., 90 mg.
109	F	36	26	GM, PM, Pm, falls	Aug. 82	Active: 1X/week	Tegretol, 800 mg; Phenobar., 120 mg.
112	M	42	7	GM, auras	Sep. 82	Active: 1X/week	Dilantin, 300 mg; Phenobar., 200 mg.
116	F	24	4	GM, PM, Pm, auras	Dec. 82	Withdrew: Jan. 83	Dilantin, 200 mg; Tegretol, 1200 mg.
117	M	37	17	GM, Pm, paresthesia	Feb. 83	Active: 1X/week	Dilantin, 200 mg; Phenobarb., 2 gr.

GM: grand mal; PM: petit mal; Pm: psychomotor.

SUBJECT: EEG
DATE:05/11/83 11;05;28 32

FREQ.	— AMP.	FREQ.	— AMP.
1 HZ	192.325815	11 HZ	109.807568
2 HZ	125.287543	12 HZ	105.289783
3 HZ	130.461157	13 HZ	61.9704227
4 HZ	80.357783	14 HZ	54.2577993
5 HZ	78.4201743	15 HZ	32.0075306
6 HZ	66.016668	16 HZ	38.922279
7 HZ	59.216572	17 HZ	32.8028577
8 HZ	51.2415154	18 HZ	22.3965271
9 HZ	53.494154	19 HZ	26.3989878
10 HZ	73.597481	20 HZ	41.08746

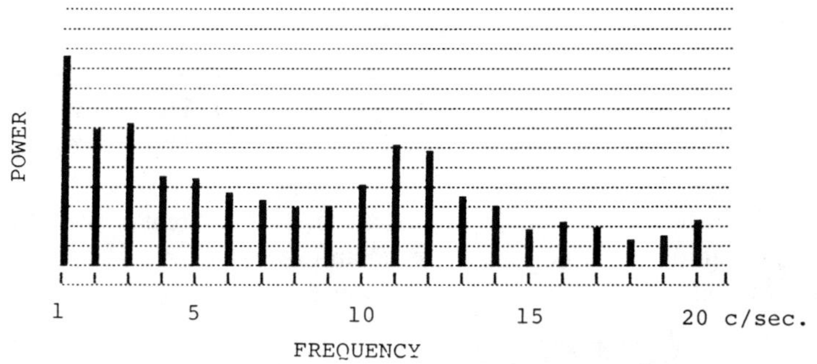

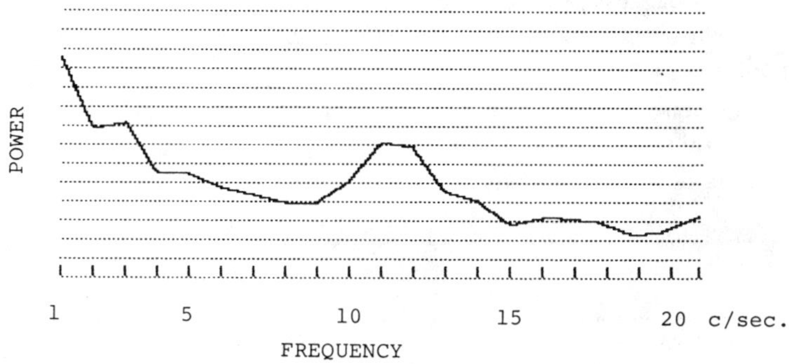

FIG. 2.7. Computer analysis and graphic representation of the power spectral composition of the EEG in an asymptomatic control subject.

abdominal breathing movements. The breathing methods adapted from various yoga techniques (Fried, 1987a, 1987b, 1990, 1993; Fried et al., 1984, 1990) to produce a specific breathing pattern employing the diaphragm—a more or less sinusoidal waveform on the video monitor with two to three peaks per screen update (20 sec). This pattern is approximately equivalent to normal breathing at about six to nine breaths per min. A horizontal line, set at 5% CO_2, was used as the $PETCO_2$ criterion. Thus, the subjects could observe the rate, rhythm, and end-tidal CO_2.

Results. Subject 109F showed a dramatic pre- to posttreatment reduction over a 6-month period, whereas the others showed a moderate reduction (chi-square significant at $p = .01$).

Figure 2.8 shows the EEG power spectral composition in 2 asymptomatic, non-HV controls subjects. Figure 2.9 shows the average power spectral composition of the EEG of 15 control subjects (10 women and 5 men, ranging in age between 22 and 53 years). Note the elevation at *alpha,* peaking at 12 Hz. Figures 2.10–2.14 show the EEG power spectra of each subject and the temporally coinciding polygraphic trace of $PETCO_2$:

- 107M dropped from 15 breaths per min on the first to 12 breaths per min on the 19th pretraining session. The EEG shows overall power elevation with a relative increase in *alpha* and a decrease at 4 and 5 Hz. Seizures decreased from 3 to 1 per month.
- 109F decreased from 18 breaths per min on the first to 11 breaths per min on the 14th pretraining session. EEG showed an increase at 8, 11, and 14 Hz. Seizures decreased from over 150 to 12 per month.
- 112M dropped from 19 breaths per min on the first to 16 breaths per min on the 23rd pretraining session. The EEG shows overall power elevation, especially in the low frequencies, peaking at 8 Hz. Seizures dropped from 5 to 3 per month.
- 116F slowed from 18 breaths per min on Session 1 to 8 breaths per minute on the 19th pretraining session. The EEG shows a slight elevation with an increase peaking at 12 Hz. Seizures dropped from 6 to 4 per month.

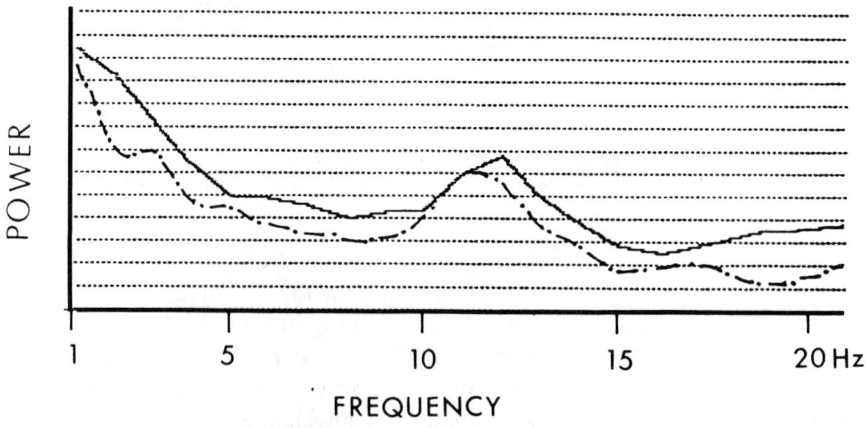

FIG. 2.8. EEG power spectral composition in two asymptomatic control subjects.

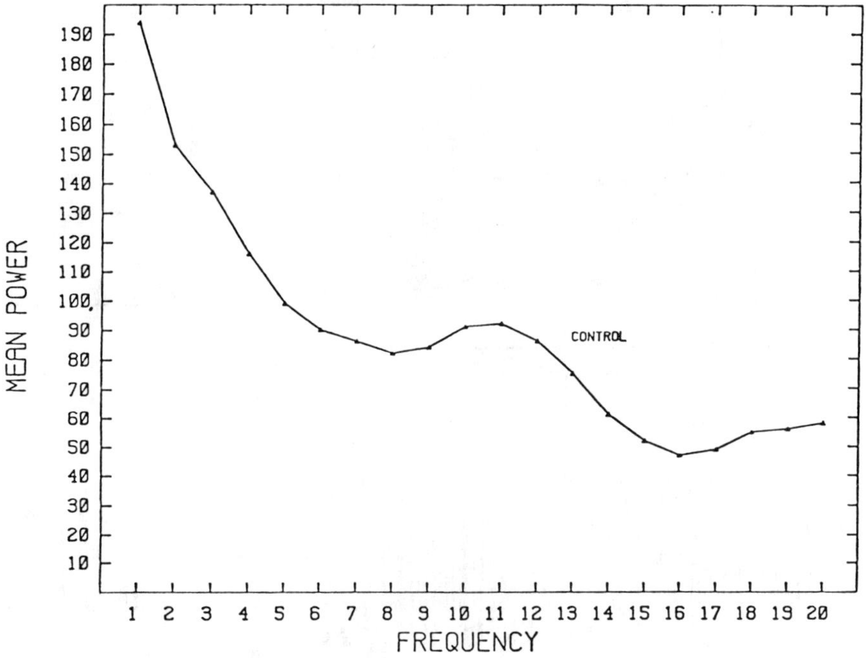

FIG. 2.9. Mean EEG power spectral composition in 15 asymptomatic control subjects.

- 117M dropped from 19 breaths per min on the first to 8 breaths per min on the 14th pretraining session. The EEG shows a pretraining elevation between 4 and 7 Hz, with a decreased elevation and increased *alpha* after 14 training sessions.

To get a better picture of alveolar ventilation, a respiration rate and $PETCO_2$ ratio (RR/CO_2) index was computed (Fig. 2.15). The index mean was 4.2 on the first and 2.56 on the last pretraining record. This difference was statistically significant (ANOVA, $p = .05$). The normal value would be about 2.4 in an average person at rest, breathing normally at 12 breaths per min, and $PETCO_2$ at 5.0% (Comroe, 1974).

DISCUSSION

These preliminary data showed that idiopathic seizure sufferers can learn diaphragmatic breathing with instructions and biofeedback, and that breathing training has an immediate and predictable effect on brain waves and seizure inci-

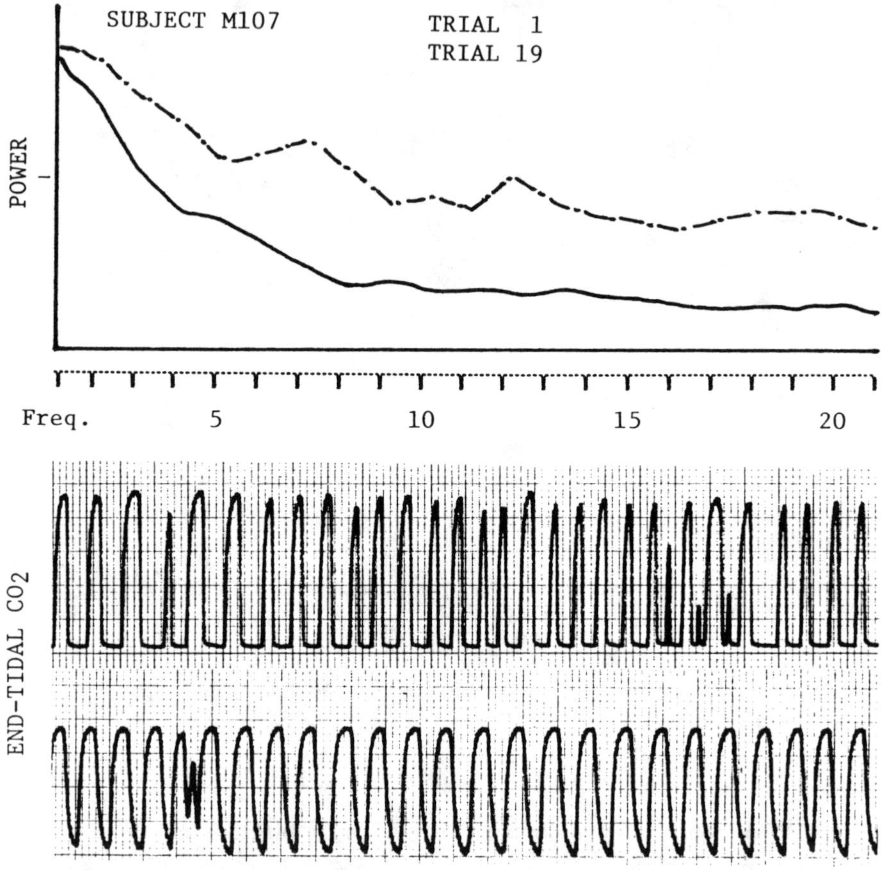

FIG. 2.10. Subject 107M: EEG power spectral composition and $PETCO_2$ trace before Trials 1 and 19.

dence. The breathing pattern in this sample of seizure sufferers was exactly like that described in previous reports (Cobb et al. 1938; Engel et al., 1947), showing varying degrees of HV, a frequent absence of EEG *alpha,* and elevation in the seizure-critical frequencies prior to training.

Following diaphragmatic respiration training with $PETCO_2$ biofeedback, breathing became somewhat slower and more regular, progressing from session to session (it was observed *before* each training session to avoid short-term training effects). A consistent after-training increase in EEG power also was observed. It could explain either increased SMR, increased *alpha,* or the change in the slope of the power spectrum envelope (i.e., normalization). Depending on how low-frequency filters are set, and the criterion for change in the EEG is the increase in power in a segment of the spectrum, then all three of these observations qualify.

In 3 of the 5 subjects in this preliminary study, EEG *theta* associated with seizures did not attenuate, yet seizure frequency decreased. Dilantin showed the same effect (i.e., seizure reduction without EEG change). Encouraged by the results of this preliminary study, we continued the procedure with these subjects and expanded the sample.

PHASE II: THE EXPANDED STUDY

Subjects. Twenty-four persons, intractable to anticonvulsant medication (see Table 2.2) and presenting chronic HV and grand mal, petit mal, psychomotor, and akinetic seizures were admitted to the program. They ranged in age from 22

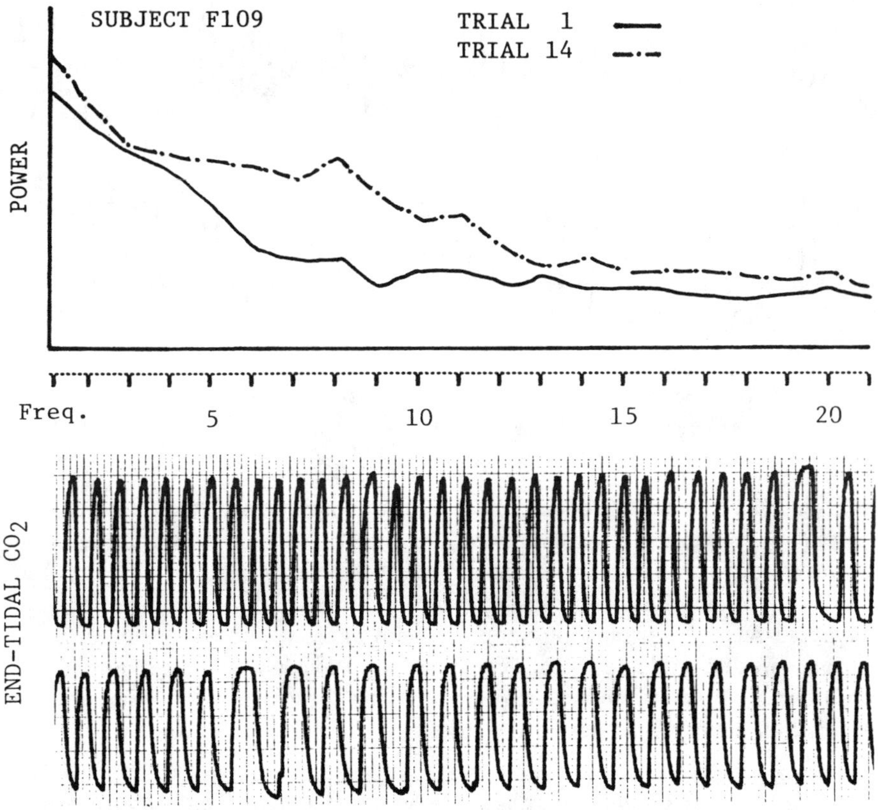

FIG. 2.11. Subject 109F: EEG power spectral composition and $PETCO_2$ trace before Trials 1 and 14.

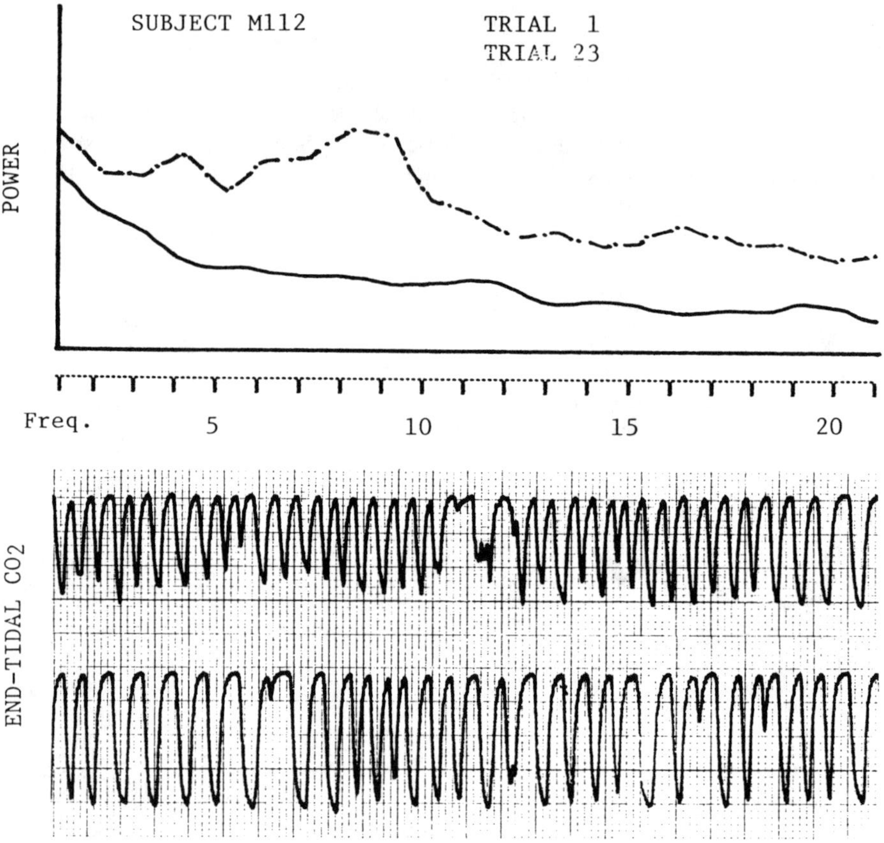

FIG. 2.12. Subject 112M: EEG power spectral composition and $PETCO_2$ trace before Trials 1 and 23.

to 53 years. Of these 24 persons, 18 stayed in the program for several months; 11, at least 7 months (10 of them with grand mal). We added an asymptomatic control group with 5 men and 10 health-service professionals and office staff at ICD, and an additional comparison group of 8 men and 7 women psychiatric outpatient referrals, presenting variously with anxiety, phobias, panic attacks, vertigo, dizziness, depression, alcohol abuse, Raynaud's disease, migraines, respiratory complaints, and vague psychosomatic chest symptoms. There was no evidence of psychosis in any of the subjects.

Results. $PETCO_2$ and EEG observations were based on data obtained during a 10-min observation and recording session preceding each biofeedback training session. During training and posttraining, observations also were made, but these data were considered limited to interpretation as short-term effects and are not included here.

The Effect of Respiration Training on Respiration. Table 2.3 summarizes the statistics for respiratory measures obtained from the training and biofeedback treatment group and the control group of asymptomatic subjects. There was a statistically significant difference between the first pretraining breathing rate (RR) and that of the controls ($F = 7.59$, $p < .05$), between the first and last pretreatment RR ($t = 4.16$, $p < .05$), and between the controls and the last pretreatment RR ($F = 3.80$, $p < .05$). No significant difference was found between any combination of groups when comparing mean $PETCO_2$ only.

In view of the compensatory relationship between end-tidal CO_2 and RR changes in chronic HV, the RR/CO_2 index was used. A statistically significant difference was found between the first pretraining and the control RR/CO_2 ($F =$

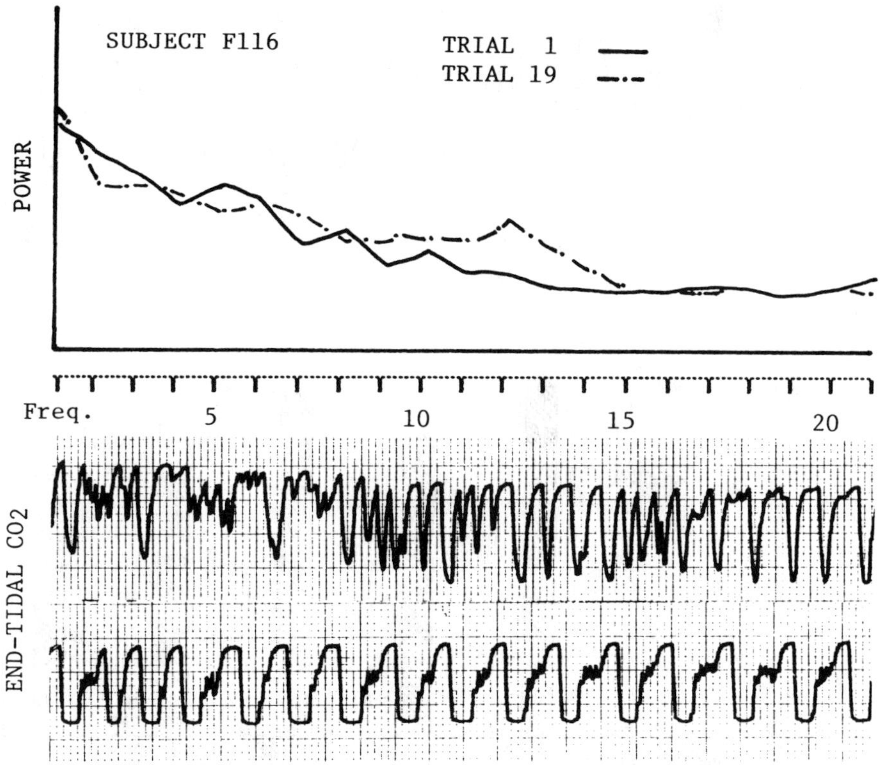

FIG. 2.13. Subject 116M: EEG power spectral composition and $PETCO_2$ trace before Trials 1 and 19.

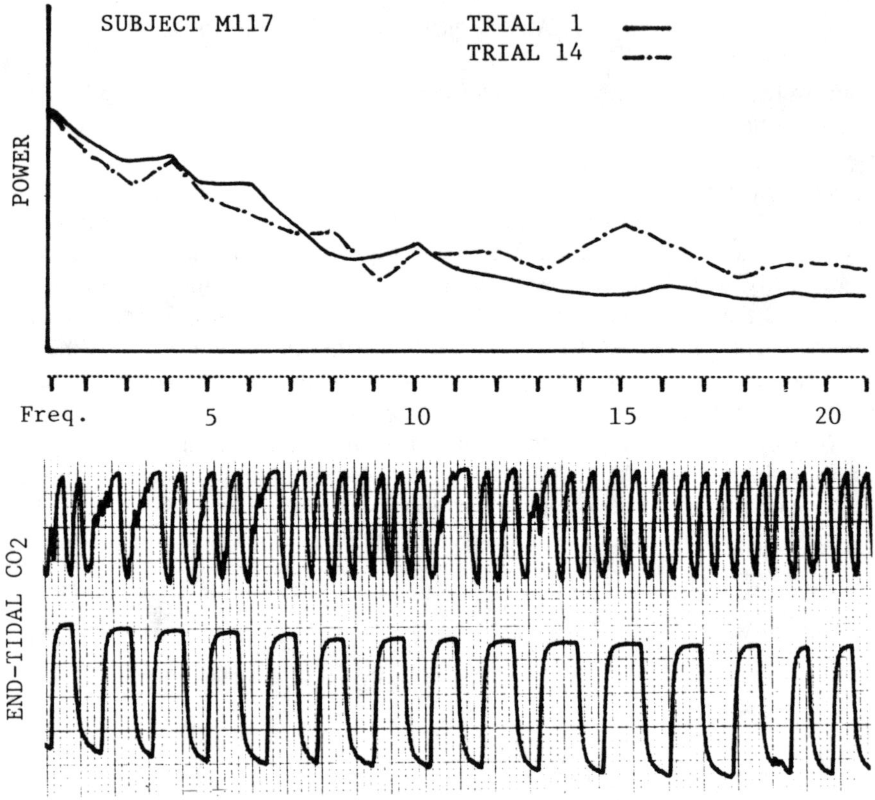

FIG. 2.14. Subject 117M: EEG power spectral composition and $PETCO_2$ trace before Trials 1 and 14.

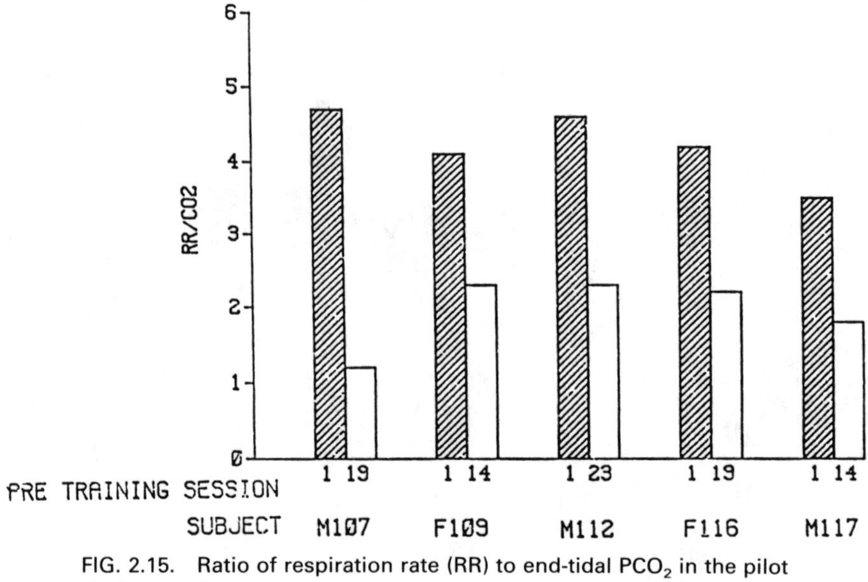

FIG. 2.15. Ratio of respiration rate (RR) to end-tidal PCO_2 in the pilot study sample.

TABLE 2.2
Description of the Subjects in Phase II, the Expanded Sample

Subject No.	*Sex*	*Age*	*Age of Onset*	*Seisure Type*	*Entered Program*	*Disposition*	*Medication*
102	F	24	13	GM, PM, Pm, blackouts	Jun. 82	Active: 1X/week	Tegretol, 1,800 mg
103	F	27	14	GM, Pm	Jun. 82	Active: 1X/week	Mysoline
104	F	31	10	GM, muscle fasciculation	Jul. 82	Active: 1X/week	Dilantin, 200 mg
105	M	36	13	GM, Pm	Aug. 82	Withdrew: April 83; reinstated Jul. 83	None
106	F	27	13	Akinetic (Syncope?)	Aug. 82	Active: 1X/week	Dilantin, 400 mg; Tegretol, 1,000 mg; Mysoline, 500 mg; Clonazepin, 2 mg; Inderal, 5 mg
107	M	39	21	GM, PM, Pm, blackouts	Jul. 82	Withdrew: Jan. 83	Dilantin, 600 mg; Phenobarbital, 90 mg
108	M	10	5	PM	Aug. 82	Withdrew: Sep. 82	Depakene, 250 mg; Clonopin, 0.5 mg
109	F	36	26	GM, PM, Pm, falls	Aug. 82	Active: 1X/week	Tegretol, 800 mg; Phenobarbital, 120 mg
110	F	30	28	GM	Aug. 82	Withdrew: after 3 weeks	Depakene, 1,000 mg; Tegretol, 800 mg; Phenobarbital, 96 mg
111	F	35	—	Migraine, EEG dysrhythm	Aug. 82	Withdrew: after 3 weeks	None
112	M	42	7	GM, auras	Sep. 82	Active: 1X/week	Dilantin, 300 mg; Phenobarbital, 200 mg
113	F	31	5	PM, Pm	Sep. 82	Suspended: medical problems	Tegretol, 200 mg

(*continued*)

TABLE 2.2 (*Continued*)

Subject No.	*Sex*	*Age*	*Age of Onset*	*Seisure Type*	*Entered Program*	*Disposition*	*Medication*
114	F	35	17	GM, PM, auras, paresthesia	Sep. 82	Active: 1X/week	Dilantin 100 mg
115	M	31	13	GM, PM	Sep. 82	Active: 1X/week	Mysoline, 1,250 mg; Mesantoin, 300 mg
116	F	24	4	GM, PM, Pm, auras	Dec. 82	Withdrew: Jan. 83	Dilantin, 200 mg; Tegretol, 1,200 mg
117	M	37	17	GM, Pm, paresthesia	Feb. 83	Active: 1X/week	Dilantin, 200 mg; Phenobarbital 2 gr
118		(unassigned)					
119		(unassigned)					
120	F	38	18	GM	Jan. 83	Withdrew: Jul. 83	Dilantin, 200 mg; Phenobarbital, 60 mg
121	F	34	5	GM, PM, Pm	Jan. 83	Dismissed: unmanageable	Dilantin, 400 mg; Depakene, 1,000 mg
122	M	34	19	GM, PM, Pm	Jan. 83	Active: 1X/week	Tegretol, 200 mg; Dilantin 100 mg
123	M	28	12	GM	Jan. 83	Dismissed: aggressive	Depakene, 1,250 mg
124	F	34	16	PM, Pm, amnesia	Feb. 83	Active: 2X/week	Zarohtin, 250 mg
125	M	40	18	GM, PM	Mar. 83	Withdrew: after 3 weeks	None

Note. From "Behavioral Control of Intractable Idiopathic Seizures: I. Self-Regulation of End-Tidal Carbon Dioxide" by R. Fried, S. R. Rubin, R. M. Carlton, and M. C. Fox, 1984, *Psychosomatic Medicine, 46,* pp. 316–331.

GM: grand mal; PM: petit mal; Pm: psychomotor.

TABLE 2.3
Comparison of the Respiratory Measure of the Seizure and Control Group in the Expanded Sample

		First pretraining			Last pretraining	
	RR	*$\bar{X}CO_2$*	*RR/CO_2*	*RR*	*$\bar{X}CO_2$*	*RR/CO_2*
Treatment	$\bar{X}$ = 17.06	4.28	4.00	12.61	4.39	2.90
Group	S = 2.62	0.41	0.64	3.70	0.61	0.81
Control	$\bar{X}$ = 14.54	4.55	3.29			
Group	S = 7.22	0.56	1.76			

Note. From "Behavioral Control of Intractable Idiopathic Seizures: I. Self-Regulation of End-Tidal Carbon Dioxide" by R. Fried, S. R. Rubin, R. M. Carlton, and M. C. Fox, 1984, *Psychosomatic Medicine, 46,* pp. 316–331. Copyright 1984 by *Psychosomatic Medicine.* Reprinted by permission.

7.56, $p < 0.05$), and between the control and the last pretraining RR/CO_2 (F = 3.82, $p < .05$). Figure 2.16 shows the change in RR/CO_2 index between the first and last pretraining sessions in the biofeedback treatment group.

The Effect of Normalization of Respiration on the EEG Power Spectrum. Figure 2.17 compares average EEG power spectra in the control subjects to that of 10 biofeedback treatment group subjects who were in the program at least 7 months and to that of the psychiatric group. In the control group, spectral distribution is typical, showing a deceleration from dc to *alpha,* then a slight rise to *beta.* A test for parallel trends (ANOVA) was statistically significant ($F = 9.62$, $p < .05$), indicating that power differences at each ordinate are not constant along the spectrum.

Spectral composition on the first and last pretraining sessions of the seizures-group are shown in Fig. 2.18. *Theta* is elevated considerably, relative to *alpha,* on the first pretreatment. On the last, the curve looks almost normal.

Normalization of Respiration and Seizure Frequency. The seizure frequency data were obtained from 10 subjects who were in the study at least 7 months. The best account of the pretreatment seizure frequency is that they averaged 56 per month. The distribution is skewed ($s = 69.88$). At the end of the first month of training, mean seizure frequency dropped to 7 per month, also skewed (s = 7.89). See Table 2.4.

Because these distributions do not meet criteria for parametric analysis, a chi-square test was used to compare them against chance occurrence. The observed seizure frequency differences were not due to random variation ($x^2 = 38.0$, $p <$ .05). Seizure frequency dropped initially to an average of seven, followed by a decrease to about three and then a stabilization at about four per month. This pattern is shown in Fig. 2.18.

The pretreatment (estimated and actual) frequency of grand mal seizures,

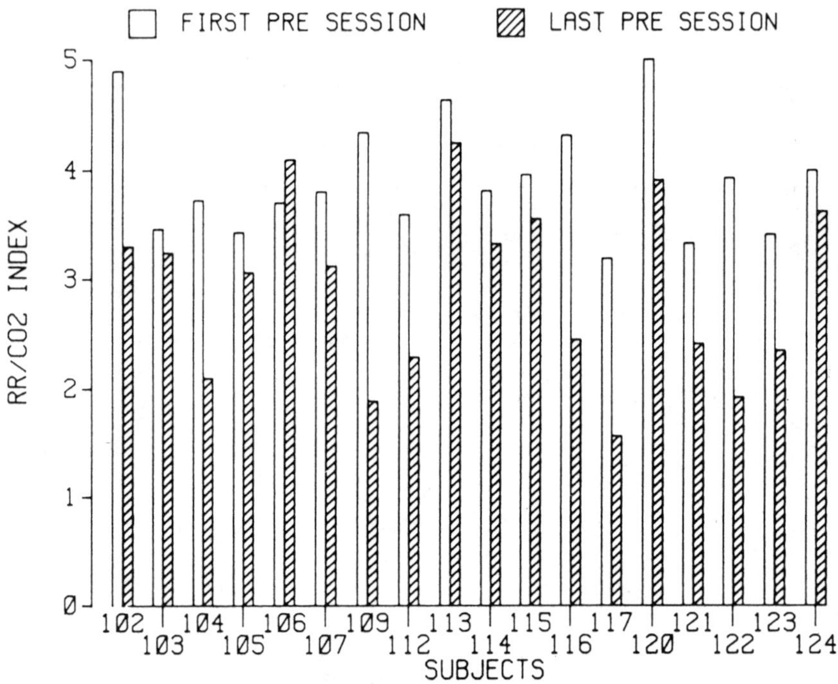

FIG. 2.16. Comparison of the pretraining respiratory output index (RR/CO_2) on the first and last sessions for the expanded sample of seizure sufferers. From "Behavioral Control of Intractable Idiopathic Seizures: I. Self-Regulation of End-Tidal Carbon Dioxide" by R. Fried, S. R. Rubin, R. M. Carlton, and M. C. Fox, 1984, *Psychosomatic Medicine, 46,* pp. 316–331. Copyright 1984 by *Psychosomatic Medicine.* Reprinted by permission.

taken separately, averaged about six per month. After the first month in the program, average frequency dropped to about two per month and, subsequently, to an average of less than one per month for the next 6 months. This distribution also is skewed, but in 8 of the 10 subjects who experienced such seizures, 4 had none at all for at least 6 months. The difference between the pre- and posttreatment seizure frequency is determined by the distribution of seizures during the 7 months observed. There is a statistically significant difference in the incidence of seizures during those 7 months ($x^2 = 27.7$, $p < .05$).

DISCUSSION

We have replicated the observation that chronic HV and seizure activity overlap. There was not a single instance in which persons with idiopathic epilepsy did not also show moderate to severe chronic HV. Of course, the reverse is not the case: The control group held a number of subjects with moderate to severe HV who did not have seizures. There is strong evidence that abdominal breathing training with $PETCO_2$ biofeedback can correct abnormal respiration. But, simply adjusting rate of respiration is inadequate. In a previously cited study, there was no indication that self-regulation of breathing produced a lasting outcome. Furthermore, in the numerous previous studies of the effects of HV and its treatment, no data were presented on the outcome of training subjects in diaphragmatic respiration.

It has been found empirically, in pilot studies prior to the present report, that awareness of the need for diaphragmatic respiration does not come until the subject can see the difference in output resulting from this type of respiration in comparison to thoracic breathing. Thus, the lasting benefits of our respiration training are believed to be related to the kind of "knowledge of results" that $PETCO_2$ biofeedback provides.

The Effect of Respiration Training on Respiration

It was impossible to maintain uniform adherence to protocols in this study—a common complaint in similar studies reviewed. There are too many human

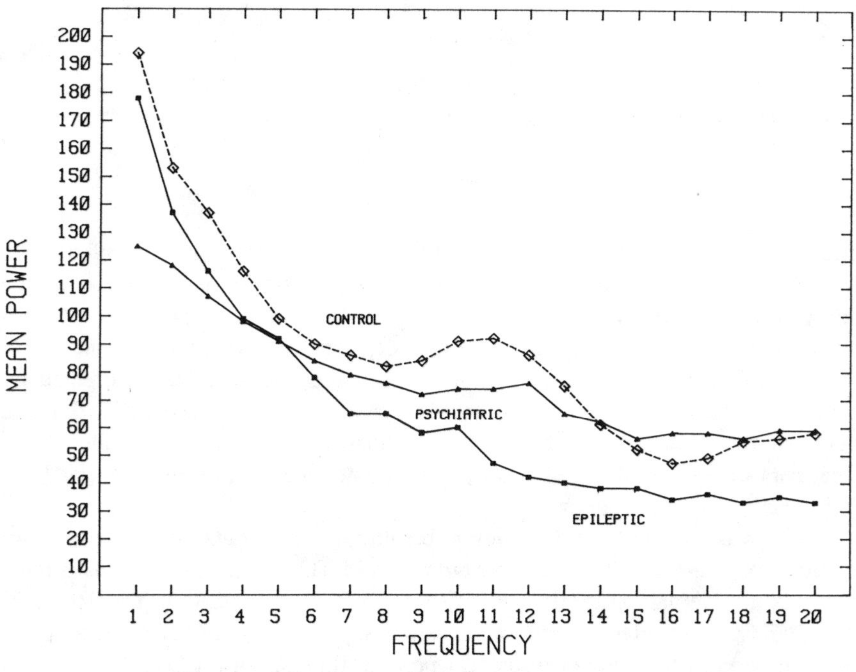

FIG. 2.17. Mean EEG power spectra of the control, psychiatric, and seizure subjects in the expanded sample. From "Behavioral Control of Intractable Idiopathic Seizures: I. Self-Regulation of End-Tidal Carbon Dioxide" by R. Fried, S. R. Rubin, R. M. Carlton, and M. C. Fox, 1984, *Psychosomatic Medicine, 46,* pp. 316–331. Copyright 1984 by *Psychosomatic Medicine.* Reprinted by permission.

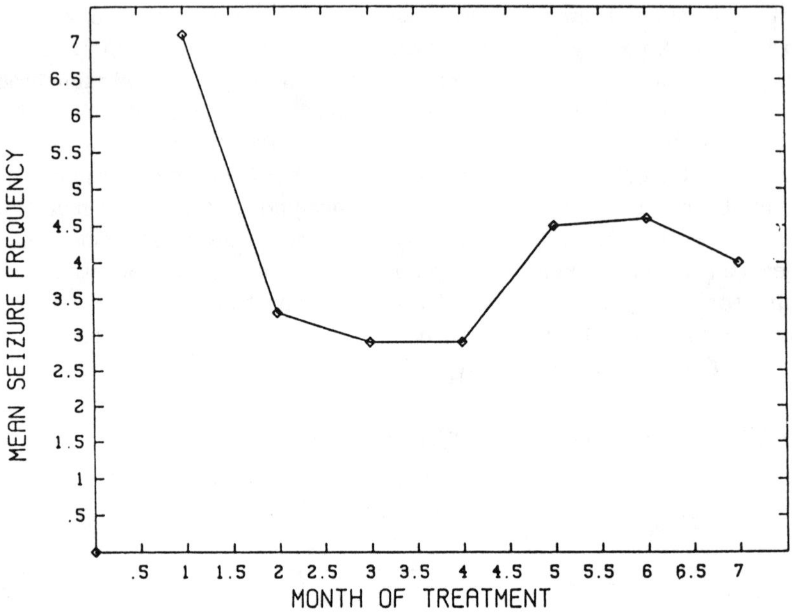

FIG. 2.18. Mean number of seizures (all types combined) in the subjects in the expanded sample who remained in the study at least 7 months.

circumstances that affect patient compliance and attendance in clinical studies: Subjects underwent a different number of training sessions; they did not enter the study at the same time; and, in some instances, I had to report the earliest record available when the first record was technically useless. These errors make statistical significance more difficult to attain, because later data were affected by change in the direction of the outcome. This tends to reduce the difference between first and last observations and underestimates the magnitude of the treatment effect. On the other hand, there was enough conformity so that I did not exactly "wing it" either.

There was a significant reduction in breathing rate (RR) because of diaphragmatic respiration, which lowers rate but not in $PETCO_2$. This must be interpreted in terms of alveolar ventilation (RR/CO_2). All factors equal, changing RR must alter $PETCO_2$: If metabolic rate is constant, the proportion of CO_2 dissipated will be a function of the number of breaths per unit time because CO_2 buildup in the lungs will be constant. Thus, the fact that no dramatic change in end-tidal CO_2 was noted over wide changes in RR indicates that there is an adjustment of CO_2 dissipation that occurs automatically with rate change. If that were not what the subjects were experiencing, they would be increasing their CO_2 dissipation as

RR decreased. That is precisely what happens if only *rate* is controlled in thoracic breathers, and that is why it does not help. The clearest indication of the breathing change is seen in the comparison of the output index RR/CO_2, which shows a dramatic change in all but Subject 106F.

The Effect of Respiration Training on the EEG

The EEG power spectrum in epileptics is categorically different from that of nonseizure sufferers. They typically have an elevation between 4–7 Hz, which was observed in this study. EEG analysis, unlike that for respiratory data, includes only data from those of the seizure subjects who remained in the study and received treatment for at least 7 months. Lubar & Bahler (1976) and Lubar et al. (1981) referred to posttraining changes in the EEG as normalization, meaning that *theta* drops as *alpha* rises in amplitude/time. It is observed here also.

The finding of abnormal EEG in moderate and severe chronic HV is consistent with our present understanding of the relationship between epileptiform EEG activity evoked routinely in EEG examination by HV. But, it is not clear how relieving HV reduces seizures. Figure 2.19 compares the EEG power spectra of the control subjects to the pre- and posttraining spectra of the epileptic subjects

TABLE 2.4
Mean Number of Seizures Experienced by the Subjects in the Expanded Sample in the First 7 Months in Treatment and Percent Improvement in RR/CO_2 Index from the First to the Last Pretraining Session*

Subject No.	*Month of Treatment* 1	2	3	4	5	6	7	*Percent Improved BPM/CO_2 Index*	*Average Seizure Frequency (per mo.)*
F102	3	4	5	5	10	0	9	33	5.14
F103	4	1	3	8	3	9	9	6	5.29
F104	10	5	2	2	9	17	8	44	7.71
M105	0	3	0	0	6	0	0	11	1.29
F109	22	7	6	6	6	7	6	67	8.57
M112	2	4	3	0	0	3	—	67	1.71
F114	16	0	1	1	1	1	1	28	3.00
M115	0	0	0	0	1	0	0	7	0.14
F116	14	8	8	7	—	—	—	38	7.40
M117	0	1	1	0	—	—	—	64	0.50
$\bar{X}$:	7.1	3.3	2.9	2.9	4.5	4.6	4.0	36.5	4.10

Note. From "Behavioral Control of Intractable Idiopathic Seizures I. Self-Regulation of End-Tidal Carbon Dioxide" by R. Fried, S. R. Rubin, R. M. Carlton, and M. C. Fox, 1984, *Psychosomatic Medicine, 46,* pp. 316–331. Copyright 1984 by *Psychosomatic Medicine.* Reprinted by permission.

*All seizures combined.

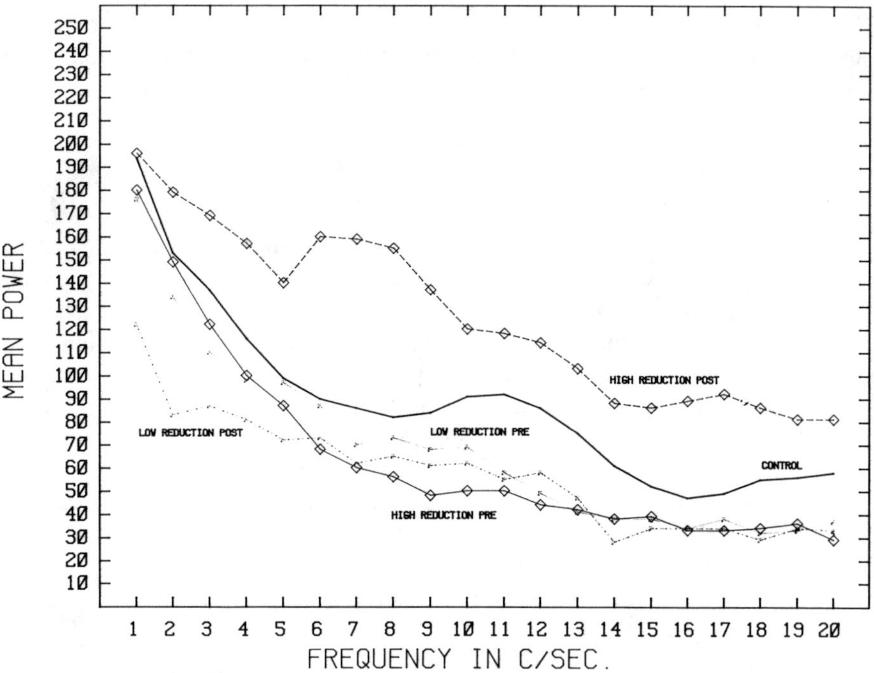

FIG. 2.19. Mean EEG power spectra in the expanded sample: Comparison of the power spectral composition before and after training in the subjects with high- and low-seizure reduction posttreatment, and power spectral composition in asymptomatic controls.

divided into two groups: those who had high- and those who had low-seizure reduction.

The subjects with low-seizure reduction, as well as those with high-seizure reduction after training, did not differ significantly from each other, nor from the controls, in the EEG power spectral composition before training. But those with high-seizure reduction after training were significantly different from the others in their EEG spectral composition. Any hypothesis about this result must, in the absence of direct evidence, be highly speculative. But, in view of the known relationship between EEG and PCO_2, it may be inferred that, in these subjects, there was a significant increase in brain blood flow, as evidenced by the exaggerated increase in overall power in the system. Those individuals with low-seizure reduction posttraining were the lowest in overall power. This conclusion is consonent with studies of constant-current rheoencephalography (Laitinen, Johansson, & Sipponen, 1966; Lechner, Geyer, & Rodler, 1967), which, by showing its direct relationship to brain blood flow, encouraged interpretation of power changes as changes in cross section of the vascular bed of the brain and, therefore, increased brain blood flow.

The Effect of Respiration Training on Seizure Activity

Correction of HV was followed by a significant diminution in seizure activity in these subjects. The reduction was not uniform, nor was the distribution of seizure types, frequency, and severity. After 7 months of training, no one had no seizure at all. However, the frequency and severity of the seizures, as well as seizure type for any subject, underwent considerable modification. Although all the subjects were intractable to therapeutic serum levels of a multitude of anticonvulsant medications, remarkably, 4 of the 8 out of 10 who experienced grand mal seizures had none during the 7-month period.

This study supports the contention that correcting HV in idiopathic seizure sufferers reduces, through the multiple pathways described, the tendency to convulsions by reducing the chronic hypoxia, which has been shown to cause abnormal EEG and to lower the seizure threshold.

SUMMARY

Breathing rate (RR), $PETCO_2$, and EEG were observed in three groups: (a) idiopathic seizures sufferers; (b) psychiatric referral subjects with stress, anxiety, and emotional, psychological, and psychophysiological disorders; and (c) asymptomatic controls. Virtually all the noncontrol subjects showed moderate to severe HV and EEG dysrhythmia. The seizure group was taught diaphragmatic breathing with $PETCO_2$ biofeedback. The training normalized their respiration and EEGs, and reduced seizure frequency and severity.

ACKNOWLEDGMENTS

This chapter was based on studies conducted at the *Rehabilitation Research Institute,* ICD-International Center for the Disabled, NY, between 1979 and 1984, when I was on leave from The City University of New York (CUNY). The studies were supported in part by the J. M. Foundation, the Clark Foundation, the Leon Lowenstein Foundation, the Gilder Foundation, and the Alcoa Foundation. I wish to express my gratitude to all the persons who contributed significantly to this research, including David J. Reynolds, Ph.D., assistant director, ICD; Richard M. Carlton, M.D., project physician; Mary C. Fox, and Sherry R.

Rubin, research associates; Helen Stonehill, chief librarian, ICD; and Stewart Riegler, M.C. (*computer maven*).

REFERENCES

Aird, R. B. (1983). The importance of seizure-inducing factors in the control of refractory epilepsy. *Epilepsia, 24,* 567–583.

Altura, B. M. (1982). Magnesium and regulation of contractility of vascular smooth muscle. In B. M. Altura, E. Davis, & H. Harders (Eds.), *Advances in microcirculation* (Vol. II, pp. 77–113). Basel: Karger.

Altura, B. M., & Altura, B. T. (1982). Mg, Na, and K interactions and coronary heart disease. *Dietary Minerals & Cardiovascular Disease Symposium, 1,* 241–265.

Badawi, K., Wallace, R. K., Orme-Johnson, D., & Rouzere, A. A. (1984). Electrophysiological characteristics of respiratory suspension periods occuring during practice of the transcendental meditation program. *Psychosomatic Medicine, 46,* 267–276.

Barolin, G. S. (1966). Migraines and epilepsies—A relationship? *Epilepsia, 7,* 53–66.

Batt, A. M., Siest, G., Khodjet el Khil, R., Le Perron, B., Weber, M., & Tridon, P. (1975). Drugs and references values in clinical chemistry. III. Effects of anticonvulsant drugs on plasma enzymes and metabolites: Correlation studies. *Drug Interference and Drug Measurement in Clinical Chemistry, Proceedings of the Third International Colloquium on Prospects in Biology* (pp. 33–41). Basel: Karger.

Bear, D. M., Freeman, R., & Greenberg, M. (1985). Psychiatric aspects of temporal lobe epilepsy. In R. E. Hales & A. J. Frances (Eds.), *Psychiatric update: American Psychiatric Association annual review* (pp. 31–37). Washington DC: American Psychiatric Association.

Berger, H. (1929). Uber das elektrenkephalogramm des menschen [Concerning the human electroencephalograph]. *Archives of Psychiatry, 87,* 527–570.

Bernstein, D. A., & Borkovec, T. D. (1973). *Progressive relaxation.* Champaign, IL: Research Press.

Bohr, C., Hasselbach, K., & Krogh, A. (1904). Ueber einen biologischer betziehung wichtigen einfluss, den die kohlensauerspannung des blutes auf dessen sauerstoff-bindung ubt [Concerning the biological consequences of the influence of carbon dioxide level on oxygen binding in blood]. *Scandinavian Archives of Physiology, 16,* 402.

Bowersox, S. S., & Sterman, J. B. (1981). Changes in sensorimotor sleep spindle activity and seizure susceptibility after somatosensory deafferentation. *Experimental Neurology, 74,* 814–828.

Brain, L. (1965). *Diseases of the nervous system.* London: Oxford University Press.

Bremer, F. (1938). L' activite electrique de l'ecorce cerebrale [The electrical activity of the cerebral cortex]. *Actualites Scientifique et Industrielles, 658,* 46.

Brewer, G. J. (1974). Red cell metabolism and function. In D. M. Surgenor (Ed.), *The red blood cell* (2nd ed., Vol. I., pp. 473–508). New York: Academic Press.

Brick, H. (1958). Carbon dioxide therapy in prison with some comparisons in private practice. In L. J. Meduna (Ed.), *Carbon dioxide therapy* (2nd ed., pp. 54–65). Springfield, IL: Charles C. Thomas.

Brill, N. G., & Seidman, H. (1942). Electroencephalographic changes during hyperventilation in epileptic and non-epileptic disorders. *Annals of Internal Medicine, 16,* 451.

Brodsky, L., Zuniga, J. S., & Casenas, E. R. (1983). Refractory anxiety: A masked epileptiform disorder? *Psychiatric Journal of the University of Ottawa, 8,* 42–45.

Brody, B. S., & Dusser de Barenne, J. G. (1932). Effects of hyperventilation on the excitability of the motor cortex in cats. *Archives of Neurology & Psychiatry, 28,* 571–585.

Brown, B. (1975). *New mind, new body.* New York: Harper & Row.

Bunn, H. F., & Jandi, J. H. (1970). Control of hemoglobin function within the red blood cell. *New England Journal of Medicine, 282,* 1414–1421.

Canelas, H. M., Marques de Assis, L., & Dejorge, F. B. (1965). Disorders of magnesium metabolism in epilepsy. *Journal of Neurology & Neurosurgery, 28,* 378–381.

Carlton, R. M., & Fried, R. (1983). Intracellular magnesium deficiencies in epilepsy. Abstract 48. *Journal of the American College of Nutrition, 2,* 288.

Caspers, H., & Simmich, W. (1966). D.C. shifts associated with seizure activity. *Excerpta Medica International Congress Series, 124,* 151–162.

Caspers, H., & Speckmann, E. J. (1972). Cerebral pO_2, pCO_2, and pH: Changes during convulsive activity and their significance for spontaneous arrest of seizures. *Epilepsia, 13,* 699–725.

Chanutin, A., & Curnish, R. R. (1967). Effect of organic phosphates on the oxygen equilibrium of human erythrocytes. *Archives of Biochemistry & Biophysics, 121,* 96–102.

Chase, M. H., & Harper, R. M. (1971). Somatomotor and visceromotor correlates of operantly conditioned 12–14 c/sec. sensorimotor cortical activity. *EEG & Clinical Neurophysiology, 31,* 85–92.

Cobb, S., Sargant, W. W., & Schwab, R. S. (1938). Simultaneous respiratory and electroencephalographic recording in petit mal. *Archives of Neurology & Psychiatry, 42,* 1189–1191.

Cogan, D. G., Schulman, J., Porter, R. J., & Mudd, S. H. (1980). Epileptiform occular movements with methylmalonic acidurea and homocystinurea. *American Journal of Ophthalmology, 90,* 251–253.

Comroe, J. H., Jr. (1974). *Physiology of respiration* (2nd ed.). Chicago: Year Book Medical Publishers.

Comroe, J. H., Jr., Forster, R. E., Dubois, H., Briscoe, A. B., & Carlsen, E. (1962). *The Lung: Clinical physiology and pulmonary function tests* (2nd ed.). Chicago: Year Book Medical Publishers.

Dahl, J., Melin, L., & Lund, L. (1987). Effects of a contingent relaxation treatment program on adults with refractory epileptic seizures. *Epilepsia, 28,* 125–132.

Darrow, C. W., & Graf, C. C. (1945). Relation of electroencephalogram to photometrically observed vasomotor changes in the brain. *Journal of Neurophysiology, 8,* 449–461.

Davis, H., & Wallace, W. (1941). Factors affecting the electroencephalographic changes induced by hyperventilation. *American Journal of Physiology, 133,* 258.

Davis, H., & Wallace, W. (1942). Factors affecting changes produced in electroencephalogram by standardized hyperventilation. *Archives of Psychiatry & Neurology, 47,* 606–625.

DeLorenzo, R. J. (1980). Phenytoin: Calcium- and calmodulin-dependent protein phosphorilation and neurotransmitter release. In G. H. Glaser, J. K. Penry, & D. M. Woodburry (Eds.), *Antiepileptic drugs: Mechanisms and action.* New York: Raven Press.

Deutsch, F., Ehrentheil, O., & Pierson, O. (1941). Capillary studies in Raynaud's disease. *Journal of Laboratory & Clinical Medicine, 26,* 1729–1750.

Durlach, J., Verdeaux, G., & Henrotte, J. G. (1973). Nouvelles recherches sur les relations entre taux de magnesium sanguin et la morphologies des traces E.E.G. chez l' homme [New investigation into the relationship between blood level of magnesium and EEG waveform]. *Revue EEG Neurophysiologique et Clinique, 3,* 269–274.

Engel, G. L., Ferris, E. B., & Logan, M. (1947). Hyperventilation: Analysis of clinical symptomatology. *Annals of Internal Medicine, 27,* 683–704.

Faurbye, A. (1943). *Blodets reaktion ved epilepsi* [The reaction of blood in epilepsy]. Unpublished doctoral dissertation, University of Copenhagen, Denmark.

Feldman, R. G., & Paul, N. L. (1976). Identity of emotional triggers in epilepsy. *Journal of Nervous & Mental Disease, 162,* 345–353.

Finley, W. W. (1977). Operant conditioning of the EEG in two patients with epilepsy: Methodologic and clinical consideration. *Pavlovian Journal of Biological Science, 12,* 93–111.

Fried, R. (1987a). *The hyperventilation syndrome—Research and clinical treatment*. Baltimore, MD: The Johns Hopkins University Press.

Fried, R. (1987b). Relaxation with biofeedback-assisted guided imagery: The importance of breathing rate as an index of hypoarousal. *Biofeedback & Self-Regulation, 12,* 273–279.

Fried, R. (1990). *The breath connection*. New York: Insight/Plenum.

Fried, R. (in press). *The psychology and physiology of breathing in behavioral medicine, clinical psychology, and psychiatry.* New York: Plenum.

Fried, R., Fox, M. C., & Carlton, R. M. (1990). Effect of diaphragmatic respiration with end-tidal CO_2 biofeedback on respiration, EEG, and seizure frequency in idiopathic epilepsy. *Annals of the New York Academy of Sciences, 602,* 67–96.

Fried, R., Rubin, S. R., Carlton, R. M., & Fox, M. C. (1984). Behavioral control of intractable idiopathic seizures: I. Self-regulation of end-tidal carbon dioxide. *Psychosomatic Medicine, 46,* 315–331.

Gastaut, H. (1970). Clinical and electroencephalographic classification of epileptic seizures. *Epilepsia, 11,* 102–113.

Gastaut, H. (1975). Comments on "Biofeedback in epileptics: Equivocal relationship of reinforced EEG frequency to seizure reduction" by B. Kaplan. *Epilepsia, 16,* 477–485.

Gastaut, H., & Tassinari, C. A. (1966). Triggering mechanisms in epilepsy—The electroclinical point of view. *Epilepsia, 7,* 85–138.

Gellhorn, E. (1953). The physiological basis of carbon dioxide therapy of the psychoneuroses. *Journal of Mental Science, 99,* 357–373.

George, W. K., George, W. D., Smith, J. P., Gordon, F. T., Baird, E., & Mills, G. C. (1964). Change in serum calcium, serum phosphate, and red cell phosphate during hyperventilation. *New England Journal of Medicine, 270,* 726–728.

Gersch, W., & Goddard, G. (1970). Locating the site of epileptic focus by spectral analysis methods. *Science, 169,* 71–72.

Gibbs, E. L., Lennox, W. G., & Gibbs, F. A. (1940). Variations in carbon dioxide content of blood in epilepsy. *Archives of Neurology & Psychiatry, 43,* 223–239.

Gibbs, F. A., Davis, H., & Lennox, W. G. (1935). The electroencephalogram in epilepsy and in conditions of impaired consciousness. *Archives of Neurology & Psychiatry, 43,* 1133–1148.

Gibbs, F. A., Williams, D., & Gibbs, E. L. (1949). Modification of the cortical frequency spectrum by changes in CO_2, blood sugar and O_2. *Journal of Neurophysiology, 3,* 49–58.

Ginter, E. L. (1955). Cerebral chemistry and convulsions. *Journal of the American Medical Women's Association, 10,* 365–372.

Glaser, G. H. (1979). Convulsive disorders (epilepsy). In H. H. Merritt (Ed.), *A textbook of neurology* (6th ed.) Philadelphia: Lea & Febiger.

Gotoh, F., Meyer, J. S., & Takagi, Y. (1965). Cerebral effects in hyperventilation in man. *Archives of Neurology, 12,* 410–423.

Gowers, W. R. (1881). *Epilepsy and other chronic convulsive diseases*. London: J & A Churchill.

Gowers, W. R. (1901). *Epilepsy and other chronic convulsive diseases*. Philadelphia: P. Blakiston's Sons.

Groen, J. J. (1975). The measurement of emotion and arousal in the clinical physiology laboratory. In L. Levi (Ed.), *Emotions—Their parameters and measurement* (pp. 724–746). New York: Raven Press.

Harper, R. M., & Sterman, M. B. (1972). Subcortical unit activity during conditioned 12–14 Hz sensorimotor rhythm in cats. *Federation Proceedings, 31,* 404.

Hauptmann, A., & Meyerson, A. (1948). Studies of finger capillaries in schizophrenia and manic-depressive psychoses. *Journal of Nervous & Mental Disease, 108,* 81–108.

Heistad, D. D., Marcus, M. L., & Abboud, F. M. (1978). Experimental attempts to unmask the effects of neural stimuli on cerebral blood flow. In M. J. Purves (Ed.), *Cerebral vascular smooth muscle and its control*. Amsterdam: Elsevier Exerpta Medica.

Himwich, H. E. (1951). *Brain metabolism and cerebral disorders*. Baltimore, MD: Williams & Wilkins.

Holcombe, V., Sterman, M. B., Goodman, S. J., & Fairchild, J. D. (1979). The immobilization response in rhesus monkey: A behavioral and electroencephalographic study. *Experimental Neurology, 63*, 420–435.

Holmberg, G. (1953). The electroencephalogram during hypoxia and hyperventilation. *EEG & Clinical Neurophysiology, 5*, 371–379.

Hughlings Jackson, J. (1931). Epilepsy and epileptiform convulsions. In J. Taylor, (Ed.), *Selected writings of John Hughlings Jackson*. London: Hoder & Stoughton.

Ikonomoff, S. I. (1970). Anticholinesterase drugs and epileptic seizures. *British Journal of Psychiatry, 117*, 679–680.

Ingvar, D. H., Siesjo, B., & Hertz, C. H. (1959). Measurement of tissue PCO_2 in the brain. *Experientia, 15*, 306–308.

Kamiya, J. (1969). Operant control of EEG alpha rhythm and some of its reported effects on consciousness. In C. Tart (Ed.), *Altered states of consciousness*. New York: Wiley.

Kaplan, B. J. (1975). Biofeedback in epileptics: Equivocal relationship of reinforced EEG frequency to seizure reduction. *Epilepsia, 16*, 477–485.

Kasamatsu, A., & Hirai, T. (1969). An electroencephalographic study of zen meditation (Zazen). *Psychologia, 12*, 205–225.

Kerr, W. J., Dalton, J. W., & Gliebe, P. A. (1937). Some physical phenomena associated with anxiety states and their relationship to hyperventilation. *Annals of Internal Medicine, 11*, 961–992.

Kesterton, J., & Clinch, N. (1985). Peripheral and central control mechanisms during respiratory suspension in transcendental meditation as evidenced by latency, hypoxia, and RQ changes. *Society for Neurosciences Abstract, 11*, 1144.

Kety, S. S., & Schmidt, C. F. (1948). The effect of altered arterial tensions of carbon dioxide and oxygen on cerebral blood flow and cerebral oxygen consumption of normal young men. *Journal of Clinical Investigation, 27*, 484–492.

Kuhlman, W. N. (1979–80). EEG feedback training of epileptic patients: Clinical and electroencephalographic analysis. In D. Shapiro, J. Stoyva, J. Kamiya, T. X. Barber, N. E. Miller, & G. E. Schwartz (Eds.). *Biofeedback and Behavioral Medicine* (pp. 466–477). New York: Aldine Press.

Kuhlman, W. N., & Allison, T. (1977). EEG feedback training in the treatment of epilepsy: Some questions and answers. *Pavlovian Journal of Biològical Science, 2*, 112–122.

Laidlaw, J., & Richens, A. (1976). *A textbook of epilepsy*. Edinburgh: Churchill Livingstone.

Laitinen, L., Johansson, G. G., & Sipponen, P. (1966). Recording of cerebral circulation by an impedance method: A preliminary report. *Brain Research, 2*, 184–186.

Latham, A. N. (1975). Effects of in vitro change in urinary pH on the enzymatic measurement and daily variation in excretion of D-glucaric acid. *Journal of Pharmacology*, 27, 612–615.

Lechner, H., Geyer, N., & Rodler, H. (1967). Rheography of function. *EEG & Clinical Neurophysiology, 23*, 185.

Lennox, W. G. (1928). The effect on epileptic seizures of varying the composition of inspired air. *Journal of Clinical Investigation, 6*, 23.

Lennox, W. G., Gibbs, F. A., & Gibbs, E. L. (1936). Effect on the electro-encephalogram of drugs and conditions which influence seizures. *Archives of Neurology & Psychiatry, 36*, 1236–1245.

Lennox, W. G., Gibbs, F. A., & Gibbs, E. L. (1938). The relationship in man of cerebral activity to blood flow and blood constituents. *Journal of Neurology & Psychiatry, 1*, 221–225.

Levine B. S., & Coburn, J. W. (1984). Magnesium, the mimic/antagonist of calcium. *New England Journal of Medicine, 310,* 1253–1255.

Lowenthal, A. (1965). A clinical biochemistry of epilepsy. *Epilepsia, 6,* 198–204.

Lubar, J. F., & Bahler, W. W. (1976). Behavioral management of epileptic seizure following EEG biofeedback training, of the sensorimotor rhythm. *Biofeedback & Self-Regulation, 1,* 77–104.

Lubar, J. F., Shasbin, H. S., Natelson, S. E., Holder, G. S., Whitsett, S. F., Pamplin, W. E., & Krulikowski, D. I. (1981). EEG operant conditioning in intractable epileptics. *Archives of Neurology, 38,* 700–704.

Lubin, A. J., & Price J. C. (1942). Effect of alkalosis and acidosis on cortical electrical activity and blood flow. *Journal of Neurophysiology, 5,* 261–268.

Maccario, M., Messis, C. P., & Vastola, E. F. (1965). Focal seizures as a manifestation of hyperglycemia without ketoacidosis. *Neurology, 15,* 195–207.

Madsen, J. (1943). Further studies on the biochemistry of epilepsy. *Acta Psychiatrica & Neurologica, 18,* 257–337.

Mairbaurl, H., & Humpeler, E. (1981). In vitro influence of adrenaline on erythrocyte metabolism and on oxygen affinity of hemoglobin. In G. J. Brewer (Ed.), *The red cell: Fifth Ann Arbor Conference* (pp. 311–319). New York: Liss.

Mathew, R. J., & Wilson, W. H. (1990). Anxiety and cerebral blood flow. *American Journal of Psychiatry, 147,* 838–849.

Mattson, R. H., Henniger, G. R., Gallagher, B. B., & Glaser, B. H. (1970). Psychophysiologic precipitants of seizures in epileptics. *Neurology, 20,* 407.

Meduna, L. J. (1958). *Carbon dioxide therapy* (2nd ed.). Springfield, IL: Charles C. Thomas.

Merritt, H. H. (1979). *A textbook of neurology* (6th ed.). Philadelphia: Lea & Febiger.

Merritt, H. H., & Putnam, T. J. (1938). Sodium diphenyl hydantoinate in the treatment of convulsive disorders. *Journal of the American Medical Association, 111,* 1068–1073.

Meyer, J. S., & Gotoh, F. (1960). Metabolic and electroencephalographic effects of hyperventilation. *AMA Archives of Neurology, 3,* 539–552.

Meyer, J. S., & Waltz, A. G. (1961). Relationship of cerebral anoxia to functional and electroencephalographic abnormality. In H. Gastaut & J. S. Meyer (Eds.), *Cerebral anoxia and the electroencephalogram* (pp. 307–328). Springfield, IL: Charles C. Thomas.

Millichap, J. G., & Ulrich, J. A. (1962). Abnormal urinary excretion of amino acids in children with petit mal epilepsy: Preliminary communication. *Mayo Clinic Proceedings, 37,* 307.

Morrice, J.K.W. (1965). Slow wave production in the EEG with reference to hyperpnea, carbon dioxide, and autonomic balance. *EEG & Clinical Neurophysiology, 8,* 49–72.

Mostofsky, D. I., & Balaschak, B. A. (1977). Psychobiological control of seizures. *Psychological Bulletin, 84,* 723–750.

Parrino, J. J. (1971). Reduction in seizures by desensitization. *Journal of Behavior Therapy & Experimental Psychiatry, 2,* 215–218.

Penfield, W. (1933). The evidence for a cerebral vascular mechanism in epilepsy. *Annal of Internal Medicine, 7,* 303–310.

Penfield, W., & Jasper, H. (1954). *Epilepsy and the functional anatomy of the brain.* Boston: Little, Brown.

Pollock, G. H. (1949). Central inhibitory effects of carbon dioxide. *Journal of Neurophysiology, 12,* 315–324.

Quy, R. J., Hutt, S. J., & Forrest, S. (1979). Sensorimotor rhythm feedback training in epilepsy: Some methodological and conceptual issues. *Biological Psychology, 9,* 129–149.

Raichle, M. E., & Plum, F. (1972). Hyperventilation and cerebral blood flow. *Stroke, 3,* 566–575.

Robinson, L. J. (1944). Encephalographic study during epileptic seizures related to hyperventilation. *Diseases of the Nervous System, 5,* 87–90.

Rosett, J. (1924). The experimental production of rigidity, or abnormal involuntary movement and of abnormal states of consciousness in man. *Brain, 47,* 293–336.

Rozen, R., Goodyer, P. R., & Scriver, C. R. (1982). GABA and taurine—What are metabolites like this doing in a place like that? In N. Freinkel (Ed.), *Contemporary metabolism* (Vol. 2, pp. 189–237). New York: Plenum.

Schwab, R. S., Grunwald, A., & Sargant, W. W. (1941). Regulation of treatment of epilepsy by synchronized recording of respiration and brain waves. *Archives of Neurology & Psychiatry, 46,* 1017–1034.

Shinozaki, K., & Furutani, M. (1968). Studies on psychobiological correlation apparent in urine—Research through so-called Kraepelin-Ketoenol Test (KES) in neuropsychiatry. *Hiroshima Journal of Medical Science, 17,* 197–219.

Soulayrol, R., Mesdjian, E., Lob, H., Tassinari, C. A., & Rogers, J. (1965). The tryptophan loading test in epileptic children. *Epilepsia, 6,* 310–324.

Stafford-Clark, D. (1964). *Psychiatry for students.* London: Allen & Unwin.

Standage, K. (1972). Treatment of epilepsy by the reciprocal inhibition of anxiety. *Guys Hospital Report, 121,* 217–221.

Sterman, M. B. (1973). Neurophysiologic and clinical studies of sensorimotor EEG biofeedback and training: Some effects of epilepsy. In L. Birk (Ed.), *Biofeedback: Behavioral medicine.* New York: Grune & Stratton.

Sterman, M. B. (1977). Effects of sensorimotor EEG feedback training on sleep and clinical manifestations of epilepsy. A critical appraisal. In J. Beatty (Ed.), *Biofeedback: Theory and research.* New York: Academic Press.

Sterman, M. B. (1981). EEG biofeedback: Physiological behavior modification. *Neuroscience & Biobehavioral Review 5,* 405–412.

Sterman, M. B., & Friar, L. (1972). Suppression of seizures in an epileptic following sensorimotor EEG feedback training. *EEG & Clinical Neurophysiology, 33,* 89–95.

Sterman, M. B., & Kovaleski, R. A. (1979). Anticonvulsant effects of restraint and pyridoxine on hydrazine seizures in the monkey. *Experimental Neurology, 65,* 78–86.

Sterman, M. B., MacDonald, L. R., & Bernstein, I. (1977). Quantitative analysis of EEG sleep spindle activity in epileptic and non-epileptic subjects. *EEG and Clinical Neurophysiology, 42,* 724.

Sterman, M. B., & Wyrwicka, E. (1967). EEG correlates of sleep: Evidence for separate forebrain substrates. *Brain Research, 6,* 143–163.

Swanson, A. G., Stavney, L. S., & Plum, F. (1958). Effects of pH and carbon dioxide on cerebral electrical activity. *Neurology, 8,* 787–792.

Temkin, N. R., & Davis, G. R. (1984). Stress as a risk factor on seizures among adults with epilepsy. *Epilepsia, 24,* 450–456.

Tharp, B. R., & Gersh, W. (1975). Spectral analysis of seizures in humans. *Computers & Biomedical Research, 8,* 503–521.

Tower, D. B. (1960). *Neurochemistry of Epilepsy.* Springfield, IL: Charles C. Thomas.

Upton, A.R.M., & Longmire, D. (1975). Effects of feedback on focal epileptic discharges in man. *Canadian Journal of Neurological Science, 3,* 153–168.

Walter, D., Rhodes, J., Brown, D., & Adey, W. (1966). Comprehensive spectral analysis of human EEG generators in posterior cerebral regions. *EEG & Clinical Neurophysiology, 20,* 224–237.

Wang, R.I.H., & Sonnenschein, R. E. (1955). pH of cerebral cortex during induced convulsions. *Journal of Neurophysiology, 18,* 130–137.

Weilburg, J. B., Bear, D. M., & Sachs, G. (1987). Three patients with concomitant panic attacks and seizure disorder: Possible clues to the neurology of anxiety. *American Journal of Psychiatry 144,* 1053–1056.

Whitman, S., Dell, J., Legion, V., Eibhlyn, A., & Statsinger, J. (1990). Progressive relaxation for seizure reduction. *Journal of Epilepsy, 3,* 17–22.

Williams, D. T., Gold, A. P., Shrout, P., Shaffer, D., & Adams, A. (1979). The impact of psychiatric intervention on patients with uncontrolled seizures. *Journal of Nervous & Mental Disease, 167,* 626–631.

Withrow, C. D. (1972). Systemic carbon dioxide derangements. In D. P. Purpura, J. K. Penry, D. B. Tower, D. M. Woodburry, & R. R. Walters (Eds.), *Experimental models of epilepsy.* New York: Raven Press.

Wolfe, L. S., & Elliott, K.A.C. (1962). Chemical studies in relation to convulsive conditions. In K.A.C. Elliott, I. H. Page, & J. H. Quastel (Eds.), *Neurochemistry* (2nd ed.). Springfield, IL: Charles C. Thomas.

Wolpe, J. (1973). *The practice of behavior therapy.* New York: Pergamon.

Woodbury, D. M., & Kemp, J. W. (1970). Some possible mechanisms of action of antiepileptic drugs. *Pharmacopsychiatry & Neuropharmacology, 3,* 201–226.

Woodson, R. D. (1979). Physiological significance of the oxygen dissociation curve shift. *Critical Care Medicine, 7,* 368–373.

Wyrwicka, W., & Sterman, M. B. (1968). Instrumental conditioning of sensorimotor cortex EEG spindles in the waking cat. *Physiology & Behavior, 3,* 703–707.

Yahr, M. D., Sciarra, D., Carter, S., & Merritt, H. H. (1952). Evaluation of standard anticonvulsant therapy in three hundred nineteen patients. *Journal of the American Medical Association, 150,* 663–667.

3 Behavior Modification and Therapy in the Management of Epileptic Disorders

David I. Mostofsky
Boston University

> *We believe that the area of physiology opened by Ivan Petrovich Pavlov is pertinent and relevant to the field of epilepsy, and that there is a need to take a longer and harder look at these psychophysiological processes in epilepsy.*
>
> —*Forster, 1967, pp. 75–76*

Behavior modification, as used in this chapter, describes the body of theory and practice accounting for the relatively permanent changes in behavior that occur following repeated conditions of specified practice, without recourse to drugs, diet, or surgery. Such demonstrations of stable behavior-change outcomes have become commonplace, particularly in remedial educational settings (or, more properly, in educational environments requiring special programming) and clinical psychotherapeutics, where the activities also are labeled as *behavior therapy. Behavior modification* derives both its philosophic stance as well as its research energy from the parent discipline of *experimental psychology,* and particularly from the work of learning specialists whose continuing efforts to refine a scientific experimental analysis of behavior hold much promise for meaningful advances in *behavioral neuroscience*. The explosion of writings in this field precludes an uncomplicated summary within the limits of a single chapter; the interested reader will find numerous monographs, texts, handbooks, and annotated bibliographies easily accessible. Many examples in this literature concerned with intellectual or emotional functioning and reeducation have, in fact, been completed with epileptic patients, although their epilepsy or attempts to behaviorally control the seizure problem is usually secondary to the purpose of the report. However, the focus of this chapter is restricted to applications that offer more direct treatment options specifically for the neurologic condition.

The adaptation and extension of behavior modification as an adjunctive treatment alternative for seizure control or epilepsy only recently has begun to receive careful attention. (This chapter does not consider the distinction between controlling seizures vs. controlling epilepsy.) Although neurologists have long been aware of environmental correlations with seizure problems (both positively and negatively), few attempts were made to contrive or to engineer environmental conditions that might be of clinical value to the epileptic. In retrospect, this neglect was quite understandable, given that the traditional neurological assessment of the seizure disorder excluded the possible contribution of a learned component in the generation and maintenance of the seizure disorder and, consequently, excluded the need to consider introducing extinction, counterconditioning, stimulus control, or similar learning mechanisms in a comprehensive treatment program. But there is increasing evidence that behavior treatment programs can offer substantial relief to the epileptic patient—not only for mental health sequelae of the disorder, retarded population, seizures that are of undisputed psychogenic origin, and disorders that follow a classic TLE profile. Indeed, the argument advanced herein is that some meaningful proportion of the seizure severity, frequency, topography, or duration can be reduced by an effective program in behavior modification. This assertion is supported by the data from treatments with various patients who differ in the diagnostic categories (according to the International Classification System), including those who are refractory to medication or for whom the asymptotic level of control remains unacceptable. In the remaining sections of this chapter, I sketch the major avenues of behavior treatments that can be used and suggest how the practicing neurologist, or clinical allied health or mental health professional, can optimize most profitably and exploit behavior therapy applications in the service of the epilepsies—short of developing the necessary personal expertise to conduct such therapy as part of his or her neurological practice. A familiarity with the nature and physiological substrate of the problem before one rushes into an uncritical implementation of catalogued protocols can be quite helpful. The *epilepsies* (the more accurate substitute term for *epilepsy*) are not a disease, nor do they represent a single, unidimensional problem. Rather, the disorders are manifestations of brain disease, neurochemical imbalance, or anatomical insult. The primary diagnostic indices that are used to confirm a seizure disorder are either or both abnormal electrical discharges (as seen in an electroencephalographic record) and changes in sensory, motor, cognitive, or conscious behaviors. The stereotyped fit or tonic–clonic convulsion is one of the many forms that the expression of a seizure may take. A brief but informative summary on the basic mechanisms of the epilepsies, and a useful list of references appear elsewhere (Hosford & McNamara, 1990). The conventional drug and surgical treatment modalities, as practiced in clinical neurology, can be found in a variety of texts and monographs, particularly *The Handbook of Neurology* (Magnus & Lorenz de Haas, 1974). The careful reader of these and similar works will note that their discussions lack any mention of the role of *behavioral* treatment protocols that may be considered for primary or adjunctive control of seizures. A recent work that appeared among the trade publications reflects the newer approaches of both behavioral and traditional management for epileptic disorders (Richard & Reiter, 1990). The general area of *classification* of epileptic seizures has come under renewed scrutiny, with consideration given to the rationale and implications that classification schemes create. The dominant activity in classification has been based on the ability to accurately identify individual seizure types, the progression of seizure forms during the course of a single attack, and the repertoire of different seizures and other symptoms allowing the identification of epileptic syndromes (Dreifuss, 1989).

VARIETIES OF TREATMENT STRATEGIES

Comprehensive reviews of the published literature describing behavioral treatment applications to seizure disorders have appeared elsewhere (Goldstein, 1990; Krafft & Poling, 1982; Mostofsky, 1981; Mostofsky & Balaschak, 1977). The common denominator among the different reports on epilepsy is that the particular interventional procedure used was generally a known and accepted tactic for changing behavior usually encountered in the context of classroom activities or general behavior management. The necessary requirements for its adaptation to the seizure problem are relatively simple, given that the therapist has a competent control of the behavioral methodology and a comfortable familiarity with the nature of the epilepsies. The premise underlying the various procedures is that seizures are another kind of learned or conditioned behavior that will be responsive to environmental contingencies. If judiciously selected, new learned behaviors in the patient's repertoire will be sufficiently strong and permanent to provide a reduction of seizures, because of extinction of the unhealthy behaviors, which may be the immediate precursors in a chain leading to the seizure or a direct trigger of seizure activity. The beneficial effects also may accrue from engaging in the newly acquired skills, which are designed to be incompatible and mutually exclusive with provoking or allowing the development of epileptic seizures. In both cases, the undesired behaviors are eliminated from the patient's repertoire.

The *behavior modification protocols* (in the broadest and least restrictive sense of the term) that are available for seizure management may be grouped into three major headings: (a) reward management or reinforcement-based strategies, (b) self-control or cognitive and psychodynamic-based strategies, and (c) psychophysiological methods. This last category primarily is represented by techniques that involve desensitization and classical conditioned extinction, which is of greatest use in reflex epilepsy (Forster, 1978). Although constituting a relatively small portion of the population of epileptics, it offers meaningful relief to those whose seizures are triggered by touch, sight, or sound. Other examples in this category would include biofeedback, relaxation training, breathing, and exercise programs, all of which are treated in greater detail in other sections of this volume. In practice, any given treatment strategy often will be seen to contain features of its technique, which could easily legitimize its membership in another category. Indeed, a given protocol may be constituted with a number of separate phases and operations drawn from the different categories. The attempt to bring the behavior modification approaches under such a categorization scheme is an attempt to introduce some relatively simple order for the uninformed clinician, and should be understood to contribute to an appreciation of styles and sensitivities, rather than to provide any firm or final description of the theories or dynamics that might explain the effectiveness of any of these techniques.

Reward Management

This technique addresses the seizure problem from the same point of view as those that alter any other nonbiologically dominant learned behavior. From replicable and solid experience with human and infrahuman subjects, learning specialists argue that if reward is administered or made accessible following the execution of some behavior, the probability is increased that the behavior will be strengthened (i.e., it will reappear within a shorter latency, it will be emitted more frequently, and it will become part of the performing repertoire with some degree of permanence).

However, if the behavior is not rewarded, the predicted outcomes are reversed. The arrangement of opportunities for reward (reinforcement) can be essentially summarized by a 2 × 2 matrix (Fig. 3.1). The rules governing the availability of reward in the behavior modification schemes most always require a linkage to the subject's response. The subject finds a reward consequence (indicated by a plus or minus sign) contingent on the response. A plus represents some object or set of conditions for which the subject is likely to expend considerable time and effort to obtain or preserve. A minus represents any object or set of conditions for which the subject is prepared to expend time and effort to stop and abort (escape) or to not have to experience or encounter them (avoidance). The experimenter is able to adjust the environment to make the plus or minus conditions appear by delivering or administering them, or by preventing (withholding) their appearance. Over time and with rehearsal, the subject learns to execute the critical behaviors, as engineered by the experimenter (therapist), subject to these essential rules that govern the dispensing of rewards. Although each element of the matrix is able to generate learned behaviors, the specific selection among the alternatives most often rests with the nature of the real

	Administer	Withhold
+	Reward	Denial (time-out)
−	Punishment	Relief (avoidance/escape)

FIG. 3.1. Taxonomy of conditioning paradigms (after Woods, 1974).

environment in which the subject functions, the special limitations of the subject, as well as the training and expertise of the therapist in executing the stylistic nature of the technique. Furthermore, the protocols that derive their power from escape, avoidance, and time out procedures risk the undesirable side effects of aversive conditions that the clinician chooses to eliminate entirely during therapy. The artful considerations in the selection and execution of the behavior modification programs will be left to the many texts, handbooks, and monographs that populate the behavior modification literature.

The assumptions about applying behavior modification routines to epileptic seizures are based, in part, on the speculation that some proportion of seizure activity is learned. This does not suggest that it is necessarily voluntary or hysterical, but rather that, under specified conditions where reward for seizures is available, these conditions may constitute a disguised opportunity for secondary gain, socially acceptable acting out, or a convenient coping vehicle for avoidance of (or escape from) stress, punishment, or uncomfortableness. Hence, the seizures may tend to reoccur, and, in the course of their emission and subsequent consequences, actually continue to be rewarded. As with all learned behaviors, such an analysis can be accommodated within the physiological context in which the electrical paroxysmal events accompany the clinical expression. Classical biological functions are easily brought under the control of reward and punishment systems, as are the behaviors associated with classroom learning and control of emotions. There is nothing in the extension of such procedures to epilepsy that contradicts the role of organicity, nor do any of the data from the realm of the pathophysiology of the epilepsies deny the possible effectiveness of learning and conditioning mechanisms. The reward management procedures rely on the judicious introduction, elimination, and timing of reinforcements (both positive and negative) to effect appropriate learning. The learning goal in question may be focused on teaching the patient to efficiently discriminate environmental conditions that have a demonstrated correlation with seizures, and to then cope with those conditions without producing a seizure. Environmental conditions, as used in this context, include (but are not limited to) subtle, private, covert, sensory, or other physiological or nonverbal activity. Learning also may be effected without the patient's ability to report awareness of personal change. Therefore, in the course of arranging the environmental consequences, it is critical for one to guard against situations that will not provide undesired rewards. Often the learning objective will be to introduce a behavioral response in the patient's repertoire that, when sufficiently dominant, will compete with and exclude a seizure response. Properly selected, such a desired behavior will be mutually exclusive with seizures. The anticipated final result will be a diminution of seizures attributable to replacing the chain of antecedent preseizure behaviors, rather than by any attempt to directly attenuate or extinguish seizure processes directly. However, the latter also might comprise a legitimate behavior modification effort and would exploit the role of counterconditioning, desensitization, or habituation as a means to neutralize both the trigger mechanisms leading to seizures as well as the seizure generating systems.

As with any variety of operant conditioning or behavior therapy, the specific features of a treatment program (i.e., the protocols sketched in Fig. 3.1; e.g., reinforcers, session length, etc.) are dictated by the unique character of the patient and his or her life space. For a child, reward may take the form of money or a special privilege; for an adolescent, perhaps the eventual reduction (or even elimination) of medication; for an adult, job employment or improvement in the quality of family living. These procedures do not appear to be selectively attractive or, contrawise, selectively less preferable for any subgroups of epileptics stratified by gender, diagnosis, cognitive, or intellectual patency. Punishers and reinforcers, as well as stimuli and responses, may be of the cognitive variety in addition to the classic observable forms familiar to stricter behaviorists (Tan & Bruni, 1986), and may include covert rewards and punishers (via training of imagined events). Furthermore, the behavioral control of specific EEG rhythms may be demonstrated as products of these methodologies (Sterman, 1972, 1982, chapter 1, this volume; Wyler, Robbins, & Dodrill, 1979). The variety of clients, settings, and treatment techniques that have been used with reward conditions is broad. A convincing demonstration of the effectiveness of the *reward* condition (Fig. 3.1) may be found in the relatively simple application undertaken in a sheltered day center with a retarded male adult having generalized seizures with complex symptomatology. The patient, suffering seizure disorders attributed to a confirmed inoperable tumor and enlarged ventricles, was praised at regular intervals when seizures did not occur. When a seizure developed, he was given no attention or display of concern and, although his seizures generally would cause him to become incontinent, under the conditions mandated by the conditioning program he alone was responsible for caring for his change of clothes. After 1–2 weeks of imposing these contingencies, a 50% reduction of seizures was noted; with continuation of the program (28 weeks), the seizures were reduced to two thirds of their pretreatment level (including 13 weeks of no seizures and 6 weeks with no more than a single episode). Such a program relied on denying reward in any form on the occurrence of a seizure (*denial* cell of Fig. 3.1), coupled with the overt administration of reward (praise) for desired (no seizure) behavior (Flannery & Cautela, 1973).

This study also exemplifies the common pattern of most clinical designs, because several reinforcement schedules and contingencies are enacted concurrently. These prototypic programs may be instituted for individual control (as within a family or classroom setting) or may be extended to larger scale activities within a clinic or hospital (Berner, chapter 10, this volume; Brown & Fenwick, 1989; Dahl, Melin, Brorson, & Schollin, 1985; Dahl, Melin, & Lund, 1988; Fenwick, 1981). Other programs have incorporated penalties, time out from ongoing activities or pleasurable surroundings (*denial* in Fig. 3.1), relief or termination from uncomfortable consequences of seizures, and punishment on the occurrence of seizures. A striking example of the *relief* procedure is the prescription of a putrid, pungent, and ugly colored liquid (assafetida), dressed up with a host of placebo labels (to imply medicinal authenticity) and given with solemn instructions that the potion is an experimental miracle, except for its terrible taste and odor. The patient is required to drink 3 tablespoons of this concoction T.I.D. or until the seizures stop. The vile drink is risk-free and is not known to have any health benefits (except perhaps as a carminative), but certainly has no anticonvulsant properties. When administered, most patients cease their seizure bouts, at least for a while. Even such a temporary interruption may be useful if only to reinstate some longer term program of control. Other forms of relief rely on the promise of avoiding or preventing less drastic consequences.

Variations in schedule parameters of the reinforcement program allow for other choices in the menu of paradigms available for treatment. For example, in our own work we have met with some guarded success in establishing a contract program with patients, which stipulates that if an agreed upon minimum number of seizures occurs in any week, some valued consequence decided upon by both patient and parent will be forthcoming. In this case, the patient provided his or her own technique for seizure control and the consequences of seizures are rewarded, not with each occurrence, but rather upon the cumulation of desired behaviors distributed over a longer period of time.

Success with reward management programs frequently are reported anecdotally, with only a limited number of unquestionably quality research designs. Admittedly, the practical difficulties for properly carrying out idealized and methodologically sound investigations in this area are real and serious, but the problems of confoundations of variable effects and the imprecise or erroneous inferences that are concluded from clinical studies requires critical readings of research reports. Given the questionable reliability with such reports, it would be presumptuous to ascribe major behavioral and biobehavioral alterations solely to some specific reward or punishment that is identified in the treatment protocol, without further clarification of the prevailing conditions of the experiment. When patient improvement does result, it may be better understood in the countless other conditions of the patient's life space, which have benefitted from the multiplier effect that originated with the restricted objectives of the experimental treatment. If we accept that some arrangement of reward conditions is effective in bringing about a meaningful reduction of seizure frequency, the patient's personal and interpersonal functioning may improve simultaneously along with the neurological change, and a host of other unprogrammed sources of rewards enter (self-esteem, peer interaction, job opportunity, etc.).

Multiple baseline designs can be useful in delineating such instances, but usually will not be sufficient to rule out all sources of error. It may be the collection of the various components that contributes to rewarding nonseizure behavior and that may ultimately be deserving of credit in both the acquisition and maintenance of health behaviors, rather than a simplistic attribution of control mechanisms via the limited therapy program alone. But the opportunity for rigorous research is clearly possible, as in the well-designed and well-executed effort of Cataldo, Russo, and Freeman (1979). In this report—a case of high-rate myoclonic seizures in a 5-year-old child—the application of the behavior modification methodology was followed. A behavioral analysis of the seizures was undertaken and was evaluated both on a hospital ward and in a controlled experimental setting. A program of contingent rest was applied, which resulted in a reduction in seizure frequency and "the apparent prevention of several grand mal episodes" (Cataldo et al., 1979). A reasonable question arises at this point: Why not design a program that attempts to condition the seizures directly rather than the awkward redesign of the surrounding environment? This question suggests that the conditionability of seizures would permit the creation of an epileptic model in human and animal, and that the extinction of seizures offers a direct treatment option. Unfortunately, the overwhelming evidence points to an inability to condition a true behavioral or electrical seizure, whether in a kindled preparation or via any other strategy (Mostofsky & Myslobodsky, 1982).

Such issues are important to recognize in the formulation of theory development in this area. However, the essential message for the practicing clinician is that there is a reliable body of data that provides support for the initiative to incorporate the learning reinforcement prototype of behavior modification protocols in the comprehensive medical management of the epilepsies.

Self-Control

The treatment styles in this category control behavior via intrapersonal and psychodynamic processes that may be either learned or innate. Patients may be taught how to implement auto suggestion or self-instruction and thought-stopping techniques. A convenient and simple way to regard *self-control* is to consider the patient as his or her own therapist (i.e., the patient rather than some external therapist becomes the dispenser of rewards, punishers, and discriminative stimuli). The essential features of all the behavior therapies change little, and the differences among techniques and procedures rest with the nature of the therapist, the form of the various stimuli, and responses such as overt or covert and sensorimotor or cognitive. Indeed, one of the mainstream variants among the behavior therapies is cognitive behavior therapy, a system that conceptually, philosophically, and procedurally differs from the more orthodox operant behavior therapy. Cognitions, self-control, coping, and similar mediating behaviors are regarded as critical operative variables in bringing about necessary changes (Pritchard, Holmstrom, & Giacinto, 1985; Tan & Bruni, 1986).

The practical translation of this approach ranges from relatively simple training in relaxation exercises and stress reduction (with or without biofeedback assistance) to the various forms of psychotherapy sessions. The patient is directed to monitor his or her thought processes and emotional state, to appreciate on a rational level the role of subconscious conflicts and anxieties, and to deal appropriately with situations that are suspect in being provocative, threatening, or catalytic in precipitating seizures. Recent reports have suggested successful results in seizure management among patients who cannot report prodromal or aura symptoms (including petit mal conditions), as well as for those who verbally report an ability to initiate thought stopping or other self-control techniques in time to prevent a developing seizure. A most interesting application of a technique representative of this class of behavior modification was reported by Feldman and Paul (1976). In this instance, the patient was videotaped during an otherwise conventional psychotherapy session, during which time she experienced a seizure. Replay of the tape to the patient, accompanied by the therapist's interpretation and guiding, enabled a reconstruction of the contextual dialogue and its clinical psychiatric significance, which may have contributed to triggering the seizure and which would otherwise not have been available as a conscious and aware event. There seems to be clear and convincing evidence that major life events, whether remembered or not, constitute serious risk factors in the generation and maintenance of epileptic attacks (Webster & Mawer, 1989).

The gains achieved by self-control techniques have been utilized largely to deal with mental health sequelae of epilepsy, but only insignificantly applied to attempt to reduce the seizure problem. The techniques are indeed effective in providing clinical support for a broad range of health-related goals, including lifestyle adjustment, coping with the difficulties attending a chronic disorder and compliance with drugs and other medical orders that are often frequent accompaniments to seizure disorders (Dodrill & Batzel, chapter 12, this volume; Hermann & Whitman, 1984). Above all, the techniques are most effective in stress reduction and anxiety elimination, the latter long regarded as a nasty culprit by psychiatric and neurologic epileptologists. Patients often report that the perception of random occurrence and the absence of their ability to "do anything about it" creates a greater disturbance than the behavioral or physiological seizures from which they suffer. Reinstatement of control is unquestionably a valued benefit that all the behavioral techniques contribute to the person with epilepsy.

Although anxiety can be viewed as a diffuse, but serious intruder among the contraindications for a epileptic, and although an acceptable scientific understanding of anxiety and its role in epileptogenesis is yet to be formulated, it is important to give some consideration to its mode of action in exacerbating seizures among patients in whom the background pathophysiological system is ever present. Currently, only sparse empirical data can be offered in support of such theoretical speculations, but it is reasonable to propose at least four mechanisms to account for anxiety effects in promoting seizures.

1. *Direct physiochemical change.* Anxiety, and its antidote relaxation, may operate on changes in corticosteroids, cerebral blood flow, or the acidosis-alkalosis and lactose levels in the blood supply to the brain. It may also accelerate neural traffic which may have the effect of supplying excessive arousal or stimulation to a system that is ill equipped to properly adjust itself to such demands.

2. *Indirect limbic cortex modulation.* The affective and emotional concomitants of anxiety may, through excitation of remote cortical sites, enervate neurophysiological propagation and stimulation of epileptogenic foci from which there ultimately will develop frank clinical seizures. Here again, the possibility of *neural traffic* (a concept that was promulgated among theoreticians in the hypnosis/anxiety areas) may play an important role in exacerbating the clinical epileptic crisis.

3. *Psychophysiological aggravation.* Consequences of anxiety states commonly are discernable by alterations in indices such as GSR, SPR, respiration, and pulse rate. Hyperventilation often may be a subtle accompaniment of anxiety and may, in its own right, provide the sufficient condition for seizure onset. In such a case, the relaxation method provides a means for eliminating the hyperventilation, and, as a consequence, the development of any seizure that would ordinarily follow it.

4. *Schedule control.* An experimental analysis of the larger behavioral space of an epileptic might model one of the many complex schedules of reinforcement in which components of the schedule interact to acquire control over behavior not directly programmed to the consequences of the schedule. For example, schedule-induced polydipsia can be induced by training an animal to work for food under certain schedules of reinforcement, with no contingencies specified for water licking. Yet the schedule will cause the animal to increase its water intake manyfold during the test session, even though it is never rewarded or punished for licking behavior. Seizures also may be subject to off-schedule

control, and the reduction of seizure occurrence may be attributable to the addition of relaxation (or some other benign response), which, having altered some unspecified schedule simply by reason of its introduction, will create a schedule that no longer supports the necessary control for seizure induction or its maintenance.

The essential nature of relaxation and its dynamic in the control of seizures requires serious examination. Fried (chapter 2, this volume) has pioneered in demonstrating the relationship of breathing-induced relaxation to shifts in the spectral composition of the EEG, in a way that effectively accomplishes the same results as SMR biofeedback procedures (Sterman, chapter 1, this volume). I propose that, in the larger sense, relaxation as a treatment entity may serve in one or more of the following capacities:

1. As a psychophysiological or somatic agent that may bring about EEG, vasovagal, or other CNS and ANS changes which, in turn, operate on the seizure-generating system(s).
2. As an attentional (cognitive) skill-improvement device that effectively provides training in (a) discrimination of private and external stimuli, (b) awareness development, (c) self control, and (d) similar skill improvements, thus enabling seizure reduction via the development of counterconditioning and extinction by mutual incompatibility.
3. By introducing an overcorrection technique that is less aversive than most and that allows for substitute behavior in the context of "coping with stress."

Psychophysiological Methods

The techniques represented in this category are essentially of several forms, including psychophysical habituation to critical parameters of a physical stimulus known to trigger a seizure (e.g., light or sound frequency, intensity, etc.). The treatment objective is to identify the trigger stimulus and then, with repeated presentations of gradual increases in the stimulus intensity or duration, to desensitize its ability to elicit the seizure activity. These procedures have been extensively studied by Forster (1978) and require long and repeated exposures to the stimuli as they are presented from subthreshold levels through the range of (now extinguished or habituated) suprathreshold values. Despite the costly and tiring limitations that these procedures entail, they are probably the treatments of choice for patients for whom the trigger may be demarcated in an external physical stimulus (e.g., startle, photosensitivity, musicogenic stimulation, etc.). These treatment procedures are less familiar to therapists, because the incidence of the idiosyncratic disorders for which they are suited, the reflex epilepsies, accounts for a fraction of a percent of the total epileptic population. However, it is remarkable that repeated publications dealing with eating epilepsy (seizures produced with swallowing or mastication of food) fail to suggest the potential benefits of behavioral treatments for this apparently familiar rarity within the epilepsies (Koul, Kousl, & Razdan, 1989; Verdu & Ruiz-Falco, 1991).

The second group within this classification is composed of the various biofeedback protocols. Following the original work by Sterman (1972), a limited number of clinical research laboratories are examining the phenomenon of cortical EEG biofeedback insofar as it provides an anticonvulsant treatment option for epilepsy management. Sterman (chapter 1, this volume) provides a detailed examination of this technique category. This class of biofeedback procedures may be seen as a variation within the total range of learning paradigms. Early studies in learning often emphasized the role of *knowledge of results* (KR). In the absence of providing a subject with the results of performance, learning will not take place. It has been argued that the effectiveness of reinforcement is to provide nothing less than a form of feedback for criterion performance. The feedback, as used in psychophysiology, is characterized by the nature of the biological information that is fed back to the subject, often with the use of elaborate electronic equipment. Nonetheless, it may be seen as variant of the general KR principle that was developed within learning methodology.

Yet another form in this category concerns the psychophysiological training with various other physiological functions that have proved effective in controlling seizure disorders. For example, hypnosis has been reported to help some patients. This procedure seems to be based largely on distraction, reassigned attention, and state of aware but relaxed concentration. Also, Fried (chapter 1, this volume) provides a detailed review of the role of breathing exercise, with and without integration with a biofeedback mode, as it may apply to the epilepsies. The results of the psychophysiological procedures at times are unclear, difficult to interpret, and costly, but indisputably remarkable. Improvement seems to be a consistent finding, but as Neal Miller—a mentor in the abused field of biofeedback—often has reminded us, we should be "bold in what we try, but cautious in what we say." The elephant's trunk is in the tent, and it is highly likely that, with advances in hardware technology and cost reductions, biofeedback treatments will be admitted to routine clinical practice. At this time, however, because of the taxing investment of time, personnel, and costs, it is not possible to expect programs such as EEG biofeedback to provide a waiting service for the interested consumer, or for clinical neurologists to consider such treatment as a practical alternative for all of their patients.

> For centuries the contribution of psychological and social forces to disease has been widely assumed and accepted as a truism. . . . To some extent progress in biobehavioral studies has been hampered because the evidence sought has been restricted to a Procustean mold not suited to the study of people functioning in their social milieu, but to far less complex interacting paradigms. New combinations of physiologic, behavioral and social approaches should provide not only quantifiable

data but data on configuration, the arrangement of circumstances in relation to the peculiarities of affected individuals. (Wolf, 1982, p. 100)

INTEGRATION IN CLINICAL PRACTICE

Although it is rare for a clinical neurologist to undertake the direct administration of the behavioral treatment strategies, it is the position of this chapter that the incorporation of behavior modification in the comprehensive medical treatment plan deserves to be accorded prominent consideration. Neurologists have come to value the services of psychologists, but generally have limited the exploitation of their services to psychometric, psychodiagnostic, or mental health and educational therapy. Even in neurological centers, where behaviorally trained and oriented personnel are assigned to the unit, they are often peripheral in the general medical treatment plan. To be sure, such behavioral therapists may be sought by the patient and asked to provide services without involvement of the medical staff. Successful outcomes, however, more often are realized and sustained when the neurologist's activities are orchestrated in consort with the behavioral treatment plan. The clinician should be aware that family or other factors often present overwhelming adverse conditions that constrain, and perhaps exclude, the suitability of properly executed treatment protocols. However, if behavior therapy is deemed appropriate, there remain many decisions to be made, many steps to be taken, and many demands to be met. The therapist must decide the priority of behaviors to be addressed, which often will determine which of the particular techniques is to be chosen. The multifactoral nature of sickness and the distinction among the facets of disease, illness, and predicament, as they relate to diagnosis, treatment, and patient care, have been discussed elsewhere (Mostofsky, 1981). These dimensions of sickness are different in important ways, and provide additional clarification for appreciating the domain of behavior modification as it relates to the treatment of the epilepsies.

The responsibilities for assuring a successful behavior modification program in epileptic treatment is shared. The patient is requested to monitor carefully—hour by hour perhaps over a 2- to 3-month period—the baseline of symptoms and other behaviors prior to implementation of a treatment course. The physician is requested to refrain from adjusting the drug program (unless critically warranted), and perhaps to consider agreeing to reduce medications contingent on demonstrated clinical improvement (an important reinforcer meaningful to many patients). The therapist might recommend some residential or other facility where intensive monitoring and environmental control may be carried out reliably, if such options exist in the community. Together with the social worker, human resource agency, psychiatrist, or clinical psychologist, the therapy team may invite participation by family members, school personnel, or employer. Frequently, special education, family therapy, and the resolution of other patient complaints are part of the final behavior modification plan. Often the services of competent behavior therapy are obtained by referral to those who maintain private practice, but such services are available. The neurologist should be critical, supportive, realistic, and optimistic as the program proceeds. The neurologist must become familiar with resources available in the community, among local academic centers and from the various agencies, foundations, and support groups in the epilepsy movement and its network of state and local chapters. If time and temperament permit, the physician can advocate social and medical change; support basic and clinical research in behavioral medicine enterprises; and encourage better training, research, and comprehensive treatment. Above all, the clinician should appreciate that behavior modification offers a real opportunity to provide relief for the individual epileptic, and thereby to contribute to better medicine.

REFERENCES

Brown, S. B., & Fenwick, P.B.C. (1989). Evoked and psychogenic seizures:2. Inhibition. *Acta Neurologica Scandinavica, 80,* 535–540.

Cataldo, M. F., Russo, D. C., & Freeman, J. M. (1979). A behavior analysis approach to high rate myoclonic seizures. *Journal of Autism and Developmental Disorders, 9,* 413–427.

Dahl, J., Melin, L., Brorson, L. A., & Schollin, J. (1985). Effects of a broad spectrum behaviour modification treatment program on children with refractory epilepsy seizures. *Epilepsia, 26,* 303–309.

Dahl, J., Melin, L., & Lund, L. (1988). Effects of a behavioural intervention on epileptic behaviour and paroxysmal activity: A systematic replication of three cases of children with intractable epilepsy. *Epilepsia, 29,* 172–183.

Dreifuss, F. E. (1989). Classification of epileptic seizures and the epilepsies. *Pediatric Clinics of North America, 39,* 265–279.

Feldman, R. G., & Paul, N. G. (1976). Identity of emotional triggers in epilepsy. *Journal of Nervous and Mental Disorders, 162,* 345–352.

Fenwick, P.B.C. (1981). Precipitation and inhibition of seizures. In E. H. Reynolds & M. R. Trimble (Eds.), *Epilepsy and psychiatry* (pp. 306–321). Edinburgh: Churchill Livingstone.

Flannery, R. B., Jr., & Cautela, J. R. (1973). Seizures: Controlling the uncontrollable. *Journal of Rehabilitation, 39,* 34–36.

Forster, F. M. (1967). Conditioned reflex therapy in epilepsy. *Georgetown Medical Bulletin, 21,* 69–76.

Forster, F. M. (1978). *Reflex epilepsy, behavioral therapy, and conditional reflexes.* Springfield, IL: Charles C. Thomas.

Goldstein, L. H. (1990). Behavioural and cognitive–behavioural treatments for epilepsy: A progress review. *British Journal of Clinical Psychology, 29,* 257–269.

Hermann, B. P., & Whitman, S. (1984). Behavioural and personality correlates of epilepsy: A review, methodological critique and conceptual model. *Psychological Bulletin, 95,* 451–497.

Hosford, D. A., & McNamara, J. O. (1990). Basic mechanisms of the epilepsies. *Current Opinion in Neurology and Neurosurgery, 3,* 262–265.

Koul, R., Kousl, S., & Razdan, S. (1989). Eating epilepsy. *Acta Neurologica Scandinavica, 80,* 78–80.

Krafft, K. M., & Poling, A. D. (1982). Behavioural treatments of epilepsy: Methodological characteristics and problems of published studies. *Applied Research in Mental Retardation, 3,* 151–162.

Magnus, O., & Lorenz de Haas, A. M. (Eds.). (1974). *The epilepsies. Handbook of clinical neurology series* (Vol. 15). New York: Elsevier.

Mostofsky, D. I. (1981). Paroxysmal disorders of the central nervous system. In S. Turner, K. Calhoun, & H. Adams (Eds.), *Handbook of clinical behavior therapy.* New York: Wiley.

Mostofsky, D. I., & Balaschak, B. (1977). Psychobiological control of seizures. *Psychological Bulletin, 84,* 723–750.

Mostofsky, D. I., & Myslobodsky, M. S. (1982). Conditioning and the kindling model of epilepsy. *International Journal of Neuroscience, 16,* 75–82.

Pritchard, P. B., Holmstrom, V. L., & Giacinto, J. (1985). Self-abatement of complex partial seizures. *Annals of Neurology, 18,* 265–267.

Richard, A., & Reiter, J. (1990). *Epilepsy: A new approach.* New York: Prentice-Hall.

Sterman, M. B. (1972). Neurophysiologic and clinical studies of sensorimotor EEG biofeedback training: Some effects on epilepsy. *Seminars in Psychiatry, 5*(4), 507–525.

Sterman, M. B. (1982). EEG feedback in the treatment of epilepsy: An overview circa 1980. In L. White & B. Tursky (Eds.), *Clinical biofeedback: Efficacy and mechanisms.* New York: Guilford.

Tan, S. Y., & Bruni, J. (1986). Cognitive-behaviour therapy with adult patients with epilepsy: A controlled outcome study. *Epilepsia, 27,* 225–233.

Verdu, A., & Ruiz-Falco, M. L. (1991). Eating seizures associated with focal cortical dysplasia. *Brain and Development, 13,* 352–354.

Webster, A., & Mawer, G. E. (1989). Seizure frequency and major life events in epilepsy. *Epilepsia, 30,* 162–167.

Wolf, S. (1982). Psychosocial forces and neural mechanisms in disease: Defining the question and collecting the evidence. *The Johns Hopkins Medical Journal, 150,* 95–100.

Woods, P. J. (1974). A taxonomy of instrumental conditioning. *American Psychologist, 29*(8), 584–597.

Wyler, A. R., Robbins, C. A., & Dodrill, C. B. (1979). EEG operant conditioning for the control of epilepsy. *Epilepsia, 20,* 279–286.

4 Psychogenic Seizures

Daniel T. Williams
Thaddeus Walczak
Wolfgang Berten
Douglas Nordli
Columbia–Presbyterian Medical Center
Marcia Bergtraum
Long Island Jewish Medical Center

It has long been recognized that a significant proportion of individuals with well-documented epilepsy report that some of their seizures seem to be precipitated by emotional stress (Fenwick, 1991; Gowers, 1885; Mattson, 1991). Indeed, the phenomenon of stress-precipitated epileptic seizures has been demonstrated electroencephalographically by many workers among experimental animals (Lockard, 1980; Martinek & Hork, 1970; Swinyard, 1963) and in clinical populations (Antebi & Bird, 1992; Guey et al., 1969; Stevens, 1962).

It has also been recognized that a significant proportion of patients with well-documented epilepsy have coexisting episodes of purely psychological origin (Gates & Hemmes, 1990; Lesser, 1985; Williams, 1982). Furthermore, after careful study, a significant proportion of individuals with apparently uncontrolled seizures are discovered to have had no neurogenic seizures at all, but only episodes of purely psychological origin.

Thus, it becomes obvious that before addressing psychotherapeutic issues in the neurobehavioral treatment of epilepsy that are focused on seizure control, careful consideration is needed regarding issues of differential diagnosis.

We use the term *psychogenic seizures* to signify episodes precipitated by emotional stress within the individual and identified, at least initially, as "seizures." On further assessment, some of these will be clarified as *psychogenically precipitated epileptic seizures* and others as *purely psychogenic (nonepileptic) seizures*. We prefer to avoid the term *pseudoseizures* because its pejorative connotation can adversely complicate communication with patients and their families.

The equally important issue of other psychopathology associated with epilepsy besides that of psychogenic seizures is dealt with in several other recent publications (Neppe & Tucker, 1992; Smith, Treiman, & Trimble, 1991; Williams, Pleak, & Hanesian, 1991).

DIFFERENTIAL DIAGNOSIS

Diagnosing the presence of epilepsy and its subtypes is the primary responsibility of the neurologist. Associated neurological tasks include clarifying whether underlying treatable causes of the seizures can be discerned and initiating appropriate medical treatment (Resor & Kutt, 1992; Scheuer & Pedley, 1990). This having been done, when seizures are not controlled with standard medical management—most often including anticonvulsant medication—the possible role of psychological factors should be systematically considered, even if no obvious factors suggesting psychogenicity have been evident to that point. Sometimes strong evidence pointing to psychogenicity, present from the outset of clinical contact, may have been overlooked by the neurologist, who may focus preferentially and understandably on the primary presenting neurological symptom and its standard medical treatment. Several pertinent differential diagnostic categories are outlined.

Psychogenically Precipitated Epileptic Seizures: Psychological Factors Affecting Physical Condition

Fenwick (1991) and Antebi and Bird (1992) outlined the multifactorial determinants of the genesis of seizures in any individual. The term *seizure threshold,* viewed as relatively stable for the individual, designates a general level of vulnerability to seizures based on genetic and constitutional factors. Independent of this intrinsic attribute of the individual, more transient influences, such as biochemical, metabolic, or psychological changes, may impact on the seizure threshold. *Facilitating* influences on this threshold may increase the likelihood of seizures during the time of their impact. Alternatively, some stimuli may *evoke* seizures directly, with a high degree of chronologic proximity and predictability. Antebi and Bird classify the facilitating and evocative stimuli as either physical (motor, sensory, or visceral) or psychological (cognitive or affective).

If uncomplicated by significant independent psychopathology, psychogenically precipitated epileptic seizures may be approached therapeutically with a variety of symptom-focused psychological and/or behavioral interventions. If significant psychopathology co-exists, this clearly must be addressed as well.

Case Illustration. This 23-year-old single female college graduate was in apparent good health until she developed seizures just as she was about to start graduate school. There were three types of episodes: (a) dystonic right-arm elevations, (b) episodes of bilateral tightening of the arms and face, and (c) a single episode of pelvic thrusting during administration of phenytoin in the emergency room. The patient reported that she retained consciousness during these episodes. MRI of the brain was normal as was the spinal fluid. Several EEGs showed mild diffuse abnormality but no epileptiform activity. The suspicion that some or all of her episodes were psychogenic led to her referral for video-EEG monitoring at our medical center.

Immediately on admission, with phenytoin discontinued, multiple episodes of dystonic posturing of the right arm were noted, each lasting about 10 sec. The patient was able to recall information presented during the episode. EEG during these episodes showed a clear ictal spike & poly-spike discharge over the left parasagittal regions. The patient was loaded with carbamazepine and a level of 11 mg/l was achieved within 24 hours. This decreased the frequency of episodes from approximately 10 per hour to about 10 per day. However, it became clear that writing and many other simple motions of the right hand would consistently precipitate these events. Writing with the left hand and anxiety also precipitated the seizures.

During psychiatric consultation, the patient disclosed that her father, a successful and charismatic entrepreneur, had been abusive to her mother, had used cocaine, and had eventually abandoned the family. In a painfully analogous manner, the boyfriend whom the patient had dated seriously for the last 2 years of college abruptly abandoned the patient shortly before the onset of her seizures. This occurred about the same time that her father, whom she had contacted, refused to help her with the oppressive forthcoming expenses of graduate school.

The patient was a good hypnotic subject in formal assessment. She was asked in hypnotic trance to focus on the feelings of abandonment, demoralization, and accumulated anger inherent in the previously noted experiences. This activated dystonic posturing episodes of the right arm that were indistinguishable from those previously recorded. The next day, a therapeutic, relaxation-oriented use of hypnosis was applied; no seizures were observed during this session. The other types of previously reported seizures were not observed during 6 days of video-EEG monitoring. The patient was switched to valproic acid, 1500 mg/day, and discharged, to be followed both neurologically and in ongoing psychotherapy. Her seizures were fully controlled within a month under this regimen, and after an interval of 3 months, she was able to resume her graduate-school studies, with no recurrence of seizures over an 8-month period. Our retrospective diagnosis in this case includes:

1. Localization related epilepsy, etiology unknown: simple partial seizures with motoric manifestations. These seizures could be evoked by either motoric movements or psychogenic precipitants.

2. Possible superimposed psychogenic (nonepileptic) seizures, by history.

Somatoform Disorders

This group of disorders suggests organic illness for which there are no organic findings to explain the symptoms and for which there is positive evidence that the symptoms are linked to psychological factors (American Psychiatric Association, 1987). By definition, the symptom production in somatoform disorders is not under voluntary control. That is, the patient does not have conscious awareness of controlling the production or withdrawal of the symptoms. Two subtypes of somatoform disorder are considered here.

Conversion Disorder

This subtype of somatoform disorder is characterized by a loss or alteration of physical functioning that suggests physical disorder, but is instead an expression of a psychological conflict or a need. After appropriate investigation, the disturbance cannot be explained by any physical disorder or known pathophysiological mechanism. Psychological factors may be judged to play a primary etiological role in a variety of ways. Thus, a temporal relationship may exist between the onset or worsening of the symptom and the presence of an environmental stimulus that activates a psychological conflict or a need. Alternatively, the symptom may be noted to free the patient from a noxious activity or encounter. Finally, the symptom may enable the patient to get help from others that might otherwise not be forthcoming. The most common conversion symptoms are those suggesting neurological disease: conversion seizures are among the most common.

Case Illustration. A 47-year-old married mother of three was admitted to the hospital for video-EEG monitoring after several years of treatment with various anticonvulsants had failed to control paroxysmal symptoms that were variously diagnosed as epileptic seizures or paroxysmal dyskinesias. Previous routine EEGs had been negative. The paroxysmal movements were eventually recorded on video-EEG monitoring and disclosed to be nonepileptic. This, coupled with a consensus that the movements were not compatible with any known organic movement disorder, led to psychiatric consultation. On review of the history, it became clear that this highly intelligent woman had experienced many forms of intense and chronic stress, dating from childhood. Early stresses included harsh and repressive parenting by mother, including frequent forced enemas and observation of many episodes of paroxysmal incapacity in her father, who had severe atherosclerotic cardiovascular disease but received inadequate medical care. As an adult, the patient felt trapped in her marriage and endured repressive and hostile treatment from her husband, rebellion by two underachieving adolescent children, and inadequate recognition for her conscientious efforts at work. Appropriate psychotherapeutic intervention on a weekly basis led to clarification that, despite superior intelligence, this patient had never felt entitled to express long-standing feelings of frustration and anger, which led to a pattern of internalization and somatization. Therapeutic work on these issues, including encouragement of appropriate self-assertion, cleared her of symptoms within a few weeks (off all anticonvulsant medications) and helped her maintain a symptom-free state for over a year with follow-up weekly psychotherapy.

Somatization Disorder (formerly Called Hysteria or Briquet's Syndrome)

This subtype of somatoform disorder most often has its onset in adolescence, with only rare documentation of prepubertal diagnosis (Livingston & Martin-Connici, 1985). The essential features include recurrent multisymptomatic complaints of several years' duration beginning before the age of 30. Medical attention is sought repeatedly, but the symptoms are not based on any physical disorder. Complaints of at least 13 symptoms from the list of 35 enumerated in DMS-III-R must be elicited in order to establish the diagnosis. These include gastrointestinal symptoms, pain symptoms, cardiopulmonary symptoms, conversion symptoms psychosexual symptoms, and female reproductive system symptoms.

It has been estimated that approximately 1% of the adult female population has this disorder (Ford, 1983; G. R. Smith, Jr., 1990), whereas it is rarely diagnosed in males. There is a higher incidence of antisocial personality disorder among family members of those with somatization disorder than in the general population. The clinical course tends to be chronic but fluctuating, with extensive utilization of medical services over time and with rare incidence of spontaneous remission. A clinically important issue is the possibility that untreated, protracted, or recurrent episodes of conversion disorder or somatoform pain disorder in childhood or adolescence may predispose one to the subsequent development of somatization disorder (Williams & Hirsch, 1988).

It is commonly assumed that conversion and somatization disorders are defined not only by the absence of demonstrable organic pathology at their onset, but also by the failure of these symptoms to result in actual physical injury to the patient. Neither of these assumptions are necessarily true. We have already noted the frequently documented existence of seizures of purely emotional origin in patients with documented epilepsy. It should be added that psychogenic seizures may, on rare occasions, result in serious self-injury.

Case Illustration. A single woman, age 47, was admitted to our long-term, video-EEG monitoring unit after her third skull fracture. Abundant psychopathology, including a psychogenic gait disorder, and many other physical complaints without demonstrable organic basis had been documented. Psychotherapy had been ongoing for several years but had failed to improve her condition, even when combined with numerous successive antidepressant medication trials. There had been several negative neurological assessments and EEGs, including sleep-deprived recordings. Yet, numerous instances of serious injury as a result of falls following brief "blackouts" had resulted in fractured teeth and bones, hematuria from a renal injury, multiple lacerations, contusions, and abrasions, and two skull fractures. There was no financial benefit to the patient from any of these injuries. She continued to work as a salesperson in a retail store while living with both of her parents, who communicated with her but not with each other. The pattern of repeated serious injuries finally prompted treatment with carbamazepine. Therapeutic levels were achieved and the episodes stopped for about 1 year, but then the falling episodes recurred, ending with the patient fracturing her skull. The neurologist was able to elicit a typical episode by suggestion in the video-EEG monitoring unit, where the patient's fall was intercepted by staff, preventing injury. Neither this episode nor any other portion of the EEG recording, yielded any evidence of seizure activity. This assessment pointed strongly to the diagnosis of purely psychogenic seizures, permitted the removal of carbamazepine and pursual of more appropriate psychotherapeutic and psychopharmacologic measures, which resulted in some clinical improvement. It was the treating psychiatrist's opinion that a coexisting personality disorder with passive, dependent, depressive, histrionic, and masochistic features had led to the perpetuation and elaboration of what had initially emerged as an acute conversion disorder in response to ongoing life stresses some 25 years earlier, but which had not been adequately diagnosed or treated.

Factitious Disorders

Factitious disorders are characterized by physical or psychological symptoms that are intentionally produced or feigned, hence considered, by definition, under voluntary control (American Psychiatric Association, 1987). The sense of voluntary control is subjective and can only be inferred by an outside observer, giving rise to ready diagnostic confusion with somatoform disorders. The judgment that symptoms are voluntarily produced is based on observations of behavior suggesting dissimulation or concealment, after excluding all other possible causes of the behavior. However, it should be noted that this behavior has a compulsive quality and hence is voluntary in the sense of being deliberate and purposeful, although implying a lack of full control that is an inherent feature of a compulsive behavior. Another essential feature is the psychological need to assume the sick role, as evidenced by the absence of external incentives for the behavior, such as economic gain, avoidance of onerous responsibilities, or attaining more comfortable circumstances via the sick role. This is important in distinguishing factitious disorders from malingering.

In its more chronic forms, factitious disorder may be associated with either physical symptoms (Munchausen syndrome) or psychological symptoms (Ganser's syndrome, pseudopsychosis, or pseudodementia). These manifestations are generally associated with severe dependent, masochistic, or antisocial personality disorders. Here again, these chronic forms of maladaptation are thought to derive from uncorrected patterns, frequently dating from childhood, of using factitious symptoms as expressions of distress. Iatrogenic problems may ensue from misguided medical and surgical interventions.

Munchausen Syndrome by Proxy

This variant of factitious disorder was first reported by Meadow (1982). He reported on 19 children under 7 years of age, from 17 families, whose mothers consistently gave fraudulent clinical histories and fabricated signs that led to needless and harmful medical investigations, hospital admissions, and treatment over a period ranging from a few months to 4 years. Episodes of bleeding, neurological abnormality, rashes, fevers, and abnormal urine were commonly simulated. Often the mothers had previous nursing training and some had a history of fabricating symptoms or signs relating to themselves. Two of the 19 children died. Meadow's study of these children and their families led to a list of warning signs to consider, together with recommendations for dealing with suspected acts. He noted the need to separate the mother and child in suspect circumstances to confirm the fabrication and emphasized the subsequent need to confront the families with the deception when it was confirmed. Of the 17 survivors in his series, 8 children were taken into protective care and the other 9 remained at home after arrangements for augmented supervision were made.

Case Illustration. A single, attractive 19-year-old woman was admitted to the neurology service at our medical center with a 10-year medical history that included, among other complaints, chronic movement disorder, seizures, and blindness. During this 10-year period, the patient had 14 hospitalizations, innumerable medications, and three major surgical procedures for presumptive treatment of dystonia musculorum deformans. The surgery had involved placement of metal rods in her foot and spine, followed eventually by a craniotomy for laser thalamotomy. The last procedure occurred when the parents signed the patient out of a child psychiatry inpatient service against medical advice. Mother was a registered nurse. None of the surgical treatments had resulted in sustained clinical improvement. On careful reassessment at our medical center, no organic basis for any of the patient's complaints was found, and inconsistencies on repeated examination pointed clearly to nonphysiologically based symptoms in all three areas of presumptive neurologic impairment. On testing of visual evoked responses, the patient purposely crossed her eyes to feign blindness, documenting a volitional, conscious role in symptom formation. With this diagnostic clarification, intensive psychotherapy and associated psychopharmacologic treatment for coexisting dysthymia was initiated. The parents, living in another state, were minimally involved during inpatient evaluation and treatment. Although partial improvement was achieved during the hospital stay and maintained at one follow-up visit, the patient's current status is unknown.

Malingering

Malingering is characterized by the voluntary production and presentation of false or grossly exaggerated physical or psychological symptoms. In contrast to factitious disorder, the symptoms in malingering are produced in pursuit of a goal that is readily recognizable based on an understanding of the individual's circumstances rather than on his or her individual psychology (Kellner, 1991; Yudofsky, 1985). Examples of such readily understandable goals include the avoidance of school or work, the securing of financial compensation, the evasion of punishment, or the acquisition of drugs. Parentally induced malingering in a school-age child could occur, for example, when parents encourage their child, directly or indirectly, to persevere in reporting symptoms in the wake of an accident, for purposes of enhancing financial claims.

As with somatoform disorders and factitious disorders, a patient's volitional intent often cannot be determined with certainty by the clinician, especially at the outset of the clinical assessment. The particular characteristic of the malingerer, namely that of deceiving and manipulating the physician into unwitting compliance with a goal of the malingerer's choosing, is particularly likely to elicit strong countertransference feelings on the part of the physician when this diagnosis is suspected. Because the confrontational presentation of such suspicion to a patient will likely sabotage any prospects of a therapeutic relationship and transform it into a hostile, adversarial one, it is particularly important to refrain from such confrontation until all other differential diagnostic possibilities have been adequately considered an explored. It is important to note that somatoform disorders may include "secondary gains," which may falsely lead to the presumption of malingering. It is therefore best in ambiguous cases to give the patient—at least initially—the benefit of the doubt, so as to preserve the clinician's therapeutic leverage with a view toward symptom alleviation. Failure of the patient (and/or parents in the case of child patients) to respond cooperatively to exhaustive supportive measures at appropriate psychotherapeutic intervention would be a reason for revising one's initial diagnostic premise.

Cormorbidity

To illustrate the differential diagnostic complexity that may pertain, consider a patient with uncontrolled seizures who is referred by a neurologist for psychiatric consultation because of apparent emotional precipitant of at least some of the seizures. The referring and consulting clinicians must discern what proportion of the seizures represent uncontrolled neurogenic seizures, a somatoform disorder, a factitious disorder, malingering, or psychologically precipitated neurogenic seizures (psychological factors affecting a physical condition). Furthermore, they must consider whether some undiagnosed physical condition (e.g., CNS infection, tumor, or degenerative disease) may be contributory. They must be aware that two or more of these conditions may coexist in the same patient. Finally, quite apart from clarification of the nature of the seizure problem, there may be considerable psychopathology that may or may not impact on the seizures, but may clinically merit independent diagnostic assessment and treatment. The result can be and often is a diagnostic and therapeutic challenge that taxes the resources of even the most seasoned neurologists and psychiatrists (Williams et al., 1978, 1979, 1991; Williams & Mostofsky, 1982).

Case Illustration. A 9-year-old girl with an above-average IQ and a history of complex partial (gelastic) seizures came to our medical center after numerous failed treatment trials on virtually every plausible anticonvulsant. She had been referred for seizure surgery, which was not performed after extensive EEG monitoring that repeatedly documented spike and wave abnormalities, because a circumscribed seizure focus accessible to surgical removal could not be delineated. During the last of many hospitalizations, the nursing staff remarked to the neurologist about the girl's histrionic and manipulative style, as well as the fact that her seizures were more numerous when the parents or physicians were present. The seizures, as recorded by the patient and observers, numbered more than 300 per day. In the absence of a plausible pharmacological or surgical intervention and in light of suggestive clinical observations, the consulting psychiatrist postulated the presence of psychogenic seizures, superimposed on a well-documented neurogenic seizure substrate. During the course of a 2-week hospital stay, intensive psychotherapeutic evaluation and treatment was pursued, including individual, parental, and family sessions, behavior modification, and hypnosis. With evidence of improvement in seizure control, anticonvulsant medication was gradually tapered. Within 2 weeks, seizure frequency had diminished to zero and the girl was discharged from the hospital. She promptly returned to school and continued to be seizure-free as her anticonvulsants were progressively tapered to zero by her neurologist during 6 months in supportive outpatient psychotherapy. She continues seizure-free over $3\frac{1}{2}$ years in follow-up, off all anticonvulsants.

This evaluation preceded the availability of video-EEG monitoring capacity for children at our medical center. Consequently, neither the neurologist nor the psychiatrist was certain, retrospectively, as to whether psychotherapeutic intervention had impacted specifically on psychogenically precipitated epileptic seizures or (more likely) on conversion seizures which had evolved on the substrate of an epileptiform disorder that had been spontaneously developmentally abating.

DIAGNOSTIC ASSESSMENT OF PSYCHOGENIC SEIZURES

A number of clinical features may suggest the presence of nonepileptic psychogenic seizures to the neurologist. Several attempts have been made to enumerate these systematically (Gates, 1992; Lowman & Richardson, 1987; Williams, 1982). Features commonly noted in nonepileptic psychogenic seizures are outlined in Table 4.1. It is important to note that many of these may be present in patients with genuine epileptic seizures. However, EEG shows characteristic abnormalities in all generalized tonic–clonic seizures and in more than 95% of complex partial seizures.

Other psychiatric disorders which may be confused with or may coexist with epileptic seizures include panic attacks, drug intoxication, psychosis, dissociative disorder, and intermittent explosive disorder.

If, at the time of initial consultation, the confluence of clinical data convinces the neurologist that probable psychogenic factors play a role in the patient's presenting symptoms, an important part of the diagnostic assessment includes apprising the patient of this possibility in a supportive manner. We have found that discussing with the patient and family the possibility that stress may play a role in their symptoms, as it does in many medical disorders, is much more palatably accepted than prematurely introducing diagnostic terms which have more definitive psychopathological connotations. If initial neurological assessment, including EEG, is negative and the neurologist discerns that a nonepileptic psychogenic disorder probably exists without any evidence of coexisting epilep-

TABLE 4.1

Characteristics Suggesting Nonepileptic Psychogenic Events

1. The seizure events emerge under stressful circumstances (cumulative and/or proximate).
2. The EEG during the seizure event is normal and shows no post-ictal slowing.
3. There are secondary gains, such as getting attention, being excused from work, collecting financial compensation, or escaping from an intolerable social situation. In this regard, nonepileptic psychogenic events usually occur in the company of others and rarely when the patient is alone.
4. There are other conversion symptoms or other indications of significant psychopathology.
5. The seizures fail to conform to a physiologic pattern. These characteristics are more diagnostic if occurring during an apparent generalized seizure:
   a. Out-of-phase movements of upper extremities or lower extremities.
   b. Pelvic thrusting.
   c. Side-to-side head movement.
   d. Corneal relfexes are present and plantar reflexes are flexor.
   e. Patient recalls movements and/or communications during the seizure event.

sy, appropriate referral for psychotherapeutic treatment can then be made promptly. In cases of a mixed clinical picture, consultation from an appropriate mental health practitioner can allow for a combined treatment approach. In cases of continued diagnostic uncertainty, continued uncontrolled seizures, and/or the patient's continued resistance to psychotherapeutic intervention, referral for long-term video-EEG monitoring at an appropriate inpatient facility would be indicated.

Long-Term Monitoring

Long term monitoring (LTM) for epilepsy refers to the simultaneous recording of the EEG and clinical behavior over extended periods of time to evaluate patients with paroxysmal disturbances of cerebral function (Gates & Hemmes, 1990). Aside from its value in delineating epileptic seizure subtypes that are difficult to record during routine EEG sessions, LTM has particular value in the assessment of psychogenic seizures. It has been shown at epilepsy centers with inpatient LTM units that the yield of seizures can be increased if the patient is withdrawn from anticonvulsants. Although this has both diagnostic and therapeutic value for psychogenic seizure patients, it is important to note that this should be done in the hospital under the supervision of experienced personnel because of the potential danger involved. Thus, the experience of Gates' group with psychogenic seizures identified a coincidence of epilepsy and psychogenic events in 58% of the patients with psychogenic events. It should be noted that there is considerable variability in this proportion among various monitoring centers, however, with several, including our own, having a much lower concordance rate of epileptic and nonepileptic events, in the range of 10%.

Recording multiple events with video-EEG allows crucial diagnostic clarification in patients suspected of suffering from psychogenic seizures. Careful analysis of clinical and EEG features of the seizures by experienced epileptologists will usually determine whether the seizures are epileptic. It is important to be certain that the recorded events are typical examples of the events the patient suffers. Review of the videotape with family members or other observers can help confirm this.

A problem arises, however, when the patient fails to have spontaneous seizure events in the LTM unit. A variety of suggestive techniques have been reported for precipitating psychogenic seizures in such circumstances (Cohen & Suter, 1982; Guberman, 1982; Linder, 1973; Peterson, Sumner, & Jones, 1950; Riley & Berndt).

The use of saline infusion as a suggestive technique (Cohen & Suter, 1982) can be readily standardized and administered without the presence of a mental health professional. It has the additional advantage of appealing to patients who would be highly resistant to the directly presented notion of a psychological etiology of their seizure events. The major disadvantage of this procedure is that it involves some degree of dissimulation, which could potentially complicate engagement of the patient in subsequent psychotherapeutic endeavor, unless the preparation of the patient, the diagnostic procedure, and the debriefing of the patient are done most judiciously.

The use of hypnosis to induce psychogenic seizures (Peterson et al., 1950; Spiegel & Spiegel, 1978) has the advantage of directly demonstrating to the patient the phenomenon of psychogenic precipitation of seizure events, thereby establishing clearly and promptly the rationale for psychotherapeutic intervention as well as the mental health professional who can initiate the process. Disadvantages include greater difficulty in standardizing a hypnotic induction process, which is most effective when individualized, and the high likelihood of resistance and/or nonhypnotizability in some patients (e.g., those with factitious disorder, malingering, or psychosis). We are currently conducting a systematic comparison of these induction modalities at our LTM unit.

Clinician's Approach to the Patient

One's tactical approach to the patient and family is of importance in establishing a rapport that is crucial for effective diagnostic assessment and treatment for all patients with suspected psychogenic seizures. The patient with a somatoform disorder, for example, is by definition unaware of the relationship between environmental stress or intrapsychic conflict and the appearance of the presenting symptoms. In such a setting, a confrontational approach with the patient or relatives during the initial assessment is clearly counterproductive. Any inquiries that are perceived by the patient as seeking to establish such etiological connections in an accusatory tone are likely to be met with denial or distortion. A preferable approach is to begin by having the neurologist explain supportively to the patient that psychological/psychiatric consultation is being sought because of the possibility that psychological factors may play some role in the patient's presenting symptom, as they do in many commonly encountered medical problems. Most patients accept that stress may make their seizures worse. The psychotherapist reemphasizes this point on initial contact with the patient. This opens the way for a collaborative dialogue in which the patient (and family) will help the psychotherapist with two difficult tasks: first understanding potential psychogenic contributants to the seizures and then, one hopes, enabling the patient to overcome these. If available medical information at the time of initial referral is not conclusive regarding the presence or absence of epilepsy, it is important to clarify that issue with the patient and family. It should also be explained that ongoing contact will be maintained with the neurologist, as both assessments proceed concurrently. An effective "team approach" minimizes the possibility of a patient splitting the staff as a maladaptive defensive maneuver.

Psychological/psychiatric assessment should yield a detailed picture of the patient's individual strengths and weaknesses, social relationships, school or work functioning, and pattern of family interaction. The process of exploring these areas often yields additional clues as to whether there is a combination of intrinsic vulnerabilities in the patient and cumulative stressors in his or her environment that would predispose to the development of psychogenic seizures. Both patients and relatives should be questioned specifically regarding any possible history of physical or sexual abuse, because the reported incidence of such abuse in patients with psychogenic seizures is high (Lowman & Richardson, 1987). Every effort should be made to establish—as fully as possible—not only a clearly defined psychiatric diagnosis (American Psychiatric Association, 1987) but also a tentative formulation of potential psychodynamic and/or behavioral contingencies which might contribute specifically to psychogenic seizures. Formal psychological testing may be a valuable adjunct in the assessment of these patients (Batzel et al., 1991; Dodrill, Batzel, Quisser, & Temlom, 198; Lowman & Richardson, 1987).

After completion of neurological and psychological/psychiatric evaluations, it is frequently helpful to have a joint meeting, if possible, between the patient, the neurologist, and the psychotherapist, particularly if the evaluation has been done in an inpatient setting. This type of meeting expedites clarifying the diagnosis to the patient and helps avoid misunderstandings or triangularizations between the patient and different clinicians.

ETIOLOGY AND PATHOGENESIS

Clinical considerations in this domain often involve hypothesis building based on historical information elicited from the patient and/or family, with a view toward formulating a strategy of treatment intervention. Insofar as we have emphasized the possibility of multifactional contributants to psychogenic seizures, clinical hypotheses regarding etiology and pathogenesis of psychogenic seizures should be formulated with this premise in mind. This avoids having the psychotherapist fixate prematurely on a plausible hypothesis which appeals to the psychotherapist but which may alienate the patient.

Psychogenically precipitated Epileptic Seizures

Contemporary models of focal epilepsy suggest that damaged cells in the center of the focus are continually firing abnormally (Lockard, 1980). For a seizure to emerge, these cells must recruit surrounding neurons. The number of cells that can be recruited may be influenced by a number of factors, including psychosocial influences. Using a monkey model, Lockard demonstrated that documented spike frequency and seizure frequency may vary as a function of environmental stress. Fenwick (1989, 1991) extended this demonstration and developed a conceptual model for understanding psychogenically precipitated epileptic seizures in clinical populations.

Somatoform Disorders, Factitious Disorders, and Malingering

Each of these categories is complex and multidetermined, defying a simple schema of etiology and pathogenesis. Thus, for somatoform disorders alone, one might consider the etiologic role of psychodynamically based psychosexual conflicts, gratification of dependency needs, reaction to environmental stress, the phenomenon of dissociation, neurophysiological predisposition, and the role of depression (Williams & Hirsch, 1988). Considerations with factitious disorders and malingering are similarly complex, generally requiring a thorough psychological and/or psychiatric assessment as a prelude to accurate diagnosis and treatment.

TREATMENT

Many different treatment approaches have been used with patients having psychogenic seizures. As with most psychotherapeutic interventions, controlled studies are extremely difficult to implement (Goldstein, 1990; Karasu, Conte, & Plutchik, 1984). Those therapeutic approaches that eclectic clinical experience has found useful are considered here. Each of these treatment approaches has some potential value for some patients. Often, different treatment approaches can be effectively combined in the management of a given patient. Consequently, it is advantageous for the clinician to be well informed about as many of these approaches as possible in order to structure a treatment plan that most effectively meets the unique needs of each patient.

Implicit in this discussion is the observation that no direct correlation exists between the specific type of psychogenic seizure and the specific type of treatment intervention clinically indicated. Whereas a variety of modalities are outlined, some common underlying features may be delineated:

1. Psychotherapeutic intervention provides a framework, by psychologically oriented review of the history, whereby the patient (and family) can discern and articulate postulated psychogenic contributants to the uncontrolled seizures.

2. Once postulated psychogenic contributants are identified, a strategy for their attenuation or control can be delineated. This engenders a sense of hope in the patient and family that a new level of understanding and a new treatment intervention can be brought to bear. An intrinsic calming effect on the patient is inherent in this process, if successfully applied.

3. Concomitant with the new treatment intervention, there is an implicit or explicit dealing with secondary gain features that may have significantly contributed to the development and/or perpetuation of the symptoms.

4. The patient's self-esteem is protected by judicious handling of the previously mentioned considerations. This frequently involves an emphasis on self-mastery, crediting the patient for active, collaborative participation in the treatment.

Reassurance, Placebo, and Suggestion

Variations on this theme have been used throughout history, sometimes quite successfully, by religious healers, physicians, and others to relieve the symptoms of the various somatizing disorders that may give rise to psychogenic seizures (Williams & Hirsch, 1988). This approach involves the use of reassurance, placebo, and/or suggestion to foster symptom relinquishment without generating sophisticated grasp, by contemporary psychiatric standards, of the symptom's psychogenic determinants. Traditionally, this has involved the invocation of supernatural healing forces and/or the exorcism of nefarious illness-producing forces so as to restore the patient to health. Frequently, the use of prayer or an associated religious ceremony is involved, for which the patient and/or family makes some monetary or other contribution as part of a process of expiation of sin or appeasement of the deity. In a more contemporary secular context, the use of placebo can serve a comparable function in mobilizing the positive expectation and belief of the patient that relief of illness will be forthcoming, thanks to the powerful forces of pharmacological intervention that the scientific revolution has generated. It should be noted in passing that more recent studies have clarified the capacity of placebo to affect neurophysiological functioning by activating the release of endorphins within the central nervous system, so that dismissing this process as "merely suggestion" is unwarranted (Spiegel & Albert, 1983). The use of these nonspecific modalities employed by medical practitioners prior to referral for psychological or psychiatric consultation may be effective for the relief of *acute* conversion symptoms that arise in response to a *short-term* and *self-limited* environmental stress. When used supportively and sensitively in such a setting, this approach may be effective in achieving sustained symptom relief. Further, the nonspecific effects of reassurance, placebo, and suggestion exert a powerful auxiliary influence in combination with any of the more specific treatments outlined later.

Complications may arise, however, when a physician prescribes anticonvulsant medication with or without the knowledge that a purely psychogenic seizure disorder exists. Here one may initiate a long-standing medication regimen for the patient with considerable untoward side effects that may vitiate and outweigh initial placebo benefits (Dodrill, 1991; D. B. Smith, 1991).

Additional complications may arise when a treatment approach based exclusively on reassurance, placebo, or suggestion is used indiscriminately for psychogenic seizures, including those with complex, sustained intrapsychic determinants and/or in the presence of continuing, unmanageable environmental stress. In such situations, this approach is counterproductive. Here, it will be either totally ineffective or of only short-term benefit, with prompt emergence of symptom recurrence or substitution. Furthermore, there is a loss of confidence by the patient and family in the clinician who takes such an approach. This is because an attempt is made to remove a symptom that has been serving a defensive function—albeit maladaptively—without alleviating the patient's underlying sources of distress.

Individual and Family Therapies

Only brief discussion of these approaches can be outlined here. Because a myriad of intermingling etiological factors may pertain, the clinician should address as many of the pertinent issues as possible in the course of history taking. Based on a thorough exploration of relevant factors in this context, a working hypothesis regarding the evolution of the psychogenic seizure disorder is likely to emerge. With this working hypothesis in mind, the clinician's next task is to explore possible ways to alleviate pathogenic environmental influences impinging on the patient and/or to augment the patient's capacity for mastering ongoing sources of distress.

Alleviating environmental stress often involves working with the patient's immediate family and significant others. For example, if marital conflict with an adult patient's spouse or between a child patient's parents appears to contribute to a patient's psychogenic seizures, direct counseling of the family member as well as the patient should be considered. Similarly, if a *valedictorian syndrome* exists in a school-aged child, whereby parents, teachers, and/or the patient have generated excessive demands for academic achievement relative to the youngster's actual intellectual capacity, then direct, supportive counseling of the patient and family as well as communication with teachers may be necessary to alleviate this frequent contributant to somatization. As another example, if sexual abuse or seduction has occurred as a precipitating factor, clearly the protection of the patient from the perpetrator as well as supportive alleviation of the patient's associated feelings of guilt and/or violation are essential ingredients in the treatment plan.

Dealing with the apparent dynamics of intrapsychic and family conflict in patients with psychogenic seizures requires tact and sensitivity. It is useful to view the somatizing symptom as a makeshift refuge to which the patient has intuitively and sometimes unconsciously retreated under duress. The clinician is challenged to formulate for the patient and family a safe and honorable route by which the symptom can be understood as a maladaptive defense encumbrance that can be relinquished with dignity in favor of a more effective coping method. There are many ways to do this, but the clinician commonly presents some version of his working hypothesis to the patient (and family, where appropriate) to aid the process of cognitive, emotional, and behavioral reorientation. In terms of conscious understanding of the relevant dynamics, the extent to which this process can be "worked through" with the patient and family members is variable.

In the pursuit of the previously noted therapeutic goals, several specialized treatment approaches are often helpful in the context of individual and/or family therapy.

Psychoanalysis. From the time of Freud's initial exploration of the dynamics of hysteria until recently, many believed that psychoanalysis or intensive, long-term, dynamic psychotherapy were the specific treatments of choice for somatoform disorders (Kellner, 1989). It is now apparent that only a minority of the patients with these disorders are candidates for such therapy. This is true in part because of the combined demands of time, money, and intellectual investment, which most patients and families simply do not have. Equally important, however, is the fact that for many patients, other approaches can achieve therapeutic results more rapidly at a much lower expense.

Clearly, psychiatrists who work with patients having psychogenic seizures must have a sophisticated grasp of the subtle and complex factors involved in the diverse intrapsychic, interpersonal, and environmental fields that impinge on these patients. It is not necessary, however, for each patient to attain a full level of insight in order to achieve effective and sustained symptom relief. Extended analytic work can certainly add new dimensions of self-understanding for those with the resources to use this approach. Yet, for the many who for various reasons cannot or do not wish to do so, more supportive and directive methods of treatment are appropriate.

Hypnosis. Freud's interest in developing the technique of psychoanalysis was heavily influenced by the limitations he observed in Charcot's authoritarian use of hypnosis to treat psychogenic seizures and by Freud's own use of hypnosis to treat various forms of hysteria (Freud, 1955a). These limitations included the narrow use of abreaction and suggestion without benefit of the dynamic understanding of symptom formation that Freud subsequently developed. In later years, Freud himself foresaw how public health needs would rekindle a need for hypnosis to enable more widespread therapeutic application of psychoanalytic insights in a more expeditious manner (Freud, 1955b).

Further considerations regarding the use of hypnosis with patients having psychogenic seizures and other somatizing disorders are outlined elsewhere (Williams, 1988, 1991; Williams et al., 1978, 1979). Admonitions against the use of hypnosis with such patients are sometimes based on the erroneous assumption that hypnosis necessarily involves the simplistic and heavy-handed use of direct suggestion that was the usual mode of Freud's contemporaries. Furthermore, there are some positive benefits to enabling a patient and family to learn that the patient's capacity for *dissociation* can be elicited under controlled therapeutic conditions. In this context, the dissociation that is an essential ingredient in the symptom formation of somatoform disorders can be considered a manageable psychological attribute that can be channeled, under therapeutic auspices, in the service of symptom alleviation. Teaching the patient a self-hypnosis exercise can help shift the patient's (and family's) attention away from preoccupation with the sick role and toward the mastery experience of returning to normal functioning.

The basis for advocating the use of hypnosis as a therapeutic adjunct for patients with psychogenically precipitated epileptic seizures is less clearly established. However, Spiegel (1991) reviewed the growing body of evidence pointing to the capacity of hypnosis to impact on a variety of neurophysiologic processes, providing suggestive support for this clinical intervention. Thus, highly hypnotizable subjects are capable of producing bidirectional changes in cortical-event-related potential amplitude to sensory stimuli, depending on the cognitive task employed during hypnosis. In contrast, subjects not easily hypnotized, studied under the same conditions in a controlled manner, showed no such changes. The demonstrated capacity of hypnotic trance states to influence gastric acid secretion (Klein & Spiegel, 1989), pain perception (Spiegel, Bierre, & Rootenberg, 1989), and blood pressure (Benson & Klipper, 1976) provides a plausible rationale for the therapeutic application of hypnosis for psychogenically precipitated epileptic seizures.

In the format used by our group, measurement of hypnotic capacity using the Hypnotic Induction Profile (Spiegel & Spiegel, 1978) is part of the initial assessment of all patients being evaluated for possible psychogenic seizures. If combined neurological and psychiatric assessment supports the impression of psychogenic seizures, hypnotizable patients are taught a self-hypnosis exercise as part of the treatment program. The content of this exercise is individualized, based on the history, cognitive capacity, and psychodynamic picture presented by the patient. Other aspects of the treatment are also individualized, including the frequency and format of individual and family therapy, associated behavior modification strategies, and, in some cases, psychopharmacological intervention. It is thus evident that whereas the use of self-hypnosis as a treatment intervention for psychogenic seizures incorporates many of the features of relaxation and desensitization outlined by Fenwick (1989, 1991), delineation of the specific impact of hypnosis under such varied clinical conditions is not currently feasible.

Behavior Modification

Therapeutic strategies geared to symptom alleviation in the somatizing disorders must deal with the secondary gain features of the symptoms. (In the case of malingering, these are equivalent to the primary gain features.) Especially with children, adolescents, and retarded patients, the long-range benefits of a therapeutic endeavor may be difficult for the patient to appreciate if the immediate benefits of the symptom constitute a substantial deterrent to symptom relinquishment. Therefore, it is essential that any ongoing secondary gain features of a symptom be diminished or eliminated. Indeed, this is crucial if removal of the symptom is to be sustained.

Mostofsky & Balaschak (1977) illustrated a number of ways in which behavior-modification strategies can be formulated with seizure patients, taking into account the existing contingencies of reinforcement that impinge on the patient. Many of the reports cited in this review do not distinguish clearly between patients with documented epilepsy, those with exclusive psychogenic seizures, or those with some combination of the two.

A number of recent reviews (Fenwick, 1989, 1991; Goldstein, 1990) updated the status of the behavioral treatments of epilepsy. Because these reviews are detailed and comprehensive, they will not be reoutlined here. Suffice it to say that a growing number of behavioral studies with improved methodologies provide abundant evidence of the close relationship between epileptic seizure activity and the psychological state of the patient. It follows that seizure control in many patients can be significantly influenced by altering the outlook and behavior of the patient. A variety of behavioral strategies are addressed by these reviews, with no clear delineation yet feasible of the specific correlation between the optimal behavioral intervention for specific seizure type.

Psychotropic Medication

Because somatoform disorders, factitious disorders, and malingering frequently coexist with other psychiatric disorders responding to medication, the psychiatrist should consider the potential value of psychotropic medications in treating patients with psychogenic seizures. In our experience, depression is a particularly common concommittant in these patients and appropriate use of antidepressant medication is frequently helpful (Williams & Hirsch, 1988; Williams, Pleak, & Hanesian, 1991). The additional therapeutic value of medication for many of these patients (aside from psychopharmacologic benefit) is that it permits easier acceptance of a treatment program where there is a "biological" component, for patients resistant to accepting a primary psychological explanation of their disorder. The obvious caveat of caution here is that with patients having both psychogenic and epileptic seizures, one must evaluate the potential impact of psychotropic medication on both the epileptic seizure threshold and the level of coexisting anticonvulsant medication. Clinical experience suggests that alprazolam, fluoxetine, and trimipramine are the antidepressants best tolerated in this population. Similar considerations apply to the use of other antianxiety and antipsychotic medications (Neppe & Tucker, 1992).

Special Considerations with Children, Adolescents, and Retarded Patients

The importance of effectively engaging the family or other caretakers of children, adolescents, and retarded patients cannot be overemphasized. Although this principle applies to any psychotherapeutic intervention with such patients, the additional features of dependency and disability engendered by uncontrolled seizures reinforces this. Parents and/or other caretakers should be interviewed early in the diagnostic process as important sources of relevant information that may not be available from the patient or the medical chart. Similarly, these caretakers are often crucial in formulating treatment plans that involve rearranging contingencies of reinforcement for ongoing behavior, supportively reviewing therapeutic communications with the patient, and administering medication.

Supportive Reality Testing

Even the most experienced of clinicians will encounter some patients and families where combined neurological, psychotherapeutic, and behavioral endeavors geared toward symptom alleviation are unsuccessful in establishing clinically adequate improvement in seizure control. Sometimes this may be related to the intractable nature of the epileptic disorder which resists available options of pharmacologic and/or surgical intervention. In such circumstances, psychotherapeutic support is often needed for the patient and family struggling to cope with the patient's impaired level of functioning.

In other situations, however, efforts at clinical intervention with patients having uncontrolled psychogenic seizures are defeated by the tenacious psychological investment that the patient and/or family have made in the incurability of the presenting seizure symptoms. Clinical experience suggests that this form of failure is more common when a somatizing disorder (with or without associated epilepsy) has become chronic and has gone through a succession of failed medical and psychotherapeutic interventions. In these cases the somatizing disorder is often interwoven with an associated personality disorder in the patient and/or family, variably involving dependent, histrionic, antisocial, masochistic, or borderline features. In such situations, the degree of individual and/or family psychopathology frequently constitutes a substantial source of resistance to appropriate treatment. These circumstances are particularly common in patients with somatization disorder, factitious disorder, and malingering. In such circumstances, referral to a psychiatric inpatient service familiar with treatment of patients having psychogenic seizures may be appropriate. Such patients and/or families, initially unwilling to explore somatizing aspects of their illness, may be willing to address features of the patient's anxiety, depression, or other dysphoric symptoms that can be the starting point for therapeutic work. Some patients and families will, however, be unengageable in treatment despite the most flexible and extended efforts. If frank abuse or neglect of the patient is documented and efforts at engagement of the patient and family in treatment is unsuccessful, the involvement of appropriate legal and welfare agencies may be necessary.

CONCLUSION

Psychotherapeutically oriented assessment of patients with uncontrolled seizures may be helpful in delineating psychogenic contributants to the seizures and hence may allow formulation of a more effective treatment program. Differential diagnosis is clearly the first task, requiring an appreciation of potential multifactorial contributants to psychogenic seizures and the many different phenomenologic manifestations of psychogenic seizures. Once a reasonably informed working hypothesis regarding diagnosis is established, the therapist's task involves helping the patient to reformulate a strategy of coping with ongoing life stresses in order to achieve improved seizure control. Accumulated clinical experience points to a number of specific therapeutic techniques which may be helpful. The therapist who approaches this task will expand the potential for effective intervention by integrating those techniques that seem most pertinent to the needs of the individual patient, while effectively conveying an empathic sensitivity for the patient's struggle to improve his or her level of functioning.

ACKNOWLEDGMENTS

The authors wish to express appreciation to Drs. Arnold Gold, Nicholas Dumont, Franco Gallucci, Adreana Notarfrancesco, Stanley Resor, and Mark Scheuer and Timothy Pedley for assistance in clinical work dealt with in this chapter.

REFERENCES

American Psychiatric Association (1987). *Diagnostic and statistical manual of mental disorders (3rd rev. ed.): DSM-III-R*. Washington, DC: American Psychiatric Association.

Antebi, D., & Bird, J. (1992). The facilitation and evocation of seizures. *British Journal of Psychiatry, 160,* 154–164.

Batzel, L. W., Dodrill, C. B., Dubinsky, B. L., Ziegler, R. G., Connolly, J. E., Freeman, R. D., Farwell, J. R., & Vining, E. P. (1991). An objective method for the assessment of psychosocial problems in adolescents with epilepsy. *Epilepsia, 32,* 202–211.

Benson, H., & Klipper, M. Z. (1976). *The relaxation response*. New York: Morrow.

Cohen, R. J., & Suter, C. (1982). Hysterical seizures: Suggestion as a provocative EEG test. *Annals of Neurology, 11,* 391–395.

Dodrill, C. B. (1991). Behavioral effects of antiepileptic drugs. In D. B. Smith, D. M. Treiman, & M. R. Trimble (Eds.), *Neurobehavioral problems in epilepsy* (pp. 213–224). New York: Raven.

Dodrill, C. B., Batzel, L. W., Quisser, H. R., & Temlom, N. R. (1980). An objective method for the assessment of psychological and social problems among epileptics. *Epilepsia, 21,* 123–135.

Fenwick, P. (1989). Behavioral treatment of epilepsy. *International Review of Psychiatry, 1,* 297–306.

Fenwick, P. (1991). Evocation and inhibition of seizures: Behavioral treatment. In D. B. Smith, D. M. Treiman, & M. R. Trimble (Eds.), *Neurobehavioral problems in epilepsy* (pp. 163–184). New York: Raven.

Ford, C. V. (1983). *The somatizing disorders: Illness as a way of life.* New York: Elsevier Biomedical.

Freud, S. (1955a). An autobiographical study. In J. Strachey (Ed.), *The standard edition of the complete psychological works of Sigmund Freud* (Vol. 20, pp. 3–74). London: Hogarth Press.

Freud, S. (1955b). Lines of advance in psychoanalytic therapy. In J. Strachey (Ed.), *The standard edition of the complete psychological works of Sigmund Freud* (Vol. 17, pp. 195–168). London: Hogarth Press.

Gates, J. R. (1992). Psychogenic nonepileptic events. In S. R. Resor & H. Kutt (Eds.), *The medical treatment of epilepsy* (pp. 197–204). New York: Marcel Dekker.

Gates, J. R., & Hemmes, R. (1990). Role and implementation of long-term monitoring for epilepsy. *Seminars in Neurology, 10,* 357–365.

Goldstein, L. H. (1990). Behavioral and cognitive-behavioral treatments for epilepsy: A progress review. *British Journal of Clinical Psychology, 29,* 257–269.

Gowers, W. R. (1885). *Epilepsy and other chronic convulsive diseases.* New York: William Wood & Co.

Guberman, A. (1982). Psychogenic seizures in nonepileptic patients. *Canadian Journal of Psychiatry, 27,* 401–404.

Guey, J., Bureau, M., Dravet, C., & Roger, J. (1969). Study of the rhythm of petit-mal absences in children in relation to prevailing situations. *Epilepsia, 10,* 441–451.

Karasu, T. B., Conte, H. R., & Plutchik, R. (1984). Psychotherapy outcome research. In T. B. Karasu (Ed.), *The psychosocial therapies* (pp. 831–872). Washington, DC: American Psychiatric Association.

Kellner, R. (1989). Somatoform and facitious disorders. In American Psychiatric Association (Ed.), *Treatments of psychiatric disorders* (Vol. 3, pp. 2119–2184). Washington, DC: American Psychiatric Association.

Kellner, R. (1991). *Psychosomatic symptoms and somatic syndromes.* Washington, DC: American Psychiatric Press.

Klein, K. B., & Spiegel, D. (1989). Modulation of gastric acid secretion by hypnosis. *Gastroenterology, 96,* 1383–1387.

Lesser, R. P. (1985). Psychogenic seizures. In T. A. Pedley & B. S. Meldrum (Eds.), *Recent advances in epilepsy: No. 2.* Edinburgh: Churchill Livingston.

Linder, H. (1973). Psychogenic seizure states: A psychodynamic study. *International Journal of Clinical and Experimental Hypnosis, 21,* 261–271.

Livingston, R., & Martin-Connici, C. (1985). Multiple somatic complaints and possible somatization disorder in prepubertal children. *Journal American Academy of Child Psychiatry, 24,* 603–607.

Lockard, J. S. (1980). A primate model of clinical epilepsy: Mechanisms of action through quantification of therapeutic effects. In J. S. Lockard & A. A. Ward (Eds.), *Epilepsy: A window to brain mechanisms* (pp. 11–49). New York: Raven.

Lowman, R. L., & Richardson, L. M. (1987). Pseudoepileptic seizures of psychogenic origin: A review of the literature. *Clinical Psychology Review, 7,* 363–389.

Martinek, Z., & Hork, F. (1970). Development of so-called "genuine" epileptic seizures in dogs during emotional excitement. *Physiologia Bohemoslovaca, 19,* 185–195.

Mattson, R. H. (1991). Emotional effects on seizure occurence. In D. B. Smith, D. M. Treiman, & M. R. Trimble (Eds.), *Neurobiological problems in epilepsy* (pp. 453–460). New York, Raven.

Meadow, R. (1982). Munchausen syndrome by proxy. *Archives Diseases of Children, 57,* 92–98.

Mostofsky, D. I., & Balaschak, B. A. (1977). Psychobiological control of seizures. *Psychological Bulletin, 84,* 723–750.

Neppe, V. M., & Tucker, G. T. (1992). Neuropsychiatric aspects of seizure disorders. In S. C. Yudofsky & R. E. Hales (Eds.), *The American Psychiatric Press textbook of neuropsychiatry* (pp. 397–426). Washington, DC: American Psychiatric Press.

Peterson, D. B., Sumner, J. W., & Jones, G. A. (1950). Role of hypnosis in differentiation of epileptic from convulsive-like seizures. *American Journal of Psychiatry, 107,* 428–433.

Resor, S., & Kutt, H. (Eds.), (1992). *The medical treatment of epilepsy.* New York: Marcel Dekker.

Riley, T. L., & Berndt, T. (1980). The role of the EEG technologist in delineating pseudoseizures. *American Journal of EEG Technology, 20,* 89–96.

Scheuer, M. L., & Pedley, T. A. (1990). The evaluation and treatment of seizures. *New England Journal of Medicine, 323,* 1468–1474.

Smith, D. B. (1991). Cognitive effects of antiepileptic drugs. In D. B. Smith, D. M. Treiman, & M. R. Trimble (Eds.), *Neurobehavioral problems in epilepsy* (pp. 197–212). New York: Raven.

Smith, D. B., Treiman, D. M., & Trimble, M. R. (1991). Neurobehavioral problems in epilepsy: *Vol. 55. Advances in neurology.* New York: Raven.

Smith, G. R., Jr. (1990). *Somatization disorder in the medical setting.* Washington, DC: National Institute of Mental Health, U.S. Government Printing Office.

Spiegel, D. (1991). Neurophysiological correlates of hypnosis and dissociation. *Journal of Neuropsychiatry & Clinical Neurosciences, 3,* 440–445.

Spiegel, D., & Albert, L. (1983). Naloxone fails to reverse hypnotic alleviation of chronic pain. *Psychopharmacology, 81,* 140–143.

Spiegel, D., Bierre, P., & Rootenberg, J. (1989). Hypnotic alteration of somatosensory perception. *American Journal of Psychiatry, 146,* 749–754.

Spiegel, H., & Spiegel, D. (1978). *Trance and treatment: Clinical uses of hypnosis.* New York: Basic.

Stevens, J. (1962). Endogenous conditioning to abnormal cerebral electrical transients in man. *Science, 137,* 974–976.

Swinyard, E. A., Mijahara, J. T., Clark, L. D., & Goodman, L. S. (1963). The effect of experimentally-induced stress on pentylenetetrazol threshold in mice. *Psychopharmacologia, 4,* 343–353.

Williams, D. T. (1982). The treatment of seizures: Special psychotherapeutic and psychobiological techniques. In H. Sands (Ed.), *Epilepsy: A handbook for the mental health professional* (pp. 58–74). New York: Bruoner/Mazel.

Williams, D. T. (1988). Hypnosis. In C. J. Kestenbaum & D. T. Williams (Eds.), *Handbook of clinical assessment of children and adolescents* (Vol. 2, pp. 1129–1146). New York: New York University Press.

Williams, D. T. (1991). Hypnosis. In J. Wiener (Ed.), *Textbook of child and adolescent psychiatry* (pp. 627–636). Washington, DC: American Psychiatric Press.

Williams, D. T., Gold, A. P., Shrout, P., Shaffer, D., & Adams, D. (1979). The impact of psychiatric intervention on patients with uncontrolled seizures. *Journal of Nervous and Mental Disease, 167,* 626–631.

Williams, D. T., & Hirsch, G. (1988). The somatizing disorders: Somatoform disorders, factitious disorders and malingering. In C. J. Kestenbaum & D. T. Williams (Eds.), *Handbook of clinical assessment of children and adolescents* (Vol. II, pp. 743–768). New York: New York University Press.

Williams, D. T., & Mostofsky, D. (1982). Psychogenic seizures in childhood and adolescence. In T. Riley & A. Roy (Eds.), *Pseudoseizures* (pp. 169–184). Baltimore: Williams & Wilkins.

Williams D. T., Pleak, R., & Hanesian, H. (1991). Neurological disorders. In M. Lewis (Ed.), *Child and adolescent psychiatry: A comprehensive textbook* (pp. 629–645). Baltimore: Williams & Wilkins.

Williams, D. T., Spiegel, H., & Mostofsky, D. (1978). Neurogenic and hysterical seizures in children and adolescents. *American Journal of Psychiatry, 135*, 82–86.

Yudofsky, S. (1985). Malingering. In H. I. Kaplan & B. J. Sadock (Eds.), *Comprehensive textbook of psychiatry* (4th ed., Vol. 2, pp. 1862–1864). Baltimore: Williams & Wilkins.

5 Exercise and Epilepsy

Bjørn Ellertsen
University of Bergen, Norway

Hege R. Eriksen
Norwegian University of Sport and Physical Education, Oslo, Norway

David I. Mostofsky
Boston University

Holger Ursin
University of Bergen, Norway

PHYSICAL TRAINING AND EPILEPSY

Physical training plays an important role in modern society, both from a medical and psychosocial perspective. However, patients with a chronic disease like epilepsy often are excluded from participation for fear of high risk of injury. Although such excessive restrictions slowly are being lifted, the literature of the last decade is regretably characterized by frequent negative recommendations regarding physical activity for epileptics. Institutionalized epileptics are the most affected. In 1960, Lennox and Lennox wrote that these patients could be described in one word: *stagnant*. They are slow in movement, thinking, communication, and bowel movement. Possible causes indicated were the epileptic problem, side effects of pharmacologic treatment, general treatment policy, and lack of physical activity. The latter topic is the focus of this chapter.

We start this discussion of physical exercise and epilepsy by reviewing and discussing some of the relevant literature. Thereafter, some aspects of this complex and challenging field are illustrated with data from a recent study of medical, physiologic, psychosocial, and psychologic effects of systematic physical training of epileptics.

Lennox and Lennox (1960) maintained that activity inhibits seizures and that seizures often occur during inactivity, dozing, or sleep. However, reports on epilepsy and physical activity are contradictory. The relevant literature may be subdivided into three major categories: (a) general recommendations, (b) questionnaire surveys, and (c) empirical studies.

In general, most publications recommend that both children and adults with epilepsy should participate in physical activities (Gates, 1991; Linschoten, van Backx, Mulder, & Meinardi, 1990; Livingstone, 1971.) According to Livingstone (1971), children with epilepsy should be allowed to participate in physical activities on equal terms with their peers, provided that the seizures are controlled. In fact, the consequences of restrained physical activity may represent more serious problems than the possible negative consequences of seizures.

Important keywords are *overprotection, psychosocial problems, negative self-image, stigma* (American Academy of Pediatrics, 1983; Freeman, 1985; Livingstone 1971), *anxiety/frustrations* (Gates, 1991), and *lack of positive physiological effects from physical activity* (Linschoten et al., 1990). Recommendations often have been made on the basis of clinical experience and anecdotal data. Mendell (1984) stated that seizures seldom seem to occur in connection with physical activity, and that available research is sparse. However, the literature is characterized by reservations and rules of caution regarding participation in physical activities, despite that few methodologically sound empirical studies are available. The American Medical Association Committee on Medical Aspects of Sports (1968, 1974, 1976) published differing points of view regarding participation in collision (e.g., rugby, American football, hockey) and contact (e.g., handball, basketball) sports regarding epileptics. Their guidelines both prohibited and recommended such participation. The American Academy of Pediatrics (1968) stated that epileptics should avoid participation in activities where the person may fall and hurt him or herself. This view was supported by The Committee on Children with Handicaps of the American Academy of Pediatrics (1983), who maintained that physical activity should be prohibited in such connections. However, individual evaluations are recommended (Bower, 1969). Parachute jumping, mountain climbing, hang gliding (American Academy of Pediatrics, 1983; Spack, 1984), and riding (Livingstone, 1971) generally are not recommended, because even minor seizure may lead to major consequences.

Recommendations depend on the degree of seizure control in the individual patient. The American Medical Association Committee on the Medical Aspects of Sports (1976) stated that patients with intractable seizures should be excluded from collision, contact, and a number of other sports (swimming, cross-country skiing, volleyball, etc.). However, these recommendation were criticized strongly (Livingston, Pauli, & Pruce, 1978), and the recommendations later were revised. The American Academy of Pediatrics (1983) stated that satisfactory seizure control and adequate counseling is important in children participating in physical activities involving risk of damage. It is now generally accepted that persons with frequent seizures, causing falling and damage, should be restricted in their activites (Gates, 1991). However, some authors contradict even this point of view, with possible exceptions regarding diving and climbing (Mendell, 1984). Greensher (1985) stated that the risk of drowning is four times higher in epileptics, as compared with other children. However, professional athletes with a history of epilepsy are engaged in contact sports without any evidence of undesirable consequences.

It is not known to what extent physical training may improve seizure control. In 1978, the U.S. Department of Health, Education and Welfare's Commission for the Control of Epilepsy and Its Consequences stated that physical activity appears to play a role in seizure prevention (Bennett, 1989). This view was supposedly documented by data collected by the commission and testimony at regional hearings. However, no data supporting the conclusion were provided in this publication (Bennett, 1989).

Most publications in the second category—survey studies—reported a low degree of participation in physical activities among epileptics. Thus, Denio, Drake, and Pakalins (1989) and Albrecht (1988) reported that more than 50% of the patients questioned were physically inactive. Similar results were obtained in a comparable investigation made in Norway. The majority of patients reported low physical activity, whereas 23% participated in organized physical training (Bjørholt, Nakken, Røhme, & Hansen, 1990). Both the lack of training facilities and problems with transportation may have contributed to this (Williams, Roth, & Ruiz, 1991), as well as low motivation, reduced energy due to medication, fear of seizures/damage, and lack of qualified instructors (Bjørholt et al., 1990).

Few patients reported seizures in connection with physical training (Albrecht, 1988; Roth, Williams, Ruiz, Stewart, & Bachtler, 1991; Williams et al., 1991). However, they did report fear of having seizures during such activity (Bjørholt et al., 1990; Williams et al., 1991). It has been reported that regular physical activity does not seem to affect seizure control negatively (Nakken, Bjørholt, Johannessen, Loyning, & Lind, 1990; Roth et al., 1991). Denio et al. (1989) reported that patients who participated in physical activity had significantly fewer seizures than inactive patients. In addition, it has been reported that adult epileptics participating in such activities showed less emotional problems than inactive patients (Roth et al., 1991). With regard to empirical studies, there are few reports about positive or negative effects of physical training on patients with epilepsy. Key references regarding the effects of physical training on EEG and/or epileptic seizures are presented and categorized in Table 5.1. The table consists of 12 references covering about 600 patients. As can be seen from the table, the literature is characterized by retrospective surveys and empirical studies, with few subjects and varying short-lasting interventions.

Most available empirical data focus on abnormal EEG activity during or after physical activity. Increased epileptic EEG activity has been reported in patients exercising on an ergometer bicycle (Horyd, Gryziak, Niedzielska, & Zielinski,

TABLE 5.1
Effects of Training on EEG and/or Epileptic Seizures

				Training			*Seizures/EEG During and After Activity*	
Reference	*Design*	*No. of Participants/ Gender*	*Age*	*Frequency/ Duration*	*Intensity*	*Type*	*Seizures/EEG (Method)*	*Number of Seizures per Person*
Albrecht (1988)	Questionnaire	32♂ 10♀	12–72			Various	Five seizures during activity & one seizure after activity (R.R)	1
Denio et al. (1989)	Questionnaire	66	÷	÷	÷	Various	Trained < seizures than untrained (R.R)	÷
Esquivel et al. (1991)	Case Study Control group	7♀ 11♂	6–17	One session 15 min rest—15 min exercise—30 min recovery—3 min hyperventilation	Maximum workload 2 min	Cycle ergometer	↓ Absences D	
Götze et al. (1967)	Case study (hyperventilation)	30	Adolescents	One session	Exhaustion	Kneebend	↓ D/EEG ↓ A/EEG (EEG)	÷

Horyd et al. (1981)		43	Adolescents	One session	Moderate	Cycle ergometer	↓D/EEG 10 ↑A/EEG (EEG)	÷
Korczyn (1979)	Case R.R.	250	>10	÷	÷	Various	Five seizures during activity ♂ (R.R)	1–2
Kuijer (1978)			15–45	One session: 10 min. rest—work—20 min. recovery	Continuous work (exhaustion) intermittent work (HR < 150 b/min)	Cycle ergometer	↑A (EEG)	
Lishman et al. (1963)	Case R.R.	7♂	14–24	÷	÷	Locomotion	÷ (R.R)	Several
Nakken et al. (1990)	Pre–post (no control)	11♂ 10♀	18–39	3–5/days at 45 min. 6 weeks	60% of $\dot{V}O_{2max}$	Div.	Nonsignificant changes six seizures during activity (observed)	2–30%
Ogunyemi et al. (1988)	Case	3	7–21	One session at 7–27 min.	÷	Cycle ergometer	↑D/EEG (EEG)	÷
Roth et al. (1991)	Questionnaire	46♂ 75♀	18–77	÷	÷	÷	No difference (R.R)	÷
Simpson et al. (1989)	Case R.R	3	Adults			Jogging	↑A/seizures (R.R)	÷

÷ = not reported; R.R. = retrospective report about seizures during training; ↑D = increased seizure/EEG activity during physical exercise; ↑A = increased seizure/EEG activity after physical exercise; ↓D = decreased seizure/EEG activity during physical exercise; ↓A = decreased seizure/EEG activity after physical exercise; ♂ = male; ♀ = female.

1981; Ogunyemi, Gomez, & Klass, 1988). There are also a few reports on seizures induced by physical activity (French & Frengley, 1983; Lishman, Symonds, Whitty, & Willison, 1963; Ogunyemi et al., 1988). However, Kuijer (1978) reported a reduction in the number of seizures during physical activity. Reduced abnormal EEG activity also has been reported following physical activity (Berney, Osselton, Kolvin, & og Day, 1981; Götze, Kubicki, Munter, & Teichman, 1967; Horyd, Gryziak, Niedzielska, & Zielinski, 1981), whereas Kuijer (1978), Horyd et al. (1981), and Simpson and Grossman (1989) reported opposite findings. Kuijer (1978) also showed that degree of EEG pathology was unrelated to type of epilepsy or medication, and that the interindividual variance was considerable. Furthermore, Kuijer (1978) recorded a greater increase in the number of seizures following continuous exercise, as compared with intermittant exercise. A relationship between plasma pH and seizures also was noted with low pH following exercise or during resting periods, and being correlated with increased epileptic activity. Nakken et al. (1990) did not find any significant differences in seizure frequency before, during, or after a training period of 4 weeks. Again, considerable individual variation was noted. Seizures typically would occur during resting periods after training. They reported that 6 out of 21 patients had seizures in connection with training. Seizures were found to be unrelated to diagnosis, type of training activity, or heart rate. In comparison, Korczyn (1979) reported that 5 out of 250 patients had seizures in connection with physical training. In a study of 500 young epileptics participating in physical activities, Bianchi Saus (1981) reported no increase in seizure activity during activity and no increase in the total number of seizures in the group.

PHYSICAL TRAINING AND SEIZURES

Why should physical activity affect abnormal EEG activity and/or seizure frequency in epileptics? Several hypotheses have been offered in the literature. Swanson, Stavney, and Plum (1958) found that acute changes in serum pH in cats would affect the EEG only when these changes were followed by a change in partial CO_2 pressure (P_{CO_2}). Cerebral neuron excitability is unaffected by changes in arterial pH, unless variations in arterial P_{CO_2} occur at the same time (Millichap, 1956). Götze et al. (1967) suggested that reduced epileptic EEG activity during training may be caused by an increase in the gamma-aminobutyric acid (GABA) concentration as a consequence of metabolic acidosis. This view is supported by those who have suggested that acidosis may prevent seizures (Millichap, Jones, & Rudis, 1964), and that alkalosis may precipitate seizures (Aird, 1983). However, Kuijer (1978) did not find any relationship between low pH (acidosis) and increased epileptogenic EEG activity.

Hyperventilation generally is regarded as a seizure precipitating factor, primarily due to reduced P_{CO_2} and increased pH (Bülow et al., 1989). Reduced P_{CO_2}

causes reduced cerebral blood flow (Fazekas, McHenry, & Alman, 1961; Raichle, Bosner, & Plum, 1970). Kuijer (1978) did not find any correlation between P_{CO_2} and epileptic activity, whereas others have maintained that hypoxia secondary to hyperventilation, and decreased P_{CO_2}, can lead to epileptic phenomena and EEG changes (Aird, 1983). In short, findings and hypotheses are contradictory. Reduced calcium and magnesium in serum also has been discussed in connection with changes in EEG activity and seizure activity during physical activity (Lishman et al., 1963). Again, data are too sparse to allow any conclusions. A more detailed discussion of the role of breathing and respiration in the control of seizures is presented by Fried in this volume (chapter 2).

PHYSICAL TRAINING

It is generally accepted that physical activity is beneficial for general health. However, no consensus has been reached regarding types of activity, intensity, frequency, duration of training sessions, or number of years with regular training needed to obtain optimal health effects (Bouchard, 1990). Physical activity contributes to positive changes in lifestyle (Shepard, 1990), and level of physical activity is correlated positively with positive moods, general well-being, and reduction in symptoms of anxiety and depression (Morgan, 1985). These relationships seem stronger in females and in people younger than 40 years (Stephens, 1988). Maximum oxygen uptake ($\dot{V}o_{2max}$) is frequently used as a measure of physical fitness and a predictor of capacity for continuous performance. Thus, most training programs aiming at improved continuous performance are designed to improve $\dot{V}o_{2max}$. This is also the case in studies on aerobic training. Recording of heart rate frequently has been used as an indicator of training intensity.

Physical training has well-documented, positive effects on a number of physiologic variables (Åstrand & Rodahl, 1986; McArdle, Katch, & Katch, 1991), and aerobic training has been demonstrated to yield positive effects on cardiovascular fitness. Among these are decreased resting heart rate, increased stroke volume and reduced blood pressure in patients with hypertension, and positive changes in plasmalipids and lipoproteins (Bouchard, 1990). There also is increased capillarization in trained muscles (Saltin & Gollnick, 1983).

Aerobic training is an activity that meets the criteria set forward by American College of Sports Medicine (1978) to obtain cardiovascular fitness (Foster, 1975; Rockefeller & Burke, 1979; Vaccaro & Clinton, 1981). Differences in training procedures make comparisons between studies problematic, but the general findings reported are increases of $\dot{V}o_{2max}$ varying between 5%–40% (Williford, Scharff, & Blessing, 1989). Stress hormones (e.g., Cortisol, Prolactine, Growth Hormone; Shangold, 1988) and cathecholamines (Dienstbier, 1989; Richter, 1988) have been reported to increase during physical training, but these responses decrease as a function of repeated training (Green, 1990). Further, baseline concentrations of Norepinephrine and Cortisol are lower in trained as compared with inactive persons during submaximal work load (Green, 1990), where Epinephrine responses are more pronounced during maximum and supramaximal work load (Richter 1988), leading to more pronounced vasodilation.

Neuroendocrine properties have been proposed as permitting endurance levels of higher exertion for longer periods of time. Changes in Betaendorphin, Epinephrine, and Serotonin levels associated with vigorous exercise also may differ for Type A individuals (McMurray, Hardy, Roberts, Forsythe, & Mar, 1989). Exercise is associated with a sensation of well-being; this often-reported finding is supported by psychometric and neurophysiologic data. Although exercise may reduce anxiety and other stress reactions because of its property of distraction, there are equally strong alternative hypotheses attributable to monoamine metabolism and/or endorphin release (Morgan, 1985). Endorphins that result from physical activity might function as anticonvulsants (as was shown in some animal experiments). This theory was proposed following a rather large project in clinical psychoneuroendocrinology conducted in New Zealand (Albrecht, 1986).

A number of investigations have demonstrated improved general well-being and reduced subjective anxiety and depression following training (Folkins & Sime, 1981; Simons, Epstein, McGowan, Kupfer, & Robertson, 1985). Other effects reported are improved mood and self-confidence (Biddle & Mutrie, 1991). Martinsen, Medhus, and Sandvik (1985) demonstrated decreased depression scores after 6–9 weeks of aerobic training, 3 hours per week. Steptoe, Moses, Mathews, and Edwards (1990) compared aerobic and strength training and found that aerobic training reduced tension and anxiety more effectively than strength training. Folkins, Lynch, and Gardner, (1972) found positive correlations between physical fitness and psychologic well-being in a group of students. This effect was strongest in females. These findings were supported by a recent study by Grønningsæter, Hytten, Skauli, Christensen, and Ursin (1992), who found improved well-being in a group of insurance company employees after a period of aerobic training, again with the strongest effect in females.

In summary, physical training is beneficial for cardiovascular functions and general health. Psychosocial factors also are influenced positively. These are also factors known to affect epileptic seizure activity. Although improved physical fitness only may influence seizure frequency directly or indirectly to a limited extent, if only for the beneficial effects of improved physical fitness, it is an important objective to be pursued to benefit epileptics, perhaps even more important than providing for physical fitness for the general population.

AN EMPIRICAL STUDY

To illustrate some of the topics discussed, we present some data from an empirical study of effects of aerobic training on epileptic seizures. An aerobic training program was offered to 15 female epileptics recruited from a group of 140 female patients. Mean age was 32 years (range 18–46). Inclusion criteria were at least one epileptic seizure per month during a baseline period. Mean duration of epilepsy in the group was 22 years (range 6–37). All participants were on optimal dosages of antiepileptic medication throughout the study. The aerobic training program consisted of two sessions per week, each lasting 60 minutes, for 15 weeks.

As can be seen from Fig. 5.1, each training session consisted of warming up, stretching, training of strength, and, finally, relaxation. Training was adapted individually on the basis of baseline fitness measures, and the goal was to obtain aerobic fitness improvement in all subjects. An experimental ABA design was adhered to (i.e., subjects served as their own controls). Seizures were recorded during a baseline period of 30 weeks before start of training, during 15 weeks of training, and during a follow-up period of 15 weeks.

A number of physiologic and psychologic tests and measures were administered at the beginning of the training period, immediately following the training period, and at the end of the follow-up period. Among these were $\dot{V}o_2max$, measured with an oxygen analyzer when running on a motor driven treadmill (Versteig & Kippersluis, 1989), and continuous heart rate measurement. Blood pressure recording and blood sampling for analysis of immunoglobulines, hormones, cholesterol, and electrolytes also was included.

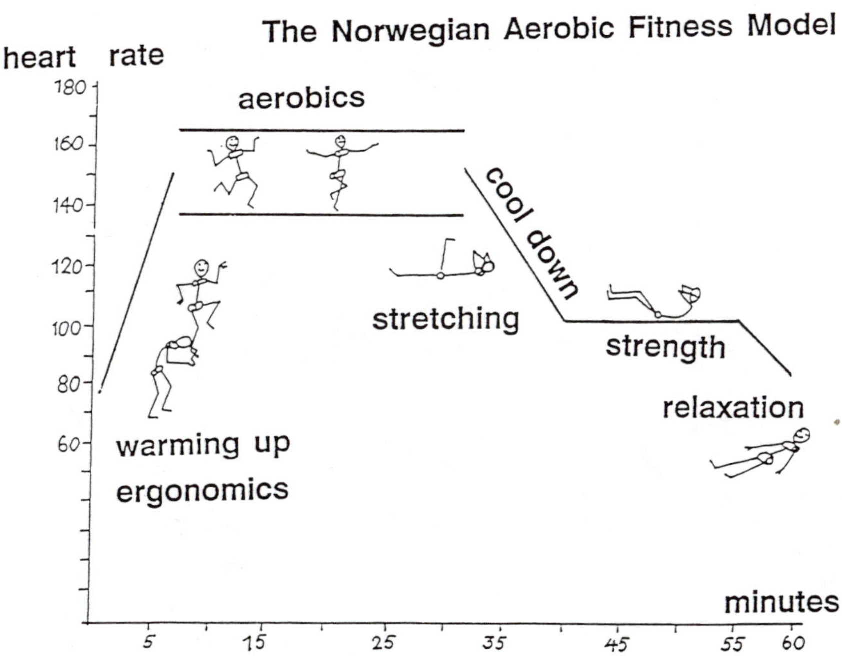

FIG. 5.1. The Norwegian Aerobic Fitness Model (Bø & Kamhaug, 1989).

The Washington Psychosocial Seizure Inventory (WPSI) (Dodrill, Batzel, Queisser, & Temkin, 1980) was administered before and after the training period, and at follow-up. WPSI is an inventory that was developed to evaluate psychologic, vocational, social, and medical problems often encountered in groups of patients with epilepsy. In addition, the Spielberger Strait-Trait Anxiety Inventory (STAI; Spielberger, Gorsuch, & Lushene, 1970), Beck's Depression Inventory (BDI; Beck, 1967), and Ursin Health Inventory (Ursin, Endresen, & Ursin, 1988) were administered. The latter questionnaire consists of 28 items concerning somatic and psychological problems. Both degree and duration of problems are evaluated in the questionnaire, yielding a sumscore index indicating degree of health problems.

Compliance was relatively high in the group (75.4%), given 30 sessions and in light of epileptic patients notoriously facing practical problems with respect to transportation. In addition, the group consisted of patients with relatively frequent and medically intractable epileptic seizures, which at times prevented them from showing up. Data on seizures are presented in Fig. 5.2. As can be seen from the figure, the median number of seizures dropped from 2.9 during the baseline period to 1.7 during training. This reduction was statistically significant and also in agreement with verbal reports from a majority of the patients. In other words, the statistical finding reflects a change in seizure frequency for most patients (i.e., a general clinical improvement in the group).

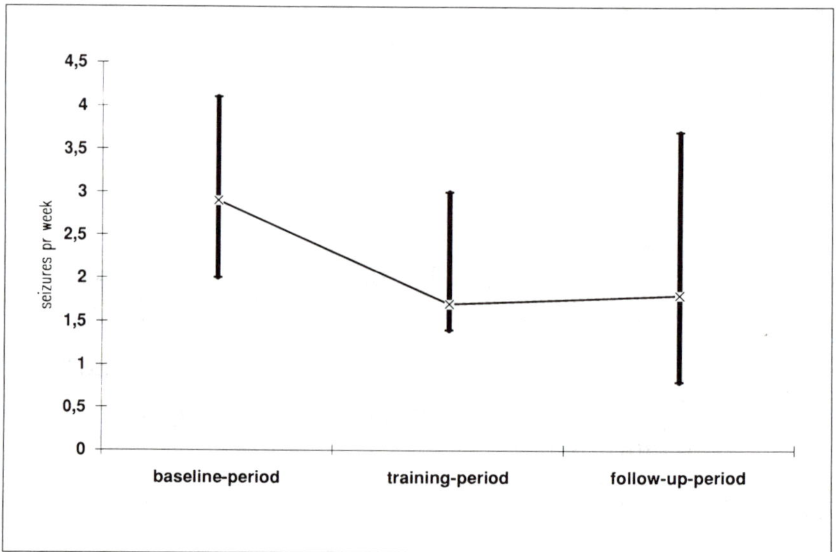

FIG. 5.2. Median and 95% confidence intervals for seizure frequency per week during baseline period (30 weeks), training period (15 weeks), and follow-up period (15 weeks).

A slight increase in median value and a considerably greater variation was observed at follow-up, as compared with the posttraining evaluation. Mean reduction in the number of seizures was 20.6%, varying between a decrease of 64.8% and an increase of 19.6% on an individual level. A significant positive correlation was found between seizure reduction and $\dot{V}o_{2max}$ during baseline ($r = .55$, $p < .05$), and a significant negative correlation between compliance and change in number of seizures ($r = -.76, p < .02$) was found. Seven persons had 27 seizures in the training room during the 30 training sessions, whereas the remaining eight patients had no seizures during the aerobic training. Most seizures occurred during the aerobics or cool down (Fig. 5.1). A significant negative correlation was found between seizures during training and $\dot{V}o_{2max}$ during baseline ($r = -.54, p < .05$). Figure 5.3 shows the increase in $\dot{V}o_{2max}$ from pre- to posttest for those who had 60% or higher compliance.

Mean increase was 8% after 30 training sessions, and this change was statistically significant. No significant changes were observed in resting heart rate or blood pressure variables. Data from the WPSI are presented in Fig. 5.4. No significant changes were found on any single WPSI scale. However, the tendencies indicated by the figure were all in favorable directions.

No significant changes were observed on The Spielberger or Beck measures

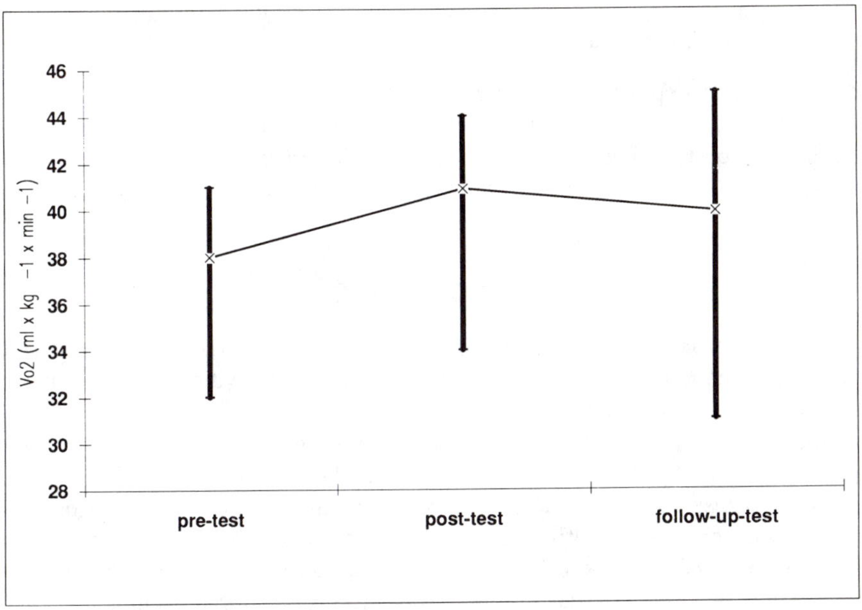

FIG. 5.3. Median and 95% confidence intervals for $\dot{V}o_{2max}$ (ml kg-1 min-1) during pretest, posttest (end of training period), and follow-up test (end of follow-up period).

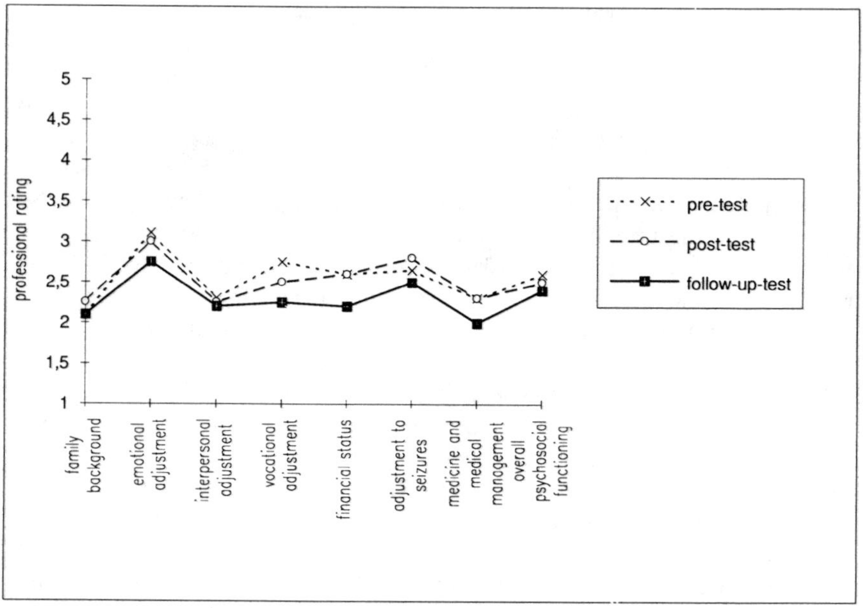

FIG. 5.4. Median scores on The Washington Psychosocial Seizure Inventory (WPSI) during pretest, posttest (end of training period), and follow-up test (end of follow-up period).

of signs and symptoms of anxiety and depression. The overall Ursin Health Inventory Index (intensity × duration) showed a significant reduction from prebaseline to posttraining. A muscle pain subindex (neck, shoulders, arms, and back) also showed a significant reduction, and this effect was maintained at follow-up testing.

CONCLUSIONS

The literature on physical training and epilepsy is characterized by reservations and rules of caution regarding participation in physical activities. However, these reservations are based on limited systematic survey data as well as limited and methodologically weak empirical evidence. The study on aerobic training on patients with partly intractable seizures presented earlier demonstrated improved physical fitness and a decreased number of seizures (without any deterious effects), as observed over a 30-week period. The positive effect on seizures seemed to be in regression at the end of the follow-up period, thus strengthening the conclusion that the physical training was responsible for the clinical effects observed. Subjectively reported health problems also were found to be decreased, whereas a tendency toward improved psychosocial functioning was indicated by the WPSI.

In conclusion, physical training represented no danger and yielded a number of positive effects in the group, including a reduction in overall number of seizures. Physical training, like the aerobic training program presented, can be recommended safely for patients with epilepsy.

REFERENCES

Aird, R. B. (1983). The importance of seizure inducing factors in the control of refractory forms of epilepsy. *Epilepsia, 24,* 567–583.

Albrecht, H. (1986). Endorphins, sport, and epilepsy: Getting fit or having one. *New Zealand Medical Journal, 99,* 915.

Albrecht, H. (1988). Physical activity, mental health and epilepsy. *The New Zealand Journal of Sports Medicine, 101,* 14–15.

American Academy of Pediatrics. Committee on Children with Handicaps and Committee on Sports Medicine. (1968). The epileptic child and competitive school athletics. *Pediatrics, 42*(4), 700–702.

American Academy of Pediatrics. Committee on Children with Handicaps and Committee on Sports Medicine. (1983). Sports and the child with epilepsy. *Pediatrics, 72*(6), 884–885.

American College of Sports Medicine. (1978). Position stand on the recommended quantity and quality of exercise for developing and maintaining fitness in healthy adults. *Medicine and Science in Sports and Exercise, 10,* vii–x.

American Medical Association Committee on Medical Aspects of Sports and the Committee on Exercise and Physical Fitness. (1968). Convulsive disorders and participation in sports and physical education. *Journal of American Medical Association, 206*(6), 1291.

American Medical Association Committee on Medical Aspects of Sports. (1974). Epileptics and contact sports. *Journal of American Medical Association, 220,* 820–821.

American Medical Association Committee on Medical Aspects of Sports of the American Medical Association. (1976). *Medical evaluation of the athlete: A guide.* Washington, DC: Author.

Åstrand, P. O., & Rodahl, K. (1986). *Textbook of work physiology, physiological bases of exercise* (3rd ed). Singapore: McGraw-Hill.

Beck, A. T. (1967). *Depression: clinical, experimental and theoretical aspects.* New York: Hober.

Bennett, D. R. (1989). Epilepsy and the athlete. In B. D. Jordan, P. Tsairus, & R. F. Warren (Eds.), *Sports neurology* (pp. 116–126). Rockville: Aspen Publishers.

Berney, T. P., Osselton, J. W., Kolvin, I., & og Day, M. J. (1981). Effects of discoteque environment on epileptic children. *British Medical Journal, 282,* 180–182.

Bianchi Saus, A. (1981). Riesgos provocados por la epilepsia. Deportes [Abstract: The risks of sports in epilepsy]. *Revista Neurologica Argentina, 7*(1), 31–37.

Biddle, S., & Mutrie, N. (Eds.). (1991). *Psychology of physical activity and exercise, a health related perspective.* Heidelberg: Springer Verlag.

Bjørholt, P. G., Nakken, K. O., Røhme, K., & Hansen, H. (1990). Leisure time habits and physical fitness in adults with epilepsy. *Epilepsia, 31,* 83–87.

Bø, K., & Kamhaug, E. L. (1989). *Gymnastikk i tiden.* Oslo, Norwegian University Press.

Bouchard, C. (1990). The consensus statement. In C. Bouchard, R. J. Shepard, T. Stephens, J. R. Sutton, & B. D. McPherson (Eds.), *Exercise, fitness and health. A consensus of current knowledge* (pp. 497–510). Champaign, IL: Human Kinetics Books.

Bower, B. D. (1969). Epilepsy and school athletics. *Developmental Medicine and Child Neurology, 2,* 244–245.

Bülow, I. V., Elbert, T., Rockstroh, B., Lutzenberger, W., Canavan, A., & Birbaumer, N. (1989). Effects of hyperventilation on EEG-frequency and slow cortical potentials in relation to an anticonvulsant and epilepsy. *Journal of Psychophysiology, 3,* 147–154.

Denio, L. S., Drake, M. E., & Pakalins, A. (1989). The effect of exercise on seizure frequency. *Journal of Medicine, 20*(2), 171–176.

Dienstbier, R. A. (1989). Arousal and physiological toughness: Implications for mental and physical health. *Psychological Review, 96*(1), 84–100.

Dodrill, C. B., Batzel, L. W., Queisser, H. R., & Temkin, N. R. (1980). An objective method for the assessment of psychological and social problems among epileptics. *Epilepsia, 21,* 123–135.

Esquivel, E. M., Chaussain, M., Plouin, P., Ponsot, G., & Arthuis, M. (1991). Physical exercise and voluntary hyperventilation in childhood absence epilepsy. *Electroencephalography and Clinical Neurophysiology, 79,* 127–132.

Fazekas, J. F., McHenry, L. C., & Alman, R. W. (1961). Cerebral hemodynamics during brief hyperventilation. *Arch. Neurology, 4,* 132–138.

Folkins, C. H., Lynch, S., & Gardner, M. M. (1972). Psychological fitness as a function of physical fitness. *Archives of Physical Medicine and Rehabilitation, 53,* 503–508.

Folkins, C. H., & Sime, W. E. (1981). Physical fitness training and mental health. *American Psychologist, 36,* 373–389.

Foster, C. (1975). Physiological requirements of aerobic dancing. *Research Quarterly, 46,* 120–122.

Freeman, J. M. (1985). Epilepsy and swimming [Letter to the editor]. *Pediatrics, 76*(1), 139.

French, J. K., & Frengley, P. A. (1983). Hypoglycemia induced seizures following a marathon [Letter to the editor]. *New Zealand Medical Journal, 96,* 407.

Gates, J. R. (1991). Epilepsy and sports participation. *The Physician and Sportsmedicine, 19*(3), 98–104.

Green, J. H. (1990). *The autonomic nervous system and exercise.* London: Chapman & Hall.

Greensher, J. (1985). Epilepsy and swimming [Letter to the editor]. *Pediatrics, 76*(1), 139.

Götze, W., Kubicki, S. T., Munter, M., & Teichman, J. (1967). Effect of physical exercise on seizure threshold. *Journal of Nervous System, 28*(10), 664–667.

Grønningsæter, H., Hytten, K., Skauli, G., Christensen, C. C., & Ursin, H. (1992). *Improved health and coping by physical exercise or cognitive behavioral stress management training in a work environment.* Manuscript submitted for publication.

Horyd, W., Gryziak, J., Niedzielska, K., & Zielinski, J. J. (1981). Exercise effect on seizure discharge in epileptics. *Neurologia Neurochirurgia Polska, 15,* 545–552.

Korczyn, A. D. (1979). Participation of epileptic patients in sports. *Journal of Sport Medicine, 19,* 195–198.

Kuijer, A. (1978). *Epilepsy and exercise—an investigation into some physiological effects of exercise in people with epilepsy: Electroencephalographic and biochemical studies.* Academisch proefschrift, Universiteit van Amsterdam.

Lennox, W. G., & Lennox, M. A. (1960). *Epilepsy and related disorders.* Boston: Little, Brown.

Linschoten, R., van Backx, F. J. G., Mulder, O. G. M., & Meinardi, H. (1990). Epilepsy and sport. *Sports Medicine, 10*(1), 9–19.

Lishman, W. A., Symonds, C. P., Whitty, C. W. M., & Willison, R. G. (1963). Seizure induced by movement. *Brain, 86,* 93–108.

Livingstone, S. (1971). Should physical activity of the epileptic child be restricted? *Clinical Pediatrics, 10*(12), 694–696.

Livingstone, S., Pauli, L., & Pruce, I. (1978). Epilepsy and sports [Letter to the editor]. *Journal of American Medical Association, 239*(1), 22.

Martinsen, E. W., Medhus, A., & Sandvik, L. (1985). Effects of aerobic exercise on depression: A controlled study. *British Medical Journal, 291,* 109.

McArdle, W. D., Katch, F. I., & Katch, V. L. (1991). *Exercise physiology, energy, nutrition, and human performance* (3rd ed). Philadelphia: Lea & Febiger.

McMurray, R. G., Hardy, C. J., Roberts, S., Forsythe, W. A., & Mar, M. H. (1989). Neuroendocrine responses of Type-A individuals to exercise. *Behavioral Medicine,15*(2), 84–92.

Mendell, J. R. (1984). The nervous system. In R. H. Strauss & W. B. Saunders (Eds.), *Sports medicine* (pp. 149–174). Philadelphia: Saunders.

Morgan, W. P. (1985). Affective beneficence of vigorous physical activity. *Medicine and Science in Sports and Exercise, 17,* 94–100.

Millichap, J. G. (1956). Anticonvulsant action of diamox in children. *Neurology, 6,* 552–559.

Millichap, J. G., Jones, J. D., & Rudis, B. P. (1964). Mechanism of anticonvulsant action of ketogenic diet. *American Journal of Disabled Children, 107,* 593–604.

Nakken, K. O., Bjørholt, P. G., Johannessen, S. I., Løyning, T., & Lind, E. (1990). Effect of physical training on aerobic capacity, seizure occurrence, and serum level of antiepileptic drugs in adults with epilepsy. *Epilepsia, 31*(1), 88–94.

Ogunyemi, A. O., Gomez, M. R., & Klass, D. K. (1988). Seizures induced by exercise. *Neurology, 38,* 633–634.

Raichle, M. E., Bosner, J. B., & Plum, F. (1970). Cerebral bloodflow during and after hyperventilation. *Arch. Neurology, 23,* 394–403.

Richter, E. A. (1988). Hormonal adaptions to exercise training. In R. S. Williams & A. G. Wallace (Eds.), *Biological effects of physical activity* (pp. 25–44). Champaign, IL: Human Kinetic Books.

Rockefeller, K. A., & Burke, E. J. (1979). Psycho-physiological analysis of an aerobic dance programme for women. *British Journal of Sports Medicine, 13,* 77–80.

Roth, D. L., Williams, V. L., Ruiz, L. L., Stewart, K. E., & Bachtler, S. E. (1991, August). *Physical exercise and emotional distress in adults with epilepsy.* Poster presented at the Annual Meeting of the American Psychological Association, San Francisco.

Saltin, B., & Gollnick, P. D. (1983). Skeletal muscle adaptability: Significance for metabolism and performance. In L. D. Peachey, R. H. Adrian, & S. R. Geiger (Eds.), *Handbook of Physiology, Section 10: Skeletal muscle* (pp. 555–631). Baltimore, MD: Waverly Press.

Shangold, M. (1988). Menstruation. In M. Shangold & G. Mirkin, (Eds.), *Women and exercise physiology and sports medicine* (pp. 129–142). Philadelphia: F. A. Davis.

Shepard, R. J. (1990). Costs and benefits of an exercising versus a nonexercising society. In C. Bouchard, R. J. Shepard, T. Stephens, J. R. Sutton, & B. D. McPherson (Eds.), *Exercise, fitness and health. A consensus of current knowledge* (pp. 49–60). Champaign, IL: Human Kinetics Books.

Simons, A. D., Epstein, L. H., McGowan, C. R., Kupfer, D. J., & Robertson, R. J. (1985). Exercise as treatment for depression: An update. *Clinical Psychology Review, 5,* 553–568.

Simpson, R. K., & Grossman, R. G. (1989). Seizures after jogging [Letter to the editor]. *The New England Journal of Medicine, 321*(12), 835.

Spack, N. P. (1984). Medical problems of the exercising child: asthma, diabetes, and epilepsy. In L. J. Micheli (Ed.), *Pediatric and adolescent sports medicine* (pp. 124–133). Boston: Little, Brown.

Spielberger, C. D., Gorsuch, R. L., & Lushene, R. (1970). *STAI manual for the state-trait anxiety inventory.* Palo Alto, CA: Consulting Psychologists Press.

Stephens, R. (1988). Physical exercise and mental health in the United States and Canada: Evidence from four populations surveys. *Preventive Medicine, 17,* 35–47.

Steptoe, A., Moses, J., Mathews, A., & Edwards, S. (1990). Aerobic fitness, physical activity, and psychophysiological reactions to mental tasks. *Psychophysiology, 27*(3), 264–274.

Swanson, A. G., Stavney, L. S., & Plum, F. (1958). Effects of blood pH and carbon dioxide on cerebral electrical activity. *Neurology, 8,* 787–792.

Ursin, H., Endresen, I. M., & Ursin, G. (1988). Psychological factors and self-reports of muscle pain. *European Journal of Applied Physiology, 57,* 282–290.

Versteig, P. G. A., & Kippersluis, G. J. (1989). Automated system of measurement of oxygen uptake during exercise testing. *International Journal of Sport and Medicine. 10*(2), 107–112.

Vaccaro, P., & Clinton, M. (1981). The effects of aerobic dance conditioning on the body composition and maximal oxygen uptake of college women. *Journal of Sports Medicine, 21,* 291–294.

Williams, V. L., Roth, D. L., & Ruiz, L. L. (1991, August). *Barriers to exercise in adults with epilepsy.* Poster presented at the annual meeting of the American Psychological Association, San Francisco.

Williford, H. N., Scharff-Olson, M., & Blessing, D. L. (1989). The physiological effects of aerobic dance. *Sports Medicine, 8*(6), 335–345.

6 Nutrition, Nutrients, and Epilepsy

Shlomo Yehuda
Bar-Ilan University, Israel

Epilepsy is a disorder that undeniably is associated with abnormal activity in the brain. An understanding of the basic anatomical, physiological, and behavioral mechanism(s) that control and influence normal brain activity is essential for an understanding of abnormal phenomena and for the development of treatment protocols that may be introduced to provide an alternative to conventional anticonvulsant medications. This chapter's aim is to review some of the findings and issues that can shed light on one of these basic mechanisms, namely, the effects of nutrients on brain biochemistry. In some instances, exaggerated claims have been made in behalf of various forms of nutritional therapies, which appear to be patently wrong. For example, the claims that diet or herbal therapy offers an effective alternative to conventional anticonvulsant therapy (e.g., the use of Datura Stramonium or Heracleum Lantum), as proposed by Lewis and Elbin-Lewis (1977), have no medical evidence to support the assertion that such therapy is useful. However, the field of nutrition offers some attractive possibilities for understanding the processes that underlie epilepsy and that may suggest reasonable directions for designing effective therapeutic protocols. This chapter briefly reviews the role of nutrients in brain biochemistry and its consequences in behavior, as seen from the perspective of the relationships among nutrition, nutrients, and epilepsy.

NUTRITION

Light and food seem to be two of the most important environmental factors that influence the health, physiology, and behavior of most vertebrates (Wurtman, Baum, & Potts, 1985; Wurtman, 1975, 1982). Although it is easy to agree with this statement, it is difficult to prove it. The relationship among nutrition, nutrients, and behavior is very complex, yet, because of the considerable interest in this field, there are many examples of unscientific (sometimes even dangerous) claims concerning the beneficial effects of certain nutrients on health and behavior. In its place, this chapter attempts to provide a realistic assessment of the status of nutritional variables that can more reasonably be expected to extend our appreciation of the link to seizure disorders.

One experimental approach to understanding the effects of nutrients is to study malnutrition, in general, and during critical phases, more specifically (such as during the prenatal and lactating periods); and to observe any resulting effects that it may exert on behavior (Brozek, 1978). Most studies of this genre have examined the effects of protein malnutrition on brain growth and morphology (e.g., Dhopeshwarker, 1983; Morgane et al., 1978; Shoemaker & Bloom, 1977; Shoemaker & Wurtman, 1971) and brain biochemistry, for example, the development of catecholamine (Shoemaker & Bloom, 1977; Wiggins, Fuller, & Enna, 1984). Other studies on lipid undernutrition have shown that it can modify significantly the brain growth and development of children and may even have long-term effects on adult behavior as well (Dhopeshwarker, 1983; Gossi et al., 1982; Lampety & Walker, 1976, 1978). Still other studies have examined dietary deficiencies in many compounds, such as niacin, folacin, thiamine, vitamin B6, magnesium, zinc, copper, and so forth, and have established that they are associated with poor learning and memory (Hamilton, Whitney, & Sizer, 1985).

On the other hand, the presence of a certain nutrient also may change behavior. For example, grain glutens have been considered major agents that evoke schizophrenia in certain genotypes (Dohan, Harper, Clark, Rodrique, & Zigas, 1984). Caffeine may improve attentional deficit disorders (Dalby, 1985), and monosodium glutamate may induce the "Chinese restaurant syndrome" (Hamilton et al., 1985). In addition, diet also may influence mood (Letherwood & Pollitt, 1983). Moreover, although brief fasting, especially skipping breakfast, was found to have adverse effects on late morning problem-solving performance by children (Pollitt, Lewis, Garza & Shulman, 1983), it nonetheless had a beneficial effect on immediate recall and short-term memory (Pollitt, Leibel, & Greenfield, 1981). Fasting for 72 hours was shown to modify the rate of bar pressing for brain self-stimulation in cats, depending on the anatomical structure being stimulated (Angyan, 1984). An interesting relationship between nutrition and cognitive function was suggested by Abalan (1985), who proposed that malnutrition is one of the etiological factors in Alzheimer's disorder.

Therefore, the concluding evidence supports a nutritional link to affective and cognitive behaviors in general. Although it would not be warranted to suggest that nutritional factors play a role in the alteration of the basic affective and cognitive systems, it seems reasonable to expect that variations in the milieu will bring about modifications within the limits of the genetic (trait) disposition of the individual person. When the behavioral profile is complicated further by the presence of a seizure disorder, the role of nutrients may take on even greater importance, and may help us to better understand, and possibly control, some of the special features of the interictal behaviors among epileptics, as revealed by numerous psychometric findings.

BRAIN NEUROTRANSMITTER PRECURSORS

Wurtman's group was the first to suggest that dietary factors can influence central neurotransmitter functions (Fernstrom & Wurtman, 1971, 1972). They showed that, under certain conditions, dietary manipulation of tryptophan (the precursor of serotonin, which is able to penetrate the brain blood barrier) causes an increase in brain serotonin level. Similarly, a dietary manipulation of tyrosine leads to an increase in dopamine or norepinephrine, and choline or lecithin, to an increase in brain acetylcholine (Anderson, 1980; Benedict, Anderson, & Sole, 1983; Fernstrom, 1981; Sved, 1983; Wurtman, 1982; Wurtman & Wurtman, 1984). The ratio between the level of tryptophan and large neutral amino acids (TRY/LNAA) in the plasma is the key factor in brain tryptophan bioavailability. An increase in the bioavailability of tryptophan was correlated with an increase in serotonin level. An additional finding showed that a carbohydrate-rich breakfast caused an increase in the TRY/LNAA ratio, whereas a protein-rich breakfast caused a decrease in this ratio (Ashley, Liardon, & Letherwood, 1985). The implications of these investigations to the problem of epilepsy are discovered shortly.

Although many studies have shown an increase in the level of certain brain neurotransmitters after appropriate dietary manipulation, the question about the effects of dietary manipulation on the functional state of the neurons that use the neurotransmitter is still open. On the one hand, attempts were made to use dietary manipulations for treating certain neurological and psychiatric disorders such as L-Dopa in Parkinson's disorder, or the use of choline or lecithin in tardive dyskinesia, Huntington's disease, Alzheimer disorders, ataxia, Tourette syndrome, and myasthenia gravis. In purely psychiatric disorders, tryptophan treatment was suggested for the treatment of depression, posthypoxic intention myoclonus, and sleep disturbances. Tyrosine has been tested as an antidepressant (Conlay & Zeisel, 1982; Wurtman, Hefti, & Melamed, 1981; Zeisel, 1981) and a nutritional approach for the treatment of pain (Seltzer, Marcus, & Stock, 1981), and for use with autistic children (Martinau, Bathelemy, Garreau, & Lelord, 1985). Furthermore, a GABA-containing diet induced a decrease in food intake (Tews, Repa, Nguyen, & Harper, 1985). Because of the relationship of this neurochemistry to neuronal activity, it seems that this approach may lead to a better understanding of epilepsy mechanisms and treatments as well.

Most of the precursors are amino acids. Taurine has some inhibitory effects on the CNS, and epilepsy is largely attributable to lack of sufficient inhibitory control in discharging neuronal populations. Lower levels of taurine indeed were found in epileptic patients (Barbeau & Donaldson, 1973). Some investigations have pointed out that L-5-hydroxytryptophan (5-HTP) can reduce posthypoxic myoclonus (Van woert, Rosenbaum, Houieson, & Bowers, 1977). Although treatment with tryptophan has been suggested, it is not an accepted option among physicians and clinical neurologists. On the other hand, the mechanisms by which the precursors modify the functional role of the presumed-to-be damaged neurotransmitter system are not clear.

For example, Trulson (1985) recently claimed that dietary tryptophan caused an increase in brain-serotonin level, whereas the activity of single serotonergic cells in an awake cat was unchanged by the diet. He concluded that dietary manipulations do not modify the functional activity of the neurons. However, these conclusions may be somewhat suspect, because the cats in this study were treated for only 3 days, and other behaviors (e.g., sleep) were not recorded. The relative failure of lecithin treatment in Alzheimer's disorder, a disorder in which a decrease in brain acetylcholine level was recorded, is yet another issue. A possible explanation is that either lecithin does not penetrate into the human brain in large enough quantities to produce salutary effects, or that the decrease in acetylcholine level is not the only, or perhaps even major, factor in the dementia associated with Alzheimer's disorder.

A novel explanation of nonprecursor dietary manipulation on cognitive functions and behavior emerged from yet another series of experiments (Yehuda, 1987). In this program of research, it was suggested that the mode of action brought about by the dietary manipulation is not explained solely by the biochemistry of the neurotransmitter system, but also involved the lipid composition of the neuronal membrane. Support for the new hypothesis will be gathered from previously known studies. A brief description of some of these newer experiments may help to appreciate the argument being advanced. The part of the axon that is responsible for the normal transfer of neuronal impulses (neuronal messages) is the axon membrane. The physical properties of the membrane are of utmost importance for the successful initiation and conduction of neuronal impulses. In the case of epilepsy, which is a state of uncontrolled firing, it is reasonable to conclude that changes in the physical or biophysical properties of the membrane have been introduced, and the contribution of lipids is essential to the process.

NEURONAL MEMBRANE LIPIDS

In addition to the precursor model for nutritional effects (e.g., via synaptic events), another approach to explain the effects of dietary manipulation is to consider the possibility that nutrients act on the lipid composition of the neuronal membrane and on membrane fluidity. Singer and Nicolson's (1972) fluid mosaic model of the biological membrane, in which both proteins and lipids are mobile within the membrane, enhanced our understanding of the functional role of the membrane (Houslay & Stanley, 1982). The composition of lipids in the membrane is very important for the normal physiological role of the membrane, especially the function of the neuronal membranes in synaptic transmission and bioelectric responses (Podlubiuk & Kleinrok, 1976; Reiman, Steinhaur, Hedler, Starke, & Hertting, 1981; Vergrossen, 1972.) The functional role of various membrane receptors seems to be dependent on normal membrane lipid composition (Kirilovsky, Steiner-Mordoch, Selinger, & Schramm, 1985; Spector & Yorek, 1985). For example, phosphotidycholine, which is produced in rat synaptosomes, is very rich in polyunsaturated fatty acids (Tacconi & Wurtman, 1985). Membrane lipid composition may change the index of membrane fluidity. At the optimal index of membrane fluidity, the ionic exchange between the cell and the outside environment is at maximum efficiency. Treatment may modify the membrane lipid composition and its fluidity. For example, an increase in cholesterol level, causes a significant decrease in membrane fluidity (Houslay & Stanley, 1982).

There are two methods to modify membrane fluidity via changes in lipid composition. One is via drug treatment. Drugs such as general and local anesthetics, certain steroids, barbiturates, alcohol, and cannabinoids cause changes in membrane fluidity (Seeman, 1982; Zubenko & Cohen, 1985). Furthermore, psychotherapeutic drugs (e.g., antipsychotic and antidepressant) also can modify the membrane fluidity index (Seeman, 1977, 1982; Zubenko & Cohen, 1985). The second method that induces changes in the lipid composition is dietary manipulation (Clandinin, Field, Hargreaves, Morson, & Zsigmond, 1985; Wahle, 1983). Certain fatty acids (mainly linolenic acid) in the diet can decrease the cholesterol (Balasubramaniam, Simon, Charg, & Hickie, 1985). Furthermore, changes in certain membrane-bound enzymes were found after lipid diet manipulation (Foot, Cruz, & Clandinin, 1983; Heger, 1979). The possibility that changes in membrane fluidity are associated with epilepsy is discussed later. The role of membrane lipid composition seems to be age-dependent, and many studies show changes in lipid composition during aging, mainly as an increase in cholesterol level (Carlile & Andras, 1985; Clandinin, Field, Hargreaves, Morson, & Zsigmond, 1985; Cohen & Zubenko, 1985; Routtenberg, 1987; Suzuki, Kobayasti, Mayakaw, & Wada, 1985b; Tappel et al., 1973). These changes may be correlated with the cognitive and behavioral changes that are observed in aging. A soybean oil diet (10%) taken for 1 month prevents the increase of plasma cholesterol level in aging rats (Suzuki, Hayakawa, Tamara, Wada, & Wada, 1985a).

LEARNING, CHOLESTEROL LEVEL, AND MEMBRANE FLUIDITY

The level of cholesterol in the neuronal membrane is one of the major factors in determining the fluidity index (Houslay & Stanley, 1982). Because cholesterol is unable to cross the brain capillaries into the brain (Dhopeshwarker, 1983), any change in cholesterol level in the neuronal membrane reflects neuronal activity in the central nervous system. An increased level of cholesterol in neuronal membrane is correlated with a decrease in the membrane fluidity index, and thereby damage to the normal physiological conduction of neuronal impulses. The specific contribution of such an insult in an epileptic patient has not been established yet, but, in the presence of poorly inhibited neurophysiological discharges, the state of the membrane structure is critical. There is no data to suggest that the management of cholesterol levels by dietary control can offer any relief in the seizure threshold, frequency, or severity to the patient with a seizure disorder.

The relationship between the level of cholesterol in the neuronal membrane and learning processes was examined recently. Instead of attempting to modify the level of cholesterol neuronal membrane level, the researchers asked the opposite question: Could learning, per se, induce changes in the level of cholesterol in neuronal membranes that are located in different regions of the brain (Kessler & Yehuda, 1985)? The changes in the level of cholesterol in different brain areas (cortex, hippocampus, hypothalamus, and brainstem) were examined in rats trained in a Y-maze. A second group of rats also was trained in a reversal learning paradigm. The results showed that one-stage learning is enough to modify the cholesterol level in preparations obtained from the hippocampus. The decrease in cholesterol level was associated with a decrease in the microviscosity index (i.e., the membrane is more fluid) in the hippocampus and the cortex. Reversal learning induced an even lower cholesterol level in the hippocampus and the cortex, as well as a parallel increase in the membrane fluidity in both brain areas. The results of these preliminary studies indicate that learning is able to induce significant changes in cholesterol level and in membrane fluidity, and therefore leads to a functional change in the neuronal membrane activity. An additional conclusion is implied—namely that the hippocampus probably is involved in mediating this type of learning. The hippocampus seems to be involved in long-term memory formations of several types of learning (e.g., in spatial learning, classical conditioning, and delay alternation tasks) (Bloom, Luzerson, & Hofstadter, 1985; Knowlton, McGowan, & Olton, 1985; Olton, Becker, & Hardelman, 1979; Wincour, 1985).

The example of the relationships between nutritional factors and learning is enlightening from several points of view. It demonstrates the possibility of utilizing dietary manipulation for bringing about changes in the brain plasma membrane composition and its associated function(s). Second, it opens the door to new approaches to antiepileptic drugs. It would be interesting to discover whether antiepileptic drugs have an effect on the neuronal membrane, and to assess cognitive functions immediately after an epileptic seizure.

CLASSICAL NEUROTRANSMITTERS

The role of benzodiazepines in epilepsy and the control of epilepsy is well known. Several attempts have been undertaken to elucidate the role of classical neurotransmitters in epilepsy. For example, Jones (1986) reviewed the role of neurotransmitters in the cerebral cortex in relation to epilepsy. He reviewed the localization and functions of serotonin, noradrenaline, dopamine, and acetylcholine, with special attention given to GABA. One of his main conclusions was that it is very difficult to find a cause-and-effect relationship between the function of a specific neurotransmitter and epileptic activity. A possible approach that might enable one to identify a given neurotransmitter as responsible for epileptic activity would be to use a selective neurotoxin. Among the best known neurotoxins are the dopaminergic neurotoxins (e.g., 6-OH-DA), yet dopamine rarely is implicated in epilepsy. Several other neurotoxins, such as kainic acid, which is a specific acetylcholine neurotoxin, had been used as a tool to investigate the role of acetylcholine in experimental models of epilepsy (Ben-Ari, Repressa, Tremblay, & Nitecka, 1986; Fariello, Golden, Smith, & Reyes, 1989). The current status of classical neurotransmitters in epilepsy is that they may have some direct effect on epilepsy; if it could be proved that any one of them is at a very low level (such as with dopamine in Parkinson), then the possibility of supplying the neurotransmitter via a precursor using a diet would provide a logical and appealing proposal (Allen, Grieve, & Griffiths, 1986).

The situation regarding the excitatory amino acids is different. It seems that these compounds play a significant role in epilepsy and epilepsy management (Foster, 1986; Heinemann, 1986; Le Fauconnier & Kratzo, 1986; Meldrum, 1986). However, the mode of action of excitatory amino acids is different from the mode of action of classical neurotransmitters, which act on receptors. In contrast, the excitatory amino acids act on the ionic concentration of calcium, potassium, sodium, and chlorine at the extracellular space near the neurons. Neuronal information is communicated along the axon as an electrical wave, where the information of the electrical wave is totally dependent on the concentration of the ionic element inside and outside the neuronal membrane. Therefore, any change in the ionic concentration will result in major changes in the ability of the membrane to carry neuronal messages (whether to facilitate or to block). Indirect support for this concept is found in reports that changes in the ionic concentration do occur during epileptic episodes (Johnston, Rutecki, & Lebeda, 1986; Stahl & Harris, 1986). The importance of the ability of the membrane to carry neuronal signals is discussed shortly.

DEFICIENCIES

Several deficiencies in nutrients or enzymes have been implicated in epilepsy. Some of them can be corrected by diet, and some surely cannot. A few examples illustrate the problem.

A disorder of nonketonic hypoglycemia is one of the many inborn metabolic errors that result in epileptic seizures, and are difficult control from the first days of life. The lack of an enzyme that catalyzes the conversion of glycine to hydroxymethyltetrahydrotolic acid, carbon dioxide, and ammonia in the liner and the brain results in an increased level of glycine in the blood (Moura-Ribeiro, Ferlin, Gallina, & Funayama, 1987). Some anticonvulsants induce a decrease in the level of folate in the red cells, and dietary intake of folate is reduced significantly among epileptic patients (Goggin, et al., 1987). The importance of deficiencies was demonstrated by Ventura, Bouget, Sartorelli, Torre, and Tommasini (1991), who described two cases of focal epilepsy with cerebral calcifications that responded poorly to medical and pharmacological treatment. In both cases, it appeared that the patients suffered from colcliac disease, and a marked decrease in folic acid was found to confirm this diagnosis. A gluten-free diet, together with a supplement of folic acid, led to marked improvement both in behavioral and physiological variables. This, of course, does not represent the majority of epileptic cases. However, it is important to realize that such cases of epilepsy do occur, and that a rather simple program of treatment derived from a nutritional perspective offers a highly significant improvement in the clinical status, even when conventional pharmacy proved to be unsatisfactory.

Several authors have shown that a magnesium deficiency may result in epilepsy. The reason is not clear. It may be that the magnesium deficiency is responsible, although it is equally possible that the deficiency may affect the calcium level, which might be the active causal factor for the condition (Leaver, Parkinson, & Schneider, 1987; Mody, Lambert, & Heinemann, 1987). Nutritional supplements of zinc or glycine did not modify the low magnesium tendency for epilepsy (Hegstad, Langmoen, & Hablitz, 1989). Iron deposits in localized brain areas also may cause epileptic seizures (Campbell, Bank, & Milgram, 1984). This observation has been supported by direct application of iron into the brain, which has been used, for many years, as a method in experimental epilepsy to create an epileptic model in an otherwise normal animal (Cśernansky et al., 1983). The epileptic effect of iron excess in the brain can be explained by the neurotoxin effect of iron creating free radicals in the brain. More specifically, a possible explanation is that iron induces an increase in lipid peroxidation, which causes damage to the neurons. In addition, lipid peroxidation causes a decrease in GABA release, which in turn decreases the inhibitory effect of GABA (Zhang, Zuo, & Wu, 1989). A similar phenomenon among trace metals may be seen in a decrease in sodium ions and an increase of potassium ions in the extracellular space, which may result in epileptic seizures (Bradbury, 1979).

BLOOD-BRAIN BARRIER

A discussion on the structure of the blood-brain barrier (BBB) is beyond the scope of this chapter. Yet, many studies have shown that changes in the functional role of the BBB do occur during epileptic seizures. The importance of the BBB relationship to nutrition is obvious. Unless uptake of compounds (dietary or therapeutic) is assured rigorously, there will be no effect on brain physiology or function. Therefore, drugs targeted to influence brain functions will not cross the BBB. On the other hand, changes in the rate of penetration to the brain may bring into the brain substances that normally do not exist in the brain and that would cause damage. Rats that received radiation to an area of 0.25 cc. at one cerebral hemisphere are clinically and electroencephalogaphically normal until there is a breakdown of the BBB at 3–6 months postradiation. This BBB lesion can be detected by transplant focal seizure activity produced by the BBB-excluded systemic convulsant biccuculine metaiodide (Remler & Marcussen, 1986). Changes in the BBB during and after epileptic activity has been demonstrated by various techniques, such as horseradish peroxidase (Bowling, 1988). Age-related changes in BBB permeability to macromolecules were investigated during seizures induced by metrazol in rats whose ages ranged from 6 to 120 days. Evans blue was used as a visual indicator of BBB integrity. Marked changes between young and old rats were found in the effect of metrazol on penetration of the BBB to different brain areas (Ziylan & Ales, 1984). Among the functions of the BBB is the regulation of nutrient availability in the brain. A better understanding of the transport mechanisms via the BBB and the discovery of special carriers, has allowed us to understand several phenomena related to BBB function (Bradbury, 1979; Pardridge, 1988). Of special interest to epilepsy research area is the discovery of carriers for glucose and insulin. The BBB transport system may serve as a rate-limiting step during seizures. Specifically, glucose availability to the seizing brain may be restricted, such that the brain glucose utilization rates are no longer independent of plasma glucose levels (Cornford & Oldendorf, 1986). It is clear that changes in glucose availability to the brain may change brain activity drastically. On the other hand, studies have shown that impairment of the glucose pathway constitutes the mode of action for some convulsants (Hevioz, Delorne, & Beauvillain, 1986).

LIPIDS

Several investigations have provided an understanding for the possible role of brain lipids in epilepsy (Schwartz, Boyes, & Aynsley-Green, 1989). The interest in brain lipids stems from the fact that lipids are important constituents of the neuronal membrane. Changes in the lipid composition of the neuronal membrane may result in corresponding changes in some functional aspect of the neuronal membrane activity as described earlier. The peroxidation of unsaturated fatty acids is changed vastly when an epileptic mirror focus is created in the rat (Rokyta, Kubik, Veliskova, & Stastna, 1989). Substances that induce epilepsy, such as iron, also increase lipid peroxidation (Zhang et al., 1989). Several studies have established that the possibility of problems with membrane fluidity may be associated with epilepsy (Nelson & Delgado-Escueta, 1986). The fact that anticonvulsant drugs induce changes in membrane fluidity is not popularly realized (Kohlschutter, Hubner, & Gartner, 1988; Stahl & Harris, 1986).

We suggest that those changes in membrane fluidity are mediated by membrane lipids. Craig and Colasanti (1989) developed a method for measuring the threshold of epileptic seizures. They injected a subacute dose of metrazol every 15 minutes until a seizure was elicited and counted the number of times an injection was administered. These trials (or equivalent times) are taken as a threshold for seizure elicitation. We recently employed the same method and found that the threshold for epileptic seizures in rats is highly dependent on the circadian cycle. When the rats were treated with a mixture of polyunsaturated fatty acids for 4 weeks, the level of the threshold for eliciting seizures was substantially elevated, namely, more injections of subacute metrazol were needed to evoke seizures (Yehuda, Carassao, & Mostofsky, in press).

To be sure, not many physicians have offered or recommended ketogenic diets for treating epilepsy. In the past, it was highly recommended. The ketogenic diet is one in which the level of fat is higher in relation to carbohydrates, such that ketosis results. Pre- and postprandial circulating concentrations of metabolic fuels and plasma insulin were documented in 59 patients with severe epilepsy while receiving either a normal diet, the classical high-fat ketogenic diet, a medium-chain triglyceride (MCT) diet, or a modified MCT diet. All three therapeutic diets improved the control of epilepsy and induced a significant increase in the concentrations of blood aceto-acetate and 3-hydroxybutyrate, the greatest elevation being seen in patients on the classic diet. The classic diet also caused a significant decrease in blood alanine values, which was not observed with other therapeutic diets. The only consistent change to occur in all patients on therapeutic diets was an increase in plasma uric acid. The mechanism by which ketogenic diets improve seizure control remains to be delineated. Whatever the reason for the beneficial effect of the diet, the link to fat and lipid is apparent.

A possible link between epilepsy and lipids may be due to the activity of prostoglandins. The production of prostoglandins is affected by seizures, and may prolong the duration of the attacks (Bazan, Birkle, Tang, & Reddy, 1986.). Furthermore, epileptic seizures commonly terminate abruptly and spontaneously, and the brain then remains refractory to further seizures for some time thereafter. The data suggest that neuronal fatigue is not involved in either of these processes, although the data concerning the role of ions and excitatory systems are unclear. Conceivably, seizure arrest and refractoriness may come about by the seizure-induced release and/or activity of multiple endogenous anticonvulsant substances. The spontaneous arrest of the seizure may involve the purine adenosine, in addition to other unknown mechanisms. Seizure refractoriness involves multiple systems, the most important of which, on available evidence, are prostaglandins (which form and originate from polyunsaturated fatty acids), opioid peptides, and, possibly, benzodiazepine systems, although other neuropeptides and the purines also may be involved (Dragunow, 1986; Dwyer, Wasterlain, Fujikawa, & Yamada, 1986).

Nutrition and nutrients are certainly not magic drugs as far as we know. Epilepsy is a condition in which the brain cells fire unpredictably in the absence of normal supra threshold stimulation. Yet the term *brain storm* has been used to describe such episodes. It is possible that these episodes are mediated by changes in the neuronal membrane, mainly in the lipid component. Furthermore, the possibility of interfering with the lipid component and other nutritional agents is very intriguing and deserving of further research. Admittedly, the history of nutritional treatment for epilepsy, as is true for other disorders, unfortunately has been colored by many false claims and outright forgery. For example, the claim made by Jarvis (1958) that "honigar" (a combination of honey and vinegar) would cure many disorders (including epilepsy) in his book *Folk Medicine* has been proved scientifically to be wrong. On the other hand, in 1951, Alexander recommended cod liver oil mixed with orange juice as a treatment for arthritis and multiple sclerosis. Although his opinion was mocked by physicians and scientists, serious studies on the effect of Omega-3 fatty acids (fish oil) are now being pursued aggressively to evaluate unambiguously the therapeutic value of those fatty acids as they may be applied for remediating the devastating consequences of various disorders, including multiple sclerosis. Therefore, it is clear that any claim for nutrition-based therapy should be studied seriously and only dismissed after careful and deliberate investigation.

ACKNOWLEDGMENTS

I thank Talia Fostick for her technical assistance in the preparation of this manuscript.

REFERENCES

Abalan, F. (1984). Alzheimer's disease and malnutrition: An new etiological hypothesis. *Medical Hypotheses, 15,* 385–393.

Abalan, F., Achiminov, A., & Pirsolie, M. (1985). Malnutrition and Alzheimer's dementia. *British Journal of Psychiatry, 147,* 320.

Alexander, D. D. (1951). *Arthritis and common sense.* New York: Hartford Pub.

Allen, I. C., Grieve, A., & Griffiths, R. (1986). Differential changes in the content of amino acid neurotransmitters in discrete regions of the rat brain prior to the onset and during the course of homocysteine-induced seizures. *Journal of Neurochemistry, 46,* 1582–1592.

Anderson, G. H. (1980). Diet, neurotransmitter and brain function. *British Medical Bulletin, 37,* 95–100.

Angyan, L. (1984). The effects of feeding and fasting on self stimulation. *Acta Physiologica Hungaria, 63,* 185–195.

Ashley, D. V. M., Liardon, R., & Letherwood, P. D. (1985). Breakfast meal composition influences plasma tryptophan to large neutral amino acid ratio of healthy young men. *Journal of Neuronal Transmission, 63,* 271–283.

Balasubramaniam, S., Simon, L. S., Charg, S., & Hickie, J. B. (1985). Reduction in plasma and increase in biliary cholesterol by diet rich in n-3 fatty acids in the rats. *Journal of Lipid Research, 26,* 684–689.

Barbeau, A., & Donaldson, J. (1973). Taruine in epilepsy. *Lancet, 2,* 387.

Bazan, N. G., Birkle, D. L., Tang, W., & Reddy, T. S. (1986). The accumulation of free arachidonic aid, diacylglycerols, prostaglandins, and lipoxygenase reaction products in the brain during experimental epilepsy. *Advances in Neurology, 44,* 879–902.

Ben-Ari, Y., Repressa, G., Tremblay, E., & Nitecka, L. (1986). Selective and non-selective seizure related brain damage produced by kainic acid. *Advances in Experimental Medicine & Biology, 203,* 647–657.

Benedict, C. B., Anderson, G. H., & Sole, M. J. (1983). The influence of oral tyrosine and tryptophan feeding on plasma catecholamines in man. *American Journal of Clinical Nutrition, 38,* 429–435.

Bloom, F. E., Luzerson, A., & Hofstadter, L. (1985). *Brain, mind and behavior.* New York: W. H. Freeman.

Bowling, T. G. (1988). Blood-brain barrier studies with special reference to epileptic seizures. *ACTA Psychiatry Scandinavia, 345*(Suppl), 15–20.

Bradbury, M. (1979). *The concept of a blood-brain barrier.* New York: Wiley.

Brozek, J. (1978). Malnutrition and behavior. *Journal of the American Dietetic Association, 72,* 17–23.

Campbell, K., Banks, S., & Milgram, N. W. (1984). Epileptogenic effects of electrolytic lesions in the hippocampus: Role of iron deposition. *Experimental Neurology, 86,* 506–514.

Carlile, C. I., & Andras, L. G. (1985). Age related changes in lipid levels and tissue lipoprotein lipase activities of the Fischer-344 rats. *Archives of Gerontology and Geriatrics, 4,* 133–140.

Clandinin, M. T., Field, C. J., Hargreaves, K., Morson, L., & Zsigmond, E. (1985). Role of diet fat in subcellular structure and function. *Canadian Journal of Physiology and Pharmacology, 63,* 546–556.

Cohen, B. M., & Zubenko, G. S. (1985). Aging and biophysical properties of cell membranes. *Life Science, 37,* 1403–1409.

Conlay, L. A., & Zeisel, S. H. (1982). Neurotransmitter precursors and brain function. *Neurosurgery, 10,* 524–529.

Cornford, E. M., & Oldendorf, W. H. (1986). Epilepsy and the blood-brain barrier. *Advances in Neurology, 44,* 787–812.

Craig, C. R., & Colasanti, B. K. (1986). GABA receptors, lipids, and gangliosides in cobalt epileptic focus. *Advances in Neurology, 44,* 379–391.

Csernansky, J. G., Holman, C. A., Bonnet, K. A., Grabowsky, K., King, R., & Mollister, L. (1983). Dopaminergic supersensitivity at distant sites following induced epileptic foci. *Life Science, 32,* 386–390.

Dalby, T. J. (1985). Will population decrease in caffeine consumption unveil attention deficit disorders in adults? *Medical Hypothesis, 18,* 163–167.

Dohan, F. C., Harper, E. H., Clark, M. H., Rodrique, R. G., & Zigas, V. (1985). Is schizophrenia rare if gain is rare? *Biological Psychiatry, 19,* 385–399.

Dhopeshwarker, G. A. (1983). *Nutrition and brain development.* New York: Plenum Press.

Dragunow, M. (1986). Endogenous anticonvulsant substances. *Neuroscience & Biobehavioral Reviews, 10*(3), 229–244.

Dwyer, B. E., Wasterlain, C. G., Fujikawa, D. G., & Yamada, L. (1986). Brain protein metabolism in epilepsy. *Advances in Neurology, 44,* 903–918.

Fariello, R. G., Golden, G. T., Smith, G. G., & Reyes, P. F. (1989). Potentiation of kainic acid epileptogenicity and sparing from neuronal damage by an NMDA receptor antagonist. *Epilepsy Research, 3*(3), 206–213.

Fernstorm, J. D., & Wurtman, R. J. (1971). Brain seratonin contents: Increase following ingestion of carbohydrate diet. *Science, 174,* 1023–1025.

Fernstrom, J. D. (1981). Effects of the diet on brain function. *Acta Astronautica, 8,* 1035–1042.

Fernstrom, J. D., & Wurtman, R. J. (1972). Brain serotonin content: Physiological regulation by plasma neutral amino acid. *Science, 174,* 414–416.

Foot, M., Cruz, T. F., & Clandinin, M. T. (1983). Effects of dietary lipid on synaptosomal acetylcholinesterase activity. *Biochemistry Journal, 211,* 507–509.

Foster, A. C. (1986). Involvement of excitatory amino acid receptors in the mechanisms underlying excitotoxic phenomena. *Advances in Experimental Medicine & Biology, 203,* 303–316.

Goggin, T., Gough, H., Bissessar, A., Crowley, M., Baker, M., & Callaghan, N. (1987). A comparative study of the relative effects of anticonvulsant drugs and dietary folate on the red cell folate status of patients with epilepsy. *Quarterly Journal of Medicine, 65*(247), 911–919.

Gossi, S., Oliverio, A., Salvati, S., Serlupi-Crescenzi, G., Tagliamonta, G., & Tomassi, G. (1982). Effects of dietary phospholipids and odd-chain fatty acids on the behavioral maturation of mice. *Food Chemistry and Toxicology, 20,* 153–157.

Hamilton, C. M. N., Whitney, E. N., & Sizer, F. S. (Eds.). (1985). *Nutrition: Concepts and controversies* (3rd ed.). St. Paul, MN: West Publishing.

Heger, H. W. (1979). Effects of dietary phospholipids on acetylcholinesterase activity in the rat brain and on phospholipid composition in liver and brain. *General Pharmacology, 10,* 427–432.

Hegstad, E., Langmoen, I. A., & Hablitz, J. J. (1989). Zinc and glycine do not modify low-magnesium-induced epileptiform activity in the immature neocortex in vitro. *Epilepsy Research, 3*(2), 174–177.

Heinemann, U. (1986). Excitatory amino acids and epilepsy-induced changes in extracellular space size. *Advances in Experimental Medicine & Biology, 203,* 449–460.

Hevioz, T. K., Delorne, P., & Beauvillain, I. C. (1986). Glycogen synthesis and immunocytochemical study of fructose-1,6, biophosphate in methionine epileptogenic rodent brain. *Journal of Cerebral Blood Flow & Metabolism, 6,* 292–297.

Houslay, M. D., & Stanley, K. K. (1982). *Dynamics of biological membranes*. New York: Wiley.

Jarvis, C. D. (1958). *Folk Medicine*. New York: Fawcett.

Johnston, D., Rutecki, P. A., & Lebeda, F. J. (1986). Synaptic events underlying spontaneous and evoked paroxysmal discharges in hippocampal neurons. *Advances in Experimental Medicine & Biology, 203,* 391–400.

Jones, E. G. (1986). Neurotransmitters in the cerebral cortex. *Journal of Neurosurgery, 65*(2), 135–153.

Kessler, R. A., & Yehuda, S. (1958). Learning induced changes in brain membrane cholesterol and fluidity: Implications for brain aging. International *Journal of Neuroscience, 26,* 73–83.

Kirilovsky, J., Steiner-Mordoch, S., Selinger, Z., & Schramm, M. (1985). Lipid requirements for reconstitution of the delipidated beta-adrenergic receptor and the regulatory protein. *FEBS Letters, 183,* 75–80.

Knowlton, B., McGowan, M., & Olton, D. S. (1985). Hippocampal stimulation disrupts spatial working memory even 8 h. after acquisition. *Behavioral and Neural Biology, 44,* 325–337.

Kohlschutter, A., Hubner, C., & Gartner, J. (1988). Decreased membrane fluidity of lymphocytes from patients with juvenile neuronal ceroid-lipofuscinosis. *American Journal of Medical Genetics, 5,* 203–207.

Lampety, M. S., & Walker, B. L. (1976). A possible essential role for dietary linolenic acid in the development of the young rat. *Journal of Nutrition, 106,* 86–93.

Lampety, M. S., & Walker, B. L. (1978). Learning behavior and brain lipid composition in rats subjected to essential fatty acid deficiency during gestation, lactation and growth. *Journal of Nutrition, 108,* 358–367.

Leaver, D. D., Parkinson, G. B., & Schneider, K. M. (1987). Neurological consequences of magnesium deficiency: Correlations with epilepsy. *Clinical & Experimental Pharmacology & Physiology, 14*(5), 361–370.

LeFauconnier, J. M., & Klatzo, I. (1986). Excitatory amino acids and the blood-brain barrier. *Advances in Experimental Medicine & Biology, 203,* 231–233.

Letherwood, P. D., & Pollitt, P. (1983). Diet-induced mood changes in normal populations. *Journal of Psychiatric Research, 17,* 147–152.

Lewis, W. H., & Elvin-Lewis, M. P. F. (1977). *Medical Botany.* New York: Wiley.

Martinau, J. C., Bathelemy, B., Garreau, B., & Lelord, G. (1985). Vitamins B6, magnesium and combined B6-Mg: Therapeutic effects in children autism. *Biological Psychiatry, 20,* 467–478.

Meldrum, B. (1986). Excitatory amino acid antagonists as novel anticonvulsants. *Advances in Experimental Medicine & Biology, 203,* 321–329.

Mody, I., Lambert, J. D., & Heinemann, U. (1987). Low extracellular magnesium induces epileptiform activity and spreading depression in rat hippocampal slices. *Journal of Neurophysiology, 57*(3), 869–888.

Morgane, P. G., Miller, M., Kemper, T., Stern, W., Forbes, W., Hali, R., Bronzino, J., Kissare, J., Mawrylewicz, E., & Resnick, O. (1978). The effects of protein malnutrition on the developing central nervous system in the rat. *Neuroscience and Biobehavioral Reviews, 2,* 137–230.

Moura-Ribeiro, M. V., Ferlin, M. L., Gallina, R. A., & Funayama, C. A. (1987). Non-ketotic hyperglycinemia. *Arquivos De Neuro-Psiquiatria, 45*(1), 67–71.

Nelson, L., & Delgado-Escueta, A. V. (1986). Fluidity of normal and epileptogenic freeze-lesioned synaptic membranes in the cat. *Brain Research, 386*(1/2), 32–40.

Nikushkin, E. V. (1987). Lipid peroxidation in the development of epileptic activity. *Patologicheskaia Fiziologiia I Eksperimentalnaia Terapiia, 6,* 19–24.

Olton, D. F., Becker, J. T., & Hardelman, G. E. (1979). Hippocampus, space and memory. *Behavior and Brain Science, 2,* 313–365.

Pardridge, W. M. (1988). Studies with isolated human brain capillaries. *Ann. New York Academy Science, 529,* 50–60.

Podlubiuk, Z. M., & Kleinrok, Z. (1976). Comparison of central action of prostoglandins A, E, E2, E alpha, and F2 alpha in the rat. *Psychopharmacology, 50,* 95–102.

Pollitt, E., Leibel, R. L., & Greenfield, D. (1981). Brief fasting, stress and cognition in children. *American Journal Clinical Nutrition, 34,* 1526–1533.

Pollitt, E., Lewis, M. L., Garza, C., & Shulman, R. J. (1983). Fasting and cognitive function. *Journal of Psychiatric Research, 17,* 169–174.

Reimann, W., Steinhaur, H. B., Hedler, L., Starke, K., & Hertting, G. (1981). Effects of prostoglandins D, E2 and E2 alpha on catecholamine release from slices of rat and rabbit brain. *European Journal of Pharmacology, 69,* 421–427.

Remler, P., & Marcussen, W. H. (1986). Systemic focal epileptogenesis. *Epilepsy, 27,* 35–42.

Rokyta, R., Kubik, V., Veliskova, & Stastna, H. (1989). The changes of peroxidation of unsaturated fatty acids in epileptic mirror focus in rats. *Activitas Nervosa Superior, 31*(3), 227–228.

Routtenberg, R. (1987). Phospholipid and fatty acid regulation of signal transduction at synapses: Potential role for protein kinase C in infirmation storage. *Journal of Neural Transmission, 24,* 239–245.

Schwartz, R. M., Boyes, S., & Aynsley-Green, A. (1989). Metabolic effects of three ketogenic diets in the treatment of severe epilepsy. *Developmental Medicine & Child Neurology, 31*(2), 152–160.

Seeman, P. (1977). Antischizophrenic drugs-membrane receptor site of action. *Biochemical Pharmacology, 26,* 1741–1748.

Seeman, P. (1982). The membrane actions of anesthetics and tranquilizers. *Pharmacological Reviews, 24,* 583–655.

Seltzer, S., Marcus, R., & Stoch, R. (1981). Perspectives in the control of chronic pain by nutritional manipulation. *Pain, 11,* 141–148.

Shoemaker, W. J., & Bloom, F. E. (1977). Effects of undernutrition on brain morphology. In R. J. Wurtman & J. J. Wurtman (Eds.), *Nutrition and the brain* (Vol. 2, pp. 147–192). New York: Raven Press.

Shoemaker, W. J., & Wurtman, R. J. (1971). Perinatal undernutrition: Accumulation of catecholamine in rat brain. *Science, 171,* 1017–1019.

Singer, B. J., & Nicolson, G. L. (1972). The fluid mosaic model of the structure of the cell membrane. *Science, 178,* 720–731.

Spector, A. A., & Yorek, M. A. (1985). Membrane lipid composition and cellular function. *Journal of Lipid Research, 26,* 1015–1035.

Stahl, W. L., & Harris, W. E. (1986). Na+, K+-ATPase: Structure, function, and interactions with drugs. *Advances in Neurology, 44,* 681–693.

Suzuki, H ., Hayakawa, S., Wada, S., & Wada, O. (1985a). Effects of the modification of plasma lipids by fish and soybean oil diets. *Biochemia et Biophysica Acta 836,* 390–393.

Suzuki, H., Kobayasti, T., Mayakaw, S., & Wada, O. (1985b). Age associated changes in rat plasma lipids, platelet fatty acids, and prostacycline release. *Biochemia et Biophysica Acta, 836,* 394–396.

Sved, A. F. (1983). Precursor control of the function of monoaminergic neurons. In R. J. Wurtman & J. J. Wurtman (Eds.), *Nutrition and behavior* (Vol. 5, pp. 223–275). New York: Raven Press.

Tacconi, M., & Wurtman, R. J. (1985). Phosphatidylcholine product in rat synaptosomes by N-methylation is enriched in polyunsaturated fatty acids. *Proceedings of the National Academy of Science, USA, 82,* 4828–4831.

Tews, J. K., Repa, J. J., Nguyen, H., & Harper, A. E. (1985). Avoidance of GABA-containing diets by olfactory Bulbectomized rats. *Physiology and Behavior, 34,* 983–986.

Trulson, M. E. (1985). Dietary affect function of brain serotonin neurons. *Life Sciences, 37,* 1067–1072.

Van woert, M. L., Rosenbaum, D., Houieson, S., & Bowers, M. B. (1977). Long term therapy of myoclonus and other neurological disorders with L-5-hydroxytrptophane ans carbidupa. *New England Journal of Medicine, 296,* 70–75.

Ventura, V., Bouget, F., Sartorelli, C., Torre, G., & Tommasini, C. (1991). Colciac diseases, folic acid deficiency and epilepsy with cerebral calcifications. *Acta Pediatrica Scandinavia, 80,* 559–562.

Vergrossen, A. J. (1972). Hypothesis for interaction between acetylcholine and prostoglandin biosynthesis: An introduction. In A. Barbeau, J. H. Growden, & R. J. Wurtman (Eds.), *Nutrition and the brain* (Vol. 5, pp. 109–112). New York: Raven Press.

Wahle, K. W. J. (1983). Fatty acid modification and membrane lipids. *Proceedings of the Nutrition Society, 42,* 273–287.

Wiggins, R. C., Fuller, G., & Enna, S. J. (1984). Undernutrition and the development of brain neurotransmitter system. *Life Sciences, 35,* 2085–2094.

Wincour, G. (1985). The hippocampus and thalamus: Their roles in short- and long-term memory and their effects of interference. *Behavioral Brain Research, 16,* 135–152.

Wurtman, R. J. (1975). The effects of light on human body. *Scientific American, 233,* 68–77.

Wurtman, R. J. (1982). Nutrients that modify brain function. *Scientific American, 246,* 50–59.

Wurtman, R. J., Baum, M. J., & Potts, J. T. (Eds.). (1985). *The medical and biological effects of light* (Vol. 453). New York: The New York Academy of Sciences.

Wurtman, R. J., Hefti, F., & Melamed, E. (1981). Precursor control of neurotransmitter synthesis. *Pharmacological Reviews, 32,* 315–335.

Wurtman, R. J., & Wurtman, J. J. (1984). Nutritional control of central neurotransmitters. In K. M. Pirke & D. Ploog (Eds.), *Psychobiology of anorexia nervosa* (pp. 4–12). Berlin: Springer.

Yehuda, S. (1987). Nutrients, brain biochemistry and behavior: A possible role for the neuronal membrane. *International Journal of Neuroscience, 35,* 21–36.

Yehuda, S., Carasso, R. L., & Mostofsky, D. T. (1993, in press). SR-3 (a mixture of fatty acids) raises the seizure threshold in rats. *European Journal of Pharmacology.*

Zeisel, S. H. (1981). Dietary choline: Biochemistry, physiology and pharmacology. *Annual Review of Nutrition, 1,* 95–121.

Zhang, Z. H., Zuo, Q. H., & Wu, X. R. (1989). Effects of lipid peroxidation on GABA uptake and release in iron-induced seizures. *Chinese Medical Journal-Peking, 102*(1), 24–27.

Ziylan, Y. Z., & Ales, N. (1984). Age related changes in regional patterns of B.B.B. breakdown during epileptic seizures. *Neuroscience Letters, 96,* 174–184.

Zubenko, G. S., & Cohen, B. M. (1985). Biophysical alterations in cell membranes associated with psychotherapeutic drug exposure, psychopathology and aging. *Psychopharmacology Bulletin, 21,* 631–640.

7 Catamenial Epilepsy

Dianne Schechter
The New York State Psychiatric Institute and Columbia University

Women with catamenial epilepsy have a predictable pattern of seizure discontrol that is associated with the menstrual cycle (Bäckström et al., 1984; Newmark & Penry, 1980). Although the existence of catamenial epilepsy remains controversial, because the reported prevalence of this disorder has ranged from 0% to 72% (Laidlaw, 1956; Newmark, 1989), there is strong support in the literature for the hypothesis that at least some epileptic women experience cyclical changes in seizure frequency in relation to the menstrual cycle. Seizures may occur only during specific phases of the menstrual cycle, or they may just be more frequent during portions of the cycle. This chapter reviews research on the timing of seizure occurrence during the menstrual cycle, mechanisms that may contribute to a catamenial seizure pattern, and potential treatment strategies.

PHYSIOLOGY OF THE MENSTRUAL CYCLE

The hormonal events leading to ovulation and menstruation involve two classes of ovarian hormones (estrogens and progestins), two pituitary hormones (follicle-stimulating hormone [FSH] and luteinizing hormone [LH]), and a hypothalamic hormone (gonadotropin-releasing hormone [GnRH]) (Martin, Reichlin, & Brown, 1977). Plasma levels of pituitary and gonadal secretions follow characteristic patterns over the course of a normal cycle (Martin et al., 1977; Turner & Bagnara, 1976). A schematic illustration of ovarian steroid and pituitary gonadotropin patterns during the menstrual cycle is provided in Fig. 7.1.

During the first half, or follicular phase, of the cycle, ovarian follicles grow and mature under the influence of FSH and LH. The developing follicles secrete increasing amounts of estrogen, which suppress FSH levels after an initial mid-

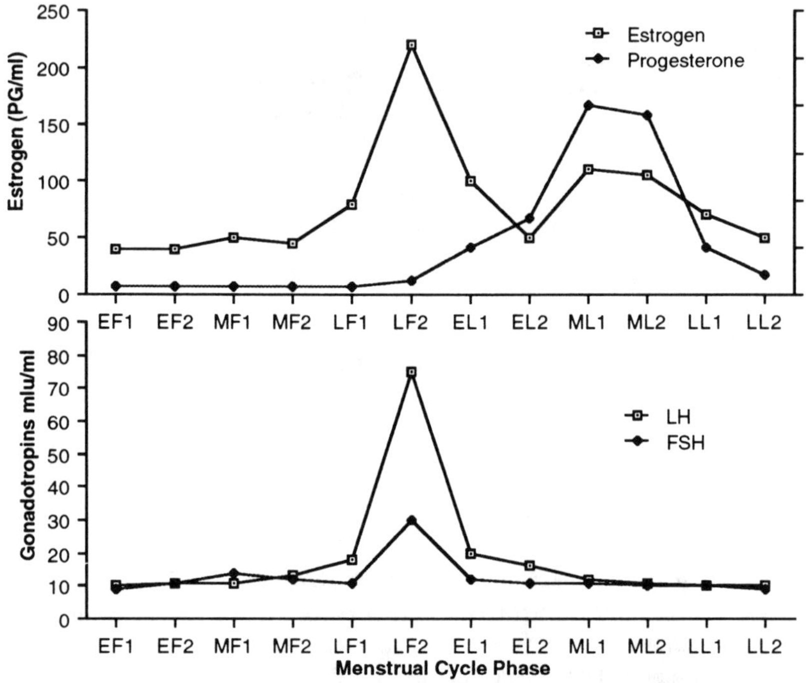

FIG. 7.1. Schematic illustration of changes in luteinizing hormone (LH), follicle stimulating hormone (FSH), estrogen, and progesterone levels during the menstrual cycle. EF = early follicular phases; MF = midfollicular phases; LF = late follicular phases; EL = early luteal phases; ML = midluteal phases; LL = late luteal phases. Ovulation occurs during LF2.

follicular rise in FSH (Vaitukaitis & Ross, 1976). A follicle destined to become a graafian follicle is selected halfway through the follicular phase, and that follicle becomes the major source of estradiol during the second half of the follicular phase. In the second half of the follicular phase, plasma concentrations of FSH decline progressively as estrogen levels reach a peak. A negative feedback relationship exists between estrogen production and FSH synthesis and secretion. Estrogen exerts a positive feedback effect on pituitary LH secretion and induces increased LH output, which culminates in a marked LH increase at midcycle. This LH peak usually is accompanied by an FSH surge (Ross et al., 1970). The midcycle surge of LH signals the onset of the second part, or luteal phase, of the menstrual cycle.

Ovulation occurs 12–36 hours after the LH peak (Yussman & Taymor, 1970). Following ovulation, the remainder of the graafian follicle is transformed into the corpus luteum, which secretes estradiol and progesterone. After a brief decline following ovulation, plasma estradiol levels reach a second, but smaller, peak before falling sharply prior to menstruation. Progesterone levels also rise swiftly following ovulation and, like estrogen, fall rapidly before menstruation.

Peak progesterone and estradiol levels usually are observed 5–8 days after the midcycle LH surge, corresponding to the 19th to 22nd day of a 28-day menstrual cycle (Vaitukaitis, 1984). If a fertilized egg is not produced, the corpus luteum proceeds through a sequence of development and regression over 14 ± 2 days (Cutler & Garcia, 1980). The consequent fall in plasma estrogens and progestins results in the onset of menstrual bleeding and the beginning of another cycle.

DOCUMENTATION OF CATAMENIAL SEIZURE PATTERNS

The majority of the research on catamenial seizure patterns has focused on the association between seizure frequency and menses. Visual inspection of seizure diaries suggests that seizure frequency may increase during a perimenstrual time period (Almqvist, 1955; Ansell & Clarke, 1956a; Dickerson, 1941; Gordon, 1909; Mattson, Lerner, & Dix, 1974; Sánchez Longo & González Saldaña, 1956). Of the 23 cases reviewed by Gordon (1909), 5 had seizures when menses began, 2 had seizures during menstruation, 2 had seizures at the end of menses, and 14 had seizures 1–2 days prior to the onset of menses. Sánchez Longo and González Saldaña (1956) reported the case of a woman whose seizures occurred during undefined premenstrual and menstrual phases. Dickerson (1941) and Almqvist (1955) reported that 9%–10% of their samples showed a relationship between seizures and menstruation. Ansell and Clarke (1956a) concluded that 63% of their sample had an increased number of seizures during menses or during the 24-hour period prior to menses. Similarly, Mattson et al. (1974) reported that 55% of their female patients had an increased number of seizures around the time of the menstrual period.

Statistical comparisons of seizure frequency during perimenstrual and non-perimenstrual portions of the menstrual cycle have supported the hypothesized increase in seizure frequency around the time of menses, but, as with visual inspection of seizure diaries, have not found good agreement about when seizures are most likely to occur. Rościszewska (1980) found a significant increase in seizures during the luteal phase with peak seizure frequency on the first day of menstrual bleeding. Mattson, Kamer, Cramer, and Caldwell (1981) also found that seizure frequency was greatest at menstruation. Taubøll, Lundervold, and Gjerstad (1991) compared seizure frequency during a 4-day premenstrual phase, a 5-day menstrual phase, and the remainder of the menstrual cycle. For most subjects, seizures were more frequent during menses than during the remainder of the cycle, and there was a trend toward increased seizure frequency during the premenstrual phase. Gueirreiro and Ramos (1991) divided menstrual cycles into six equal segments. Seizures were most frequent during the premenstrual phase, but were not significantly more likely during menstruation than during other phases of the menstrual cycle.

Several investigations found that seizure frequency fluctuates in relation to nonperimenstrual segments of the menstrual cycle (Bäckström, 1976; Bandler, Kaufman, Dykens, Schleifer, & Shapiro, 1957; Laidlaw, 1956; Schechter, Labar, Pedley, Ottman, & Endicott, 1989; Taubøll et al., 1991). Laidlaw (1956) found a reduced incidence of seizures during the midluteal phase, in addition to an increased incidence of seizures around the first day of menses. He hypothesized that the decreased seizure activity was related to high progesterone levels that characterize the midluteal phase. Bäckström (1976) tested Laidlaw's (1956) hypothesis in a pilot study of seven women by visually assessing seizure frequency in relation to ovarian steroid patterns. He found reduced seizure frequency coincident with high progesterone levels during the midluteal phase. Seizures increased when progesterone levels declined and during the few days prior to presumed ovulation coincident with high estrogen levels. Taubøll et al. (1991) also found evidence of increased seizure frequency during the mid- to late follicular phases.

In summary, the evidence of a catamenial influence on seizure frequency is strongest for an undefined perimenstrual time frame. There also is some evidence of increased seizure occurrence during the mid- to late follicular phases, and of a decreased incidence of seizures during the midluteal phase.

Although many studies suggest that the menstrual cycle may influence the occurrence of seizures in some women, methodologic problems in the research strategies used preclude making conclusions about the nature of the catamenial seizure pattern, or the consistency of the effects either within or among subjects. The inconsistent findings across studies reflect the influence of several study design problems:

1. Protocols often have been limited to visual inspection of seizure diaries.
2. The majority of research has focused exclusively on seizure frequency during or just prior to menses, rather than at points throughout the menstrual cycle.
3. Studies that have measured seizure frequency during other portions of the menstrual cycle have not used endocrine data to accurately divide menstrual cycles into phases. Menstrual cycles are heterogeneous with regard to the temporal patterning of ovarian and pituitary hormones (Mishell et al., 1971; Treloar, Boynton, & Behn, 1967). Therefore, phase definitions are most accurate when they are based on patterns of ovarian and pituitary hormones.
4. Anovulatory menstrual cycles have not been excluded from data analyses.
5. The possibility that individuals show different catamenial seizure patterns reflecting different etiologies has not been explored. However, there is some evidence that such heterogeneity exists. Bandler et al. (1957) found

that 16 of the 22 subjects experienced increased seizure frequency during at least one segment of the menstrual cycle, but phase preference was distributed across all portions of the cycle. A similar heterogeneity was found in our laboratory (Schechter et al., 1989). Eight female subjects completed a seizure diary daily for six menstrual cycles. Menstrual cycles were divided into six phases on the basis of cycle day, and seizures were aggregated by cycle phase separately for each subject across all cycles. The menstrual cycle phase influence on seizure occurrence was significant for seven subjects, but the phase associated with increased or decreased seizures varied from subject to subject.

6. The consistency of an individual's catamenial seizure pattern across different menstrual cycles has not been documented. Preliminary data analyses indicate that composite seizure patterns from up to six menstrual cycles were representative of some, but not all menstrual cycles that contributed to the summary patterns (Schechter et al., 1989).
7. Most studies have not described adequately types of seizures or antiepileptic medications.

Additional research is needed to characterize the time periods when women may be at an increased or decreased risk for seizures. Future studies should consider the entire menstrual cycle, use endocrine data to define menstrual cycle phases, and control for variables such as seizure types and antiepileptic medications.

ETIOLOGY

One or more of the following mechanisms may contribute to a catamenial influence on seizure frequency: (a) direct effects of ovarian steroids, and (b) secondary effects of ovarian steroids on such variables as water retention and plasma levels of seizure medications.

Direct Effects of Ovarian Steroids

Influence of Ovarian Steroids on Brain Excitability

Estrogens have been found to be excitatory in a wide range of laboratory models of epileptic seizures. Application of conjugated estrogens to cortical tissue activates an existing seizure focus (McQueen & Woodbury, 1975) and creates a new seizure focus in cats (Julien, Fowler, & Danielson, 1975; Marcus, Watson, & Goldman, 1966). Estradiol lowers the electroshock seizure threshold in intact (Stitt & Kinnard, 1968) and ovariectomized rats (Woolley & Timiras, 1962a). Replacement of estradiol in ovariectomized rats also increases the acquisition rate of kindled seizures in the amygdala (Hom & Buterbaugh, 1986) and anterior neocortex (Buterbaugh, 1989). In humans, intravenous injection of 20–40 mg of premarin increased electroencephalographic abnormalities in 11 of 16 epileptic women and was associated with clinical seizures in 4 (Logothetis, Harner, Morell, & Torres, 1959).

The convulsant activity of estradiol in electroshock and kindling models of epilepsy seems to occur within physiological levels of the hormone (Buterbaugh, 1989; Hom & Buterbaugh, 1986). An interesting study of electroshock seizure threshold at different points during the estrus cycle in rats also suggests that physiological levels of estrogen influence seizure threshold. Convulsive reactivity was lowest during diestrus, higher during proestrus, and highest during estrus, the portion of the cycle when estradiol is highest (Woolley & Timiras, 1962b).

In contrast to estrogen, progesterone acts as a central nervous system depressant. Progesterone induces anesthesia in large doses (Gyermek, Genther, & Flemming, 1967; Gyermek, Iriarte, & Crabbe, 1968; Merryman, Boiman, Barner, & Rothchild, 1954) and acts as an anticonvulsant against metrazol-induced seizures (Selye, 1942). One of the progesterone metabolites, 3-α-hydroxy-5-α-pregnan-20-one, is effective against metrazol-, (+)-bicuculline- and picrotoxin-induced seizures (Belelli, Bolger, & Gee, 1989). Progesterone and its 5-α and 5-β pregnanolone metabolites also depress interictal epileptiform activity from penicillin foci on the cat's cerebral cortex (Landgren, Aasly, Bäckström, Dubrovsky, & Danielson, 1987; Landgren, Bäckström, & Kalistratov, 1978). Intravenous administration of luteal phase levels of progesterone significantly reduces interictal spike activity in epileptic women with location related epilepsy (Bäckström et al., 1984).

The mechanism of action of ovarian steroids on seizure activity is not known. Logothetis et al. (1959) found that intravenous (IV) administration of conjugated estrogens increased electroencephalographic abnormalities in as little as 30 sec. Such a rapid effect suggests a direct action on neural membranes, rather than the slower indirect mechanism involving genomic activation characteristic of the ovarian steroid's influence on the reproductive system (Pfaff & McEwen, 1983). Several mechanisms have been postulated to explain the anesthetic and antiseizure properties of progesterone (Herzog, 1987). These include: (a) progesterone depresses oxygen and glucose metabolism (Gordon, 1956), (b) progesterone acts directly on neural membranes to decrease epileptiform activity (Landgren et al., 1978), (c) progesterone potentiates the effects of endogenous anticonvulsants such as adenosine (Swanson & Phillis, 1987), (d) progesterone competes with antiseizure medications for degredation by the hepatic microsomal enzyme system (Kumar, Behari, Ahuja, & Jailkhaui, 1988; Shavit et al., 1984), and (e) progesterone acts indirectly via progesterone metabolites that have direct membrane effects (Bäckström et al., 1984).

The last hypothesis is intriguing, given that the anesthetic and anticonvulsant potency of some of the progesterone metabolites is much greater than that of progesterone (Gyermek et al., 1967, 1968). The 3-α-hydroxylated pregnanes, in particular, have strong anticonvulsant and sedative properties (Belelli et al., 1989; Gyermek et al., 1967, 1968), which are thought to be separate from their hormonal effects (Belelli, Lan, & Gee, 1990; Craig, 1966; Smith, Waterhouse, & Woodward, 1987). Some of the progesterone metabolites, especially 3-α-hydroxy-5-α-pregnan-20-one, influence brain excitability by modulating a steroid recognition site on the $GABA_A$-benzodiazepine receptor complex (GBRC) in a barbituate-like manner (Belelli et al., 1990; Gee, 1988; Harrison, Majewska, Harrington, & Barker, 1987; Majewska, Harrison, Schwartz, Barker, & Paul, 1986).

Progesterone regulation of the GBRC may have physiological relevance for the modulation of brain excitability (Belelli et al., 1990). Support for this hypothesis comes from in vitro observations that some of the progesterone metabolites are stronger modulators of the GBRC than some of the benzodiazepines (Gee, Chang, Brinton, & McEwen, 1987; Morrow, Suzdak, & Paul, 1987). In addition, the most potent progesterone metabolites at the GBRC occur naturally through the enzymatic activity of 5-α- or 5-β-reductace and 3-α-oxidoreductase (Canick et al., 1986; Karavolas, Bertics, Wodges, & Rudie, 1984; Krieger & Scott, 1984, 1989). These enzymes are present peripherally and in the brain (Canick et al., 1986; Karavolas et al., 1984; Krieger & Scott, 1984, 1989).

Influence of Ovarian Steroids on Seizure Frequency

The evidence that estrogen and progesterone influence brain excitability suggests several hypotheses about the association between seizure frequency and ovarian steroids during the menstrual cycle. These include: (a) seizure frequency is related positively to estrogen level (Logothetis et al., 1959), (b) seizure frequency is related inversely to progesterone level (Laidlaw, 1956), and (c) a high estrogen to progesterone level is associated with increased seizure susceptibility (Bäckström, 1976).

Estrogen Hypothesis. If change in estrogen level were the sole mechanism contributing to catamenial epilepsy, one would expect seizures to increase in frequency throughout the follicular phase, peak just prior to ovulation, decrease briefly and reach a second lower peak during the midluteal phase, and decline precipitously just prior to menses (see Fig. 7.1). Bäckström (1976) reported increased seizure frequency concurrent with the late follicular rise in estrogen level, but other investigators have not replicated this finding (Jacono & Robertson, 1987; Rościszewska, Buntner, Guz, & Zawisza, 1986). No studies have found an association between rising estrogen level during the luteal phase and increased seizure activity. Contrary to the estrogen hypothesis, seizure frequency tends to decrease during the luteal phase rise in progesterone, and to increase during the time period when estrogen level is falling in the late luteal phase and when estrogen levels are low during menses (Almqvist, 1955; Ansell & Clarke,

1956a; Bäckström, 1976; Dickerson, 1941; Gordon, 1909; Gueirreiro & Ramos, 1991; Mattson et al., 1974; Sánchez Longo & González Saldaña, 1966; Taubøll et al., 1991).

In light of the excitatory influence of estrogen on neuronal activity, one might hypothesize that patients with catamenial epilepsy have a higher than normal estrogen level during the late follicular phase and during the mid- to late luteal phases. None of the studies reviewed found higher levels of estrogen in catamenial epilepsy patients than in epileptic or nonepileptic controls. Instead, one study found that patients with catamenial seizure patterns had lower levels of estrogen throughout the menstrual cycle than nonepileptic controls (Rościszewska et al., 1986). Three studies found no difference in estrogen levels in patients with catamenial seizure patterns than in epileptic and nonepileptic controls (Bonuccelli et al., 1989; Murri, Bonuccelli, & Melis, 1986; Narbone et al., 1990).

Some support for the estrogen hypothesis has come from evidence that seizure frequency increases when estrogen levels are highest during anovulatory menstrual cycles (Bäckström, 1976).

Progesterone Hypothesis. If change in progesterone level were the sole mechanism contributing catamenial epilepsy, one would expect seizure frequency to be stable during the follicular phase, to decrease during the early luteal phase, to be lowest during the midluteal phase, and to increase during the late luteal phase at the time of progesterone withdrawal (see Fig. 7.1). Several studies have found an association between peak luteal phase progesterone level and decreased frequency of seizures, and increased seizure frequency concurrent with progesterone withdrawal (Bäckström, 1976; Jacono & Robertson, 1987; Rościszewska et al., 1986). That these associations were evident in women who were not selected because they had a catamenial seizure pattern raises the possibility that the menstrual cycle influences seizure occurrence in a large proportion of epileptic women with uncontrolled seizures (Bäckström, 1976; Jacono & Robertson, 1987).

Given that progesterone exerts an inhibitory influence on neuronal activity, one might expect catamenial epilepsy patients to have abnormally low levels of progesterone during the luteal phase. The results of studies that compared progesterone levels in patients with catamenial seizure patterns with those in nonepileptic controls supports this hypothesis (Bonuccelli et al., 1989; Murri et al., 1986; Narbone et al., 1990; Rościszewska et al., 1986). The progesterone decrement was pronounced particularly in patients on antiepileptic drugs (AEDs) (Bonuccelli et al., 1989; Murri et al., 1986). Murri et al. (1986) found a significant progesterone deficiency in untreated and treated patients with a catamenial seizure pattern, but this deficiency was stronger in those taking AEDs. Bonuccelli et al. (1989) also found reduced levels of progesterone in the overall group of catamenial epilepsy patients in comparison with nonepileptic controls, but the progesterone deficiency was statistically significant only in patients on AEDs.

Patients with catamenial seizure patterns also have been found to have lowered luteal phase progesterone levels in comparison with noncatamenial epileptic controls, but this has been true only for patients on AEDs (Bonuccelli et al., 1989). Although Rośiszewska et al. (1986) reported that luteal phase progesterone and estrogen levels were not significantly different in catamenial epilepsy patients than in noncatamenial epileptic controls, their conclusion is limited by the lack of clearly defined catamenial and noncatamenial seizure patterns in their subjects. Visual inspection of the seizure frequency data suggests that both groups exhibited a seizure pattern associated with the menstrual cycle. Subjects had the fewest number of seizures on Day 22 and the greatest number of seizures on Day 27. The increased seizure frequency on Day 27 was slightly greater for the catamenial epilepy group.

The association between AEDs and reduced progesterone level may, in part, be a consequence of the fact that some of the AEDs (i.e., phenytoin, phenobarbitol, carbamazepine) are powerful inducers of the hepatic microsomal enzymes that also metabolize ovarian steroids (Conney, 1967; Richens, 1984).

Estrogen/Progesterone Ratio Hypothesis. A schematic illustration of changes in the estrogen to progesterone ratio during the menstrual cycle is provided in Fig. 7.2.

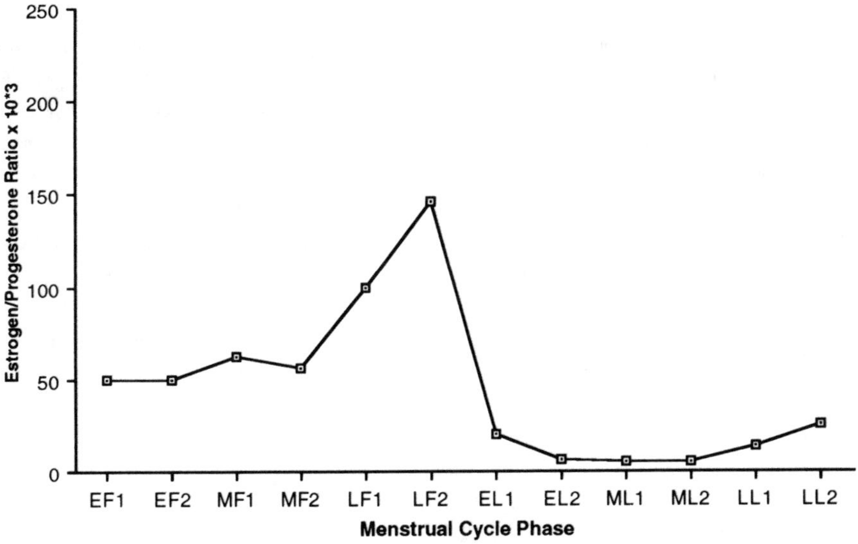

FIG. 7.2. Schematic illustration of changes in the estrogen/progesterone ratio during the menstrual cycle. EF = early follicular phases; MF = midfollicular phases; LF = late follicular phases; EL = early luteal phases; ML = midluteal phases; LL = late luteal phases. Ovulation occurs during LF2.

If change in estrogen/progesterone ratio were the sole mechanism contributing catamenial epilepsy, one would expect seizure frequency to gradually increase during the follicular phase until reaching a peak just prior to ovulation, gradually decline during the luteal phase until reaching a nadir during the midluteal phase, and then begin to increase just prior to menses. This hypothesis would not predict that seizure frequency would be increased greatly just prior to or during menses.

Only one study compared the estrogen/progesterone ratio and seizure frequency during the menstrual cycle (Bäckström, 1976). Bäckström (1976) found a positive correlation between the incidence of seizures and the estrogen/progesterone ratio. Consistent with the estrogen/progesterone hypothesis, seizure frequency was highest at the time of the late follicular phase estrogen peak and was low during the midluteal phase (Bäckström, 1976). However, a second peak in seizure frequency that occurred during menstruation is not consistent with the estrogen/progesterone ratio hypothesis. Perimenstrual increases in seizure frequency are most consistent with the hypothesized effect of progesterone withdrawal.

Indirect Effects of Ovarian Steroids

Influence of Menstrual Cycle Changes in Water Retention

It has been hypothesized that seizure activity may be exacerbated by water retention associated with the luteal phase of the menstrual cycle (Ansell & Clarke, 1956a). No support for this hypothesis has been found. Stitt and Kinnard (1968) administered desoxycorticosterone trimethylacetate to male rats to simulate a state of fluid retention that would resemble the water retention thought to occur premenstrually in women. They found no change in electroshock seizure threshold. Ansell and Clarke (1956a) measured body weight changes during the menstrual cycle in women with and without an unspecified catamenial seizure pattern. Degree of body weight change did not differ in the two groups. In addition, they found no correlation between seizure frequency and weight gain during a perimenstrual time period. Bäckström (1976) charted seizure frequency and changes in body weight in seven epileptic women and also found no relationship between body weight and seizure frequency.

Influence of Menstrual Cycle on Anticonvulsant Drug Level

It is possible that menstrual cycle changes in seizure frequency result, at least in part, from changes in the metabolism of antiepileptic drugs. Bäckström and Jorpes (1979) evaluated the stability of serum concentrations of AEDs (phenytoin, phenobarbitol, carbamazepine) during the menstrual cycle, and the association between the levels of AEDs and levels of estradiol and progesterone. The subjects included seven epileptic women for whom menstrual cycle changes associated with ovarian steroid levels had been documented (Bäckström, 1976). AEDs were stable throughout the menstrual cycle for five of the seven subjects. Neither of the other two subjects showed a drug level pattern associated with the menstrual cycle. No consistent correlations between AED and ovarian steroid levels were found. Bäckström and Jorpes (1979) concluded that the relationship between seizure frequency and plasma levels of ovarian steroids documented in a previous study (Bäckström, 1976) were not caused by changes in serum concentrations of antiepileptic medications.

Since then, three studies have found evidence that phenytoin levels fluctuate in relation to the menstrual cycle for (Kumar et al, 1988; Rościszewska et al., 1986; Shavit et al., 1984). These studies combined a group comparison design with a within subject design to assess menstrual cycle changes in phenytoin level during menses and during a presumed ovulatory time period in women with and without a perimenstrual increase in seizure frequency. Shavit et al. (1984) found that phenytoin levels were significantly lower during menses than during midcycle in both groups of women, but the degree of change was greater for patients with a catamenial seizure pattern. Kumar et al. (1988) also found a decline in phenytoin level in both groups, but the fall in drug level was statistically significant only for the group of women with a perimenstrual increase in seizure frequency. Rościszewska et al. (1986) found that phenytoin levels were consistently lower in women with a perimenstrual increase in seizures than in women with no menstrual cycle change in seizure frequency, but the group difference was statistically significant only on Day 28 of the menstrual cycle. There were no significant group differences in phenobarbitone level. Within-cycle changes in phenytoin and phenobarbitone level were not reported.

These studies suggest that altered metabolism of phenytoin, and perhaps other AEDs, may contribute to perimenstrual increases in seizure frequency. However, that fluctuations in phenytoin level generally stayed within therapeutic limits suggests that other factors also contribute to this type of catamenial seizure pattern (Bäckström & Jorpes, 1979; Kumar et al., 1988; Shavit et al., 1984).

The mechanisms that contribute to the decline in antiepileptic medications are not known fully, but the hepatic microsomal enzyme system has been implicated (Kumar et al., 1988; Shavit et al., 1984). This enzyme system is responsible for inactivation of ovarian steroid hormones and many of the AEDs (i.e., phenytoin, phenobarbitol, carbamazepine). Ovarian hormones may compete with AEDs, resulting in slowed inactivation of AEDs when hormone levels are high. Withdrawal of ovarian steroids in the late luteal phase may result in increased metabolism of antiseizure medications and, therefore, lower serum levels (Kumar et al., 1988; Shavit et al., 1984).

Influence of Menstrual Cycle Mood Changes on Seizure Frequency

Although the association between menstrual cycle mood changes and catamenial epilepsy largely has been ignored, there is suggestive evidence that women with significant perimenstrual mood changes are at an increased risk for seizures just prior to or during menses (Kamer, 1981; Rościszewska, 1980). For example, Kamer (1981) found that the degree of premenstrual negative mood significantly predicted the frequency of seizures during menstruation. In addition, Rościszewska (1980) reported that premenstrual tension was more common in women who had increased seizures during or just prior to menses (73%–84%), than in women with no catamenial seizure pattern (22%).

TREATMENT STRATEGIES

Modulation of Antiepileptic Drug Intake

Phenytoin levels may be lower during menses than during midcycle (Kumar et al., 1988; Shavit et al., 1984). In two investigations, a decline in phenytoin level was evident in patients without catamenial epilepsy, but was greater in women who had a perimenstrual increase in seizure frequency (Kumar et al., 1988; Shavit et al., 1984). Additional research is needed to determine if levels of other AEDs fluctuate in relation to the menstrual cycle. The modulation of AED levels during the menstrual cycle may a useful form of treatment for some patients with catamenial seizure patterns.

Diuretic Therapy

The diuretic acetazolamide (Diamox) has been suggested for the treatment of catamenial seizures (Ansell & Clarke, 1956b). Ansell and Clarke (1956b) reported improvement in three catamenial epilepsy patients treated with acetazolamide, but increasingly higher dosages were needed to maintain seizure control. A well-controlled investigation of acetazolamide as an adjunctive form of therapy has not been conducted. It is unlikely that diuretics are a useful form of therapy for catamenial seizure exacerbations, because water retention does not seem to contribute to perimenstrual increases in seizure frequency (Ansell & Clarke, 1956a; Bäckström, 1976).

Benzodiazepine Therapy

The benzodiazepine, clobazam, acts as an anticonvulsant (Allen et al., 1983; Gastaut & Low, 1979), but tolerance to its antiepileptic effects may develop with chronic treatment (Feely, 1983). Feely, Calvert, and Gibson (1982) suggested that intermittent clobazam therapy may control perimenstrual seizure exacerbation without the development of tolerance. In a placebo-controlled investigation, 14 of 18 patients had at least a 50% reduction in their perimenstrual seizures when clobazam was added to their antiepileptic medications (Feely et al., 1982). Clobazam was administered in doses of 20 or 30 mg per day during a 10-day perimenstrual time period that was individualized for each patient. Treatment began 2–4 days before the time period when seizure frequency increased. Long-term follow-up of 13 patients indicated that 9 benefitted from this form of therapy for time periods ranging from 6 months to 3½ years (Feely & Gibson, 1984). Side effects included increased seizure frequency between periods of clobazam therapy in three subjects and strong sedation in one subject. None of the subjects developed a tolerance to the antiepileptic effect of clobazam.

Progesterone Therapy

The strong experimental and clinical evidence of progesterone's anticonvulsant action suggests that progesterone may be a useful form of therapy for catamenial exacerbation of seizures. There are very few reports of the use of progesterone for the treatment of catamenial epilepsy. Logothetis et al. (1959) indicated that three out of five patients with catamenial seizure patterns improved on 10 mg of progesterone given three times a day, but they noted that the follow-up time period was not long enough to determine the utility of progesterone therapy. Herzog (1986) reported the successful use of progesterone therapy in a sample of women with complex partial seizures who had either anovulatory menstrual cycles or inadequate luteal phases. Subjects experienced exacerbation of seizures either prior to and during menses, during midcycle, or during the entire luteal phase. Natural progesterone suppositories were administered in dosages of 50–400 mg during the time periods when seizures were exacerbated, and progesterone dosages were adjusted to maintain luteal phase serum levels of 5–25 ng/ml. On average, seizure frequency decreased by 68%. Six of the eight women had fewer seizures with progesterone therapy. However, some of the subjects experienced an exacerbation of seizures each month following discontinuation of progesterone (Herzog, 1987). This effect was eliminated or greatly decreased when progesterone was tapered over 3 or 4 days, rather than discontinued abruptly (Herzog, 1986, 1987). Adverse side effects of progesterone overdosage included excessive fatigue, depression, and asthenia (Herzog, 1986). Additional possible side effects include weight gain, breast tenderness, and irregular vaginal bleeding (Herzog, 1991).

Progesterone therapy may be particularly appropriate for women who have a luteal phase deficiency (Herzog, 1986, 1991). Inadequate luteal phases are often, but not always, characterized by deficient progesterone production by the corpus luteum, whereas estrogen production is preserved (Goldstein et al., 1982; Jones, 1976; Sherman & Korenman, 1974). Under this circumstance, the estrogen/progesterone ratio is elevated during much of the menstrual cycle. Progesterone therapy will lower the estrogen to progesterone ratio, and therefore should be associated with a decrease in seizure frequency (Bäckström, 1976).

Women with catamenial epilepsy who do not have a reproductive endocrine disorder also may benefit from progesterone therapy (Herzog, 1991). However, a beneficial effect of natural progesterone only has been demonstrated for women with anovulatory menstrual cycles or inadequate luteal phases (Herzog, 1986). Further research is needed to determine the efficacy of this form of therapy in patients with no demonstrable reproductive endocrine disorder.

Synthetic Progestin Therapy

There have been case reports that oral synthetic progestins reduce seizure frequency in patients with catamenial seizure exacerbations (Groff, 1962; Hall, 1977). However, a double-blind, placebo-controlled clinical investigation found norethisterone was not effective in the control of seizures associated with the menstrual cycle (Dana-Haeri & Richens, 1983). There has been one case report that parenteral administration of medroxyprogesterone acetate significantly decreased seizure frequency in a patient with increased seizures during menses (Zimmerman, Holden, Reiter, & Dekaban, 1973).

Behavior Therapy

Behavioral strategies for reduction of seizure frequency may be useful for women with catamenial seizure patterns, because the likelihood that they will have a seizure is associated predictably with specific portions of the menstrual cycle. There have been no reports in the literature of behavioral treatment of catamenial epilepsy. A behavioral therapy approach to seizure reduction would include determination of an individual's seizure pattern, and may include the use of techniques such as progressive muscle relaxation, contingent relaxation, and biofeedback training (Dahl, Melin, & Lund, 1987; Mostofsky & Balaschak, 1977; Sterman, MacDonald, & Stone, 1974).

CONCLUSION

Seizure discontrol associated with the menstrual cycle is a clinically significant problem (Bäckström et al., 1984; Herzog, 1991; Mattson & Cramer, 1985) for which few interventions are available.

Methodologic problems make it difficult to determine the prevalence of menstrual cycle changes in seizure frequency. It is possible that the menstrual cycle influences seizure threshold for a large proportion of women with epileptic seizures that are not well controlled by traditional antiepileptic medications.

Visual inspection of seizure diaries only will facilitate selection of women with very dramatic catamenial seizure patterns. Statistical evaluation of well-defined segments of the menstrual cycle is needed to determine the proportion of women who have more subtle changes in seizure frequency associated with the menstrual cycle.

The majority of research has focused on the hypothesis that seizure frequency increases during a perimenstrual time period. A review of the likely mechanisms contributing to catamenial seizure patterns suggests that seizure frequency may fluctuate in relation to other segments of the menstrual cycle. Additional research is needed to define more accurately the time periods when seizure frequency is likely to decrease, as well as time periods when women may be at increased risk for seizures. Future studies also should consider the possibility that the menstrual cycle may influence the degree of spread from seizure foci.

The etiology of catamenial epilepsy seems to be directly or indirectly associated with changes in ovarian hormone levels during the menstrual cycle. Both estrogen and progesterone seem to play a role such that estrogen has an excitatory influence on seizure activity and progesterone has an opposite effect.

It is not known why some women are more affected by changes in the ovarian steroids than other women. Possibly important discriminating variables include the type of epilepsy and seizures, location of seizure foci, types of antiepileptic medications, levels and rates of change of ovarian steroids, and degree of perimenstrual mood change.

Very little research has addressed the development of treatment strategies for catamenial epilepsy. At present, potential treatment approaches include modulation of antiepileptic drug levels to minimize fluctuations related to the menstrual cycle, intermittent clobazam or progesterone therapy, and perhaps behavior therapy. Additional research in this area should address the likely mechanisms that contribute to catamenial seizure patterns. One possibility involves the use of the reduced metabolites of progesterone (Bäckström et al., 1984).

ACKNOWLEDGMENTS

This chapter was supported in part by the Research Foundation for Mental Hygiene Biomedical Research Support Program, the Epilepsy Foundation of America, the American Epilepsy Society, and the New York State Department of Mental Hygiene.

REFERENCES

Allen, J. W., Oxley, J., Robertson, M. M., Trimble, M. R., Richens, A., & Jaward, S. M. (1983). Clobazam as adjunctive treatment in refractory epilepsy. *British Medical Journal, 286,* 1246–1247.

Almqvist, R. (1955). The rhythm of epileptic attacks and its relationship to the menstrual cycle. *Acta Psychiatrica Scandanavica, 30,* 1–116.

Ansell, B., & Clarke, E. (1956a). Epilepsy and menstruation: The role of water retention. *Lancet, 2,* 1232–1235.

Ansell, B., & Clarke, E. (1956b). Acetazolamide in treatment of epilepsy. *British Medical Journal, 1,* 650–654.

Bäckström, T. (1976). Epileptic seizures in women in relation to variations of plasma estrogen and progesterone during the menstrual cycle. *Acta Neurologica Scandanavica, 54,* 321–347.

Bäckström, T., & Jorpes, P. (1979). Serum phenytoin, phenobarbitol, carbamazepine, albumin; and plasma estradiol, progesterone concentrations during the menstrual cycle in women with epilepsy. *Acta Neurologica Scandanavica, 59,* 63–71.

Bäckström, T., Landgren, S., Zetterlund, B., Blom, S., Dubrovsky, B., Bixo, M., & Södergård, R. (1984). Effect of ovarian steroid hormones on brain excitability and their relation to epilepsy seizure variation during the menstrual cycle. In R. J. Porter, A. A. Ward, Jr., R. H. Mattson, & M. Dam, M. (Eds.), *Advances in epileptology: XVth Epilepsy International Symposium* (pp. 269–277). New York: Raven Press.

Bandler, B., Kaufman, I. C., Dykens, J. W., Schleifer, M., & Shapiro, L. N. (1957). Seizures and the menstrual cycle. *American Journal of Psychiatry, 113,* 704–708.

Belelli, D., Bolger, M. B., & Gee, K. W. (1989). Anticonvulsant profile of the progesterone metabolite 5α-pregnan-3α-OH-20-one. *European Journal of Pharmacology, 166,* 325–329.

Belelli, D., Lan, N. C., & Gee, K. W. (1990). Anticonvulsant steroids and the GABA/benzodiazepine receptor-chloride ionophore complex. *Neuroscience and Behavioral Reviews, 14,* 315–322.

Bonuccelli, U., Melis, G. B., Paoletti, A. M., Fioretti, P., Murri, L., & Muratorio, A. (1989). Unbalanced progesterone and estradiol secretion in catamenial epilepsy. *Epilepsy Research, 3,* 100–106.

Buterbaugh, G. G. (1989). Estradiol replacement facilitates the acquisition of seizures kindled from the anterior neocortex in female rats. *Epilepsy Research, 4,* 207–215.

Canick, J. A., Vaccaro, D. E., Livingston, E. M., Leeman, S. E., Ryan, K. J., & Fox, T. O. (1986). Localization of aromatose and 5α-reductase to neuronal and non-neuronal cells in the fetal rat hypothalamus. *Brain Research, 372,* 277–282.

Conney, A. H. (1967). Pharmacological implications of microsomal enzyme induction. *Pharmacological Reviews, 19,* 317–366.

Craig, C. R. (1966). Anticonvulsant activity of steroids: Separability of anticonvulsant from hormonal effects. *Journal of Pharmacology and Experimental Therapy, 53,* 337–343.

Cutler, W. B., & Garcia, C. R. (1980). The psychonueroendocrinology of the ovulatory cycle of women: A review. *Psychoneuroendocrinology, 5,* 89–111.

Dahl, J., Melin, L., & Lund, L. (1987). Effect of a contingent relaxation treatment program on adults with refractory epileptic seizures. *Epilepsia, 28,* 125–132.

Dana-Haeri, J., & Richens, A. (1983). Effect of norethistrone on seizures associated with menstruation. *Epilepsia, 24,* 377–381.

Dickerson, W. W. (1941). The effect of menstruation on seizure incidence. *Journal of Nervous and Mental Disease, 94,* 160–169.

Feely, M. (1983). Long-term use of clobazam in refractory epilepsy. *IRCS Journal of Medical Science, 152,* 83.

Feely, M., Calvert, R., & Gibson, J. (1982). Clobazam in catamenial epilepsy: A model for evaluating anticonvulsants. *Lancet, 2,* 71–73.

Feely, M., & Gibson, J. (1984). Intermittent clobezam for catamenial epilepsy: Tolerance avoided. *Journal of Neurology, Neurosurgery, and Psychiatry, 47,* 1279–1282.

Gastaut, J., & Low, M. D. (1979). Antiepileptic properties of clobezam, a 1-5 benzodiazepine in man. *Epilepsia, 20,* 437–446.

Gee, K. W. (1988). Steroid modulation of the GABA/benzodiaepine receptor-linked chloride ionophore. *Molecular Neurobiology, 2,* 291–317.

Gee, K. W., Chang, W.-C., Brinton, R. E., & McEwen, B. S. (1987). GABA-dependent modulation of the Cl-ionophore by steroids in rat brain. *European Journal of Pharmacology, 136,* 419–423.

Goldstein, D., Zuckerman, H., Harpaz, S., Barkai, J., Geva, A., Gordon, S., Shalev, E., & Schwartz, M. (1982). Correlation between estradiol and progesterone in cycles with luteal phase deficiency. *Fertility and Sterility, 37,* 348–354.

Gordon, A. (1909). Epilepsy in its relation to menstrual periods. A study of twenty-three cases. *New York Medical Journal, 90,* 733–735.

Gordon, G. S. (1956). Hormones and metabolism: Influence of steroids on cerebral metabolism in man. *Recent Progress in Hormone Research, 12,* 153.

Groff, D. N. (1962). Suggestions for control of epilepsy (Letter). *New York Medical Journal, 62,* 3017.

Gueirreiro, C. A. M., & Ramos, M. C. (1991). Premenstrual seizure increase: Influence of age, duration of disease, seizure frequency, previous complaint of premenstrual accentuation, EEG, and CT scan findings. *Arquivos de Neuro-Psiquiatria, 49,* 27–32.

Gyermek, L., Genther, G., & Flemming, N. (1967). Some effects of progesterone and related steroids on the central nervous system. *International Journal of Neuropharmacology, 6,* 191–198.

Gyermek, L., Iriarte, J., & Crabbe, P. (1968). Structure-activity relationship of some steroidal hypnotic agents. *Journal of Medical Chemistry, 11,* 117–125.

Hall, S. M. (1977). Treatment of menstrual epilepsy with a progesterone-only oral contraceptive. *Epilsepsia, 18,* 235–236.

Harrison, N. L., Majewska, M. D., Harrington, J. W., & Barker, J. L. (1987). Structure-activity relationships for steroid interaction with the gamma-amniobutyric acid-A receptor complex. *Journal of Pharmacology and Experimental Therapy, 241,* 346–353.

Herzog, A. G. (1986). Intermittent progesterone therapy and frequency of complex partial seizures in women with menstrual disorders. *Neurology, 36,* 1607–1610.

Herzog, A. G. (1987). Progesterone in seizure therapy [Reply to the author]. *Neurology, 37,* 1433.

Herzog, A. G. (1991). Reproductive endocrine considerations and hormonal therapy for women with epilepsy. *Epilepsia, 32* (Suppl. 6). S27–S33.

Hom, A. C., & Buterbaugh, G. G. (1986). Estrogen alters the acquisition of seizures kindled by repeated amygdala stimulation or pentylenetetrazol administration in ovarectomized female rats. *Epilepsia, 27,* 103–108.

Jacono, J. J., & Robertson, J. M. (1987). The effects of estrogen, progesterone, and ionized calcium on seizures during the menstrual cycle of epileptic women. *Epilepsia, 28,* 571–577.

Jones, G. S. (1976). The luteal phase defect. *Fertility and Sterility, 27,* 351–356.

Julien, R. M., Fowler, G. W., & Danielson, M. G. (1975). The effects of antiepileptic drugs on estrogen-induced electrographic spike-wave discharge. *Journal of Pharmacology, 193,* 647–656.

Kamer, J. (1981). Epilepsy and the menstrual cycle. *Dissertation Abstracts International, 42,* 423.

Karavolas, H. J., Bertics, P. I., Wodges, D., & Rudie, N. (1984). Progesterone processing by neuroendocrine structures. In F. Celotti, F. Naftolin, & L. Martin (Eds.), *Metabolism of hormonal steroids in the neuroendocrine structures* (pp. 149–170). New York: Raven Press.

Krieger, N., & Scott, R. G. (1984). 3α-hyroxy steroid oxidoreductase in rat brain. *Journal of Neurochemistry, 52,* 887–890.

Krieger, N., & Scott, R. G. (1989). Non-neuronal localization for steroid converting enzyme: 3α-hyroxy steroid oxidoreductase in olfactory tubercle of rat brain. *Journal of Neurochemistry, 52,* 1866–1870.

Kumar, N., Behari, M., Ahuja, G. K., & Jailkhaui, B. L. (1988). Phenytoin levels in catamenial epilepsy. *Epilepsia, 29,* 155–158.

Laidlaw, J. (1956). Catamenial epilepsy. *Lancet, 2,* 1235–1237.

Landgren, S., Aasly, J., Bäckström, T., Dubrovsky, B., & Danielson, E. (1987). The effect of progesterone and its metabolites on the interictal epileptiform discharge in the cat's cerebral cortex. *Acta Physiologica Scandanavica, 131,* 33–42.

Landgren, S., Bäckström, T., & Kalistratov, G. (1978). The effect of progesterone on the spontaneous interictal spike evoked by the application of penicillin to the cat's cerebral cortex. *Journal of Neurological Sciences, 36,* 119–133.

Logothetis, I., Harner, R., Morell, F., & Torres, F. (1959). The role of estrogens in catamenial exacerbation of epilepsy. *Neurology, 9,* 352–360.

Majewska, M., Harrison, N., Schwartz, R., Barker, J., & Paul, S. (1986). Steroid hormone metabolites are barbituate-like modulators of the GABA receptor. *Science, 232,* 1004–1007.

Marcus, E. M., Watson, C. W., & Goldman, P. I. (1966). Effects of steroids on cerebral electrical activity. *Archives of Neurology, 15,* 521–532.

Martin, J. B., Reichlin, S., & Brown, G. M. (1977). *Clinical neuroendocrinology.* Philadelphia: F. A. Davis.

Mattson, R. H., & Cramer, J. A. (1985). Epilepsy, sex hormones and antiepileptic drugs. *Epilepsia, 26(Suppl 1),* S40–S51.

Mattson, R. H., Kamer, J. A., Cramer, J. A., & Caldwell, B. V. (1981). Seizure frequency and the menstrual cycle: A clinical study. *Epilepsia, 22,* 242.

Mattson, R. H., Lerner, E., & Dix, G. (1974). Precipitating and inhibiting factors in epilepsy: A statistical study. *Epilepsia, 15,* 271–272.

McQueen, J. K., & Woodbury, D. M. (1975). Attempts to produce spike-and-wave complexes in the electrocorticogram of the rat. *Epilepsia, 16,* 295–300.

Merryman, W., Boiman, R., Barner, L., & Rothchild, I. (1954). Progesterone 'anesthesia' in human subjects. *Journal of Clinical Endocrinology and Metabolism, 14,* 1567–1569.

Mishell, D. R., Nakamura, R. M., Grosignani, P. G., Stone, S., Kharma, K., Nagata, Y., & Thorneycroft, I. (1971). Serum gonadotropin and steroid patterns during the normal menstrual cycle. *American Journal of Obstetrics and Gynecology, 111,* 60–65.

Morrow, A. L., Suzdak, P. D., & Paul, S. M. (1987). Steroid hormone metabolites potentiate GABA receptor-mediated chloride ion flux with nanomolar potency. *European Journal of Pharmocology, 142,* 483–485.

Mostofsky, D. I., & Balaschak, B. A. (1977). Psychobiological control of seizures. *Psychological Bulletin, 84,* 723–750.

Murri, L., Bonuccelli, U., & Mellis, G. B. (1986). Neuroendocrine evaluation in catamenial epilepsy. *Functional Neurology, 1,* 399–406.

Narbone, M. C., Ruello, C., Oliva, A., Baviera, G., D'Amico, D., Bramanti, P., & Perri, R. (1990). Hormonal disregulation and catamenial epilepsy. *Functional Neurology, 5,* 49–53.

Newmark, M. E. (1989). Catamenial epilepsy: A neurologic myth persisting for more than 100 years [Abstract]. *Epilepsia, 30,* 704.

Newmark, M. E., & Penry, J. K. (1980). Catamenial epilepsy: A review. *Epilepsia, 21,* 281–300.

Pfaff, D. J., & McEwen, B. S. (1983). Actions of estrogens and progestins on nerve cells. *Science, 219,* 808–814.

Richens, A. (1984). Enzyme induction and sex hormones. In R. J. Porter, A. A. Ward, Jr., R. H. Mattson, & Dam, M. (Eds.), *Advances in epileptology: XVth Epilepsy International Symposium* (pp. 215–220). New York: Raven Press.

Rościszewska, D. (1980). Analysis of seizure dispersion during menstrual cycle in women with epilepsy. *Monographs in Neural Sciences, 5,* 280–284.

Rościszewska, D., Buntner, B., Guz, I., & Zawisza, L. (1986). Ovarian hormones, anticonvulsant drugs, and seizures during the menstrual cycle in women with epilepsy. *Journal of Neurology, Neurosurgery and Psychiatry, 49,* 47–51.

Ross, G. T., Cargelle, C. M., Lipsett, M. D., Rayford, P. L., Marshall, J. R., Strott, C. A., & Rodbard, D. (1970). Pituitary and gonadal hormones in women during spontaneous and induced ovulatory cycles. *Recent Progress in Hormone Research, 26,* 1–62.

Sánchez Longo, L. P., & González Saldaña, L. E. (1966). Hormones and their influence in epilepsy. *Acta Neurologica Latin America, 12,* 29–47.

Schechter, D., Labar, D. R., Pedley, T. A., Ottman, R., & Endicott, J. (1989). Influence of the menstrual cycle on seizures [Abstract]. *Epilepsia, 30,* 704–705.

Selye, H. (1942). The antagonism between anesthetic steroid hormones and pentamethylenetetrazol (Metrazol). *Journal of Laboratory and Clinical Medicine, 27,* 1051–1059.

Shavit, G., Lerman, P., Korczyn, A. D., Kivity, S., Bechar, M., & Gitter, S. (1984). Phenytoin pharmacokinetics in catamenial epilepsy. *Neurology, 34,* 959–961.

Sherman, B. M., & Korenman, S. G. (1974). Measurement of serum LH, FSH, estradiol and progesterone in disorders of the human menstrual cycle: The inadequate luteal phase. *Journal of Clinical Endocrinology and Metabolism, 39,* 145–149.

Smith, S. S., Waterhouse, B. D., & Woodward, D. J. (1987). Locally applied progesterone metabolites alter neuronal responsiveness in the cerebellum. *Brain Research Bulletin, 18,* 739–747.

Sterman, M. B., MacDonald, L. R., & Stone, R. K. (1974). Biofeedback training of the sensorimotor electroencephalogram rhythm in man: Effects on epilepsy. *Epilepsia, 15,* 395–416.

Stitt, S. L., & Kinnard, W. J. (1968). The effects of certain progestins and estrogen on the threshold of electrically induced seizure patterns. *Neurology, 18,* 213–216.

Swanson, T. H., & Phillis, J. W. (1987). Progesterone in seizure therapy [Letter]. *Neurology, 37,* 1433.

Tauboll, E., Lundervold, A., & Gjerstad, L. (1991). Temporal distribution of seizures in epilepsy. *Epilepsy Research, 8,* 153–165.

Treloar, A. E., Boynton, R. E., & Behn, B. G. (1967). Variation of the human menstrual cycle through productive life. *International Journal of Fertility, 21,* 844–853.

Turner, C. D., & Bagnara, J. T. (1976). *General endocrinology.* Philadelphia: W. B. Saunders.

Vaitukaitis, J. L. (1984). Premenstrual syndrome. *The New England Journal of Medicine, 311,* 1371–1373.

Vaitukaitis, J. L., & Ross, G. T. (1976). Clinical studies of gonadotropins in the female. *Pharmacology and Therapeutics, Part C, 1,* 317–329.

Woolley, D. E., & Timiras, P. S. (1962a). The gonad-brain relationship: Effects of female sex hormones on electroshock convulsions in the rat. *Endocrinology, 70,* 196–209.

Woolley, D. E., & Timiras, P. S. (1962b). Estrous and circadian periodicity and electroshock convulsions in rats. *American Journal of Physiology, 202,* 379–382.

Yussman, M. A., & Taymor, M. L. (1970). Serum levels of follicle stimulating hormone and leutinizing hormone and of plasma progesterone related to ovulation by corpus luteum biopsy. *Journal of Clinical Endocrinology and Metabolism, 30,* 396–399.

Zimmerman, A. W., Holden, K. R., Reiter, E. O., & Dekaban, A. S. (1973). Medroxyprogesterone acetate in the treatment of seizures associated with menstruation. *The Journal of Pediatrics, 83,* 959–963.

8 Neuroactive Steroids and Epilepsy

Michael S. Myslobodsky
Tel-Aviv University

Gonadal and adrenal steroids have a pivotal role in a wide range of behavioral phenomena such as sexual behavior and aggression, impregnation, pregnancy, birth, maternal behavior, anxiety, sleep, coordination of the neuroendocrine response to stress, and adaptation to environmental challenges. They play a key role in the regulation of cell development, conservation of body sodium and carbohydrate metabolism, and so forth. The failure of any or several of these functions may be sufficient to contribute to epilepsy. By the same token, many of them might be conceived of as being a part of an endogenous machinery directed at stabilizing brain reactivity. Among the more celebrated examples are the proconvulsant potency of estrogens, as well as certain anticonvulsive influences of progesterone and deoxycorticosterone metabolites that were long reproduced in experimental animals (Heuser, Ling, & Buchwald, 1965; Michael, 1965; Timiras, 1969; Woodbury, 1952; Woolley & Timiras, 1962a, 1962b). There are numerous indications of a cyclic exacerbation of adverse emotional disturbances, somatic discomfort, and seizures in females known as catamenial epilepsy (Newmark & Penry, 1980; Schechter, chapter 7, this volume). The enhanced photosensitivity and episodes of petit mal epilepsy also are occasionally subject to catamenial exacerbations (Newmark & Penry, 1979), thereby suggesting the contribution of the ovarian steroids (Rosciszewska, Buntner, Guz, & Zawisza, 1986). Yet, until very recently, no firm conclusion could be drawn regarding the nature of these effects.

Beach (1948) argued that gonadal steroids alter thresholds of synaptic events in the central nervous system. Since that time, a myriad of papers—some of them dealing with pro- and anticonvulsant effects of steroids—appeared in support of that hunch. But how is this achieved? Although steroids greatly enhance the traffic of stimuli traveling through the vastly interconnected circuits governing reproductive behavior, including the limbic system and brainstem (Pfaff, 1989), general elevation of excitatory drive is insufficient to account for the development of seizures. To the contrary, it may as well have an opposite, anticonvulsant effect, acting through other neurotransmitter systems that are implicated in epilepsy. Steroids could interact with numerous enzymatic reactions and affect the synthesis of enzyme proteins from precursors. The potent interactions of steroids with dopaminergic (Maus, Premont, & Glowinski, 1990) or norepinephrinergic neurotransmission (Axelrod, 1974; Iversen, 1971) are among such examples.

Steroids are highly lipophilic substances that might cause epileptogenic action through nonspecific alterations of lipid membranes that affect the rate by which they and other substances permeate. In this capacity, they could alter the excitability thresholds of neural, muscular, and glandular cells. Yet certain structural constraints for the central action of the steroid molecules are obvious. For example, their depressive activity required the presence of 5α- or 5β-reduced steroid A ring and a 3α-hydroxyl group; 3β-hydroxysteroids may be less ineffective (Gee, 1988), suggesting that steroid lipophilicity is an important, but not the only mechanism determining their action.

Authoritative textbooks state that steroids trigger a cascade of events initiated by protein receptors in the cytosole, which lead to genomic effects with consequent alterations of complex behaviors through the induction of the biosynthesis of proteins, hormones, and neurotransmitters. This lengthy process may take hours, and even days. This length is consistent with a classical view that steroids affect neuronal functions via their action on the genome (McEwen, Coirini, & Schumacher, 1990; McEwen, Denef, Gerlach, & Plapinger, 1974). However, it appears that pro- and anticonvulsant effects of steroids happen within seconds or a few minutes after they are administered. These central nongenomic interactions, discovered for a number of naturally occurring reduced metabolites of progestens, androgens, and corticoids, were defined as *neuroactive* (Paul & Purdy, 1992). The neuroactive potency of steroids has become a focus of growing attention within the last decade, after it was discovered that γ-aminobutyric acid (GABA) receptor is a physiological target for naturally occurring steroids (Belelli, Lan, & Gee, 1990; Majewska, Harrison, Swartz, Baker, & Paul, 1986; Paul & Purdy, 1992).

Based on this evidence, it was shown that there exists an unambiguous biochemical, molecular biological, and electrophysiological framework applicable to the clinical experience with which the central effects of steroids could be more easily understood. In this chapter, I discuss some examples of pro- and anticonvulsant effects of steroids. The reader interested in more detailed information on molecular and biochemical machinery of their action is referred to the papers cited in the text and, in particular, to the reviews by Belelli, Lan, & Gee (1990), Majewska (1987b), Miller (1992), Paul and Purdy (1992), and Gee (1988).

GABA AND NEUROACTIVE STEROIDS

The relevance of GABA to the central effects of steroids was long perceived as plausible. Bilateral adrenalectomy was shown to produce increased [^{3}H]GABA binding sites, whereas corticosterone treatment opposed the change (Kendall, McEwan, & Enna, 1982). GABA content in the amygdala and septum was decreased following castration of rats, and such changes were antagonized by testosterone or estradiol (Early & Lenard, 1978). GABA antagonists (bicuculline, picrotoxin) administered intracerebroventricularly appear to stimulate ACTH release in rats with deafferented medio-basal hypothalamus, and the effect is antagonized by a coadministration of GABA (Makara & Stark, 1978). Some ACTH-analogues or corticosterone were shown to decrease brain GABA content in rats and mice (Leonard, 1974; Sadasivudu, Rao, & Murthy, 1977). There were numerous other examples indicating that GABA-steroid bonds accompany us literally *ab ovo usque ad mala*. The ovaries have a high affinity uptake system for GABA (Erdo, 1983). The oviduct in the rat has GABA level twice as high as that of the brain (del Rio, 1981). These and other findings point to a profound involvement of GABA in neuroendocrine regulation (DeFeudis, 1984). Yet, the nature of this coupling remained obscure, perhaps because the issue was the effect of GABA and GABAergic substances on different hormones and/or hormonally dependent mechanisms, rather than hormonal effects on the system of GABAergic neurotransmission.

The first tangible clue to the mystery of the GABA-steroid coupling was provided when a potent sedative pregnane steroid, alphaxalone (3α-hydroxy-5α-pregnane-11,20-dione), was observed to augment effects of GABA and its agonists in the preparation of the rat cuneate nucleus (Harrison & Simmonds, 1984). It was shown that A-ring reduced metabolites of progesterone and deoxycorticosterone (pregnanolone; 3β-hydrox-5α-pregnan-20-one, and THDOC; 3α, 21-dihydroxy-5α-pregnan-20-one) potentiated benzodiazepine and muscimol binding (Harrison, Majewska, Harrington, & Baker, 1987; Majewska et al., 1986). These findings, seen in the context of GABAergic effects of benzodiazepines and barbiturates, helped to unveil the nature of the hypnotic potency of steroids, established over 50 years ago by Selye (1941). The question remained as to how GABA, a ubiquitous neurotransmitter, could mediate the entire spectrum of highly specialized actions of various steroids at its multiple target sites.

Only recently it appeared possible to reconcile the multitude of steroid effects with the structure of the $GABA_A$ receptor. The latter is being recognized as a complex hetero-oligomeric, membrane-bound protein. Molecular genetic techniques showed that the $GABA_A$ receptor is composed of a family of subunits (α1 to α6, β1 to β3, γ1 to γ3, δ, ρ) (Schofield, Shivers, & Seeburg, 1990). Each family is characterized by diverse extra- and intraneuronal domains, so that there may be a great number of receptors subtypes present in different brain areas.

GABA, or its agonists, cause depression of cellular excitability by prolonging

Cl^- ion conductance. Some modulators of the GABA receptor interact directly with the Cl^- ionophore, such as agonists (e.g., barbiturates) or antagonists (e.g., picrotoxin). Figure 8.1 demonstrates that the Cl^- channel is labeled by still another convulsant, structurally related to picrotoxinin, *t*-[^{35}S]-butyl bicyclophosphorothionate ([^{35}S]TBPS) that also binds preferentially to a convulsant site at or near the Cl^- channel associated with the $GABA_A$ receptor. Benzodiazepines, barbiturates, and a variety of antiepileptic agents cause sedative, anxiolytic, pro-, and anticonvulsant effects through their interaction with a number of such binding sites. Steroids apparently have their own steroid recognition site

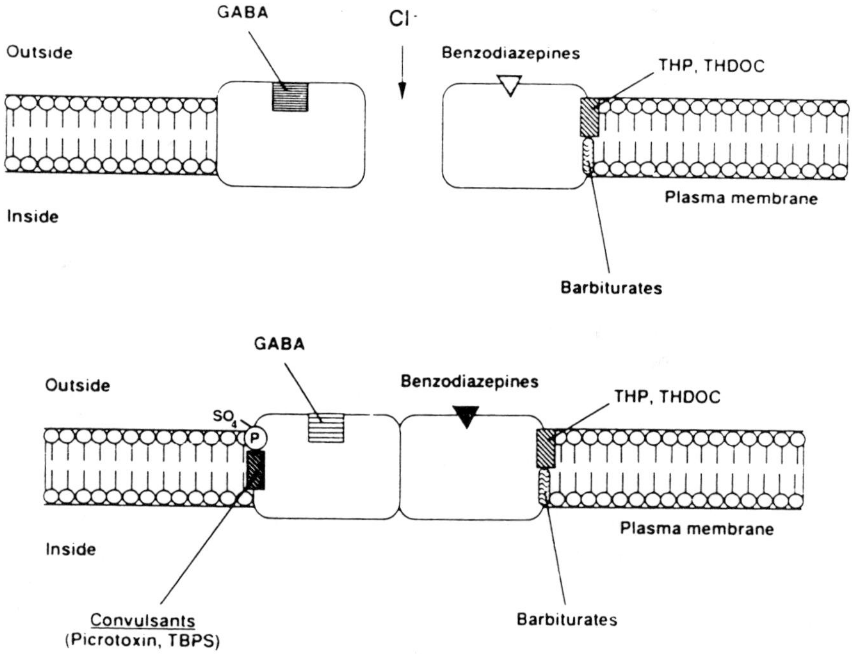

FIG. 8.1. Possible sites of steroid interaction with the $GABA_A$ receptor. THP-tetrahydroprogesterone, 5α-pregnan-3α-ol-20-one; THDOC-tetrahydrodeoxycorticosterone, 5α-pregnane-3α,21-diol-20-one; P-SO_4-pregnenolone sulphate. THP and THDOC affect the chloride channel like anesthetic barbiturates (upper diagram), whereas P-SO_4 closes the channel like the convulant picrotoxin (lower diagram). From "Steroid Regulation of the $GABA_A$ Receptor: Ligand Binding, Chloride Transport and Behavior" by M. D. Majewska, 1990, In D. Chadwick & K. Widdows (Eds.), *Ciba Foundation Symposium 153. Steroids and Neuronal Activity*. Chichester: Wiley. Copyright 1990 by John Wiley & Sons, Inc.

of the receptor (Fig. 8.1), which also seems to exist in a number of different forms (Belelli et al., 1990; Paul & Purdy, 1992).

The modulation specificity of $GABA_A$ receptor is determined by expression of its various subunits and their combinations, which make the receptor sensitive to either barbiturates, benzodiazepines, or steroids. Studies by Paul and associates (Majewska et al., 1986; Paul & Purdy, 1992) recognized that hypnotic steroids (allopregnenolone and allotetrahydroDOC) are barbiturate-like by biochemical and electrophysiological criteria. They enhanced the binding of [^{3}H]benzodiazepines to $GABA_A$ receptor in a manner similar to anesthetic barbiturates; they potentiated (in submicromolar concentration) GABA-activated Cl^- conductance and directly stimulated the latter when given in μM concentrations. A number of recently examined pregnane steroids appear to cause sedative effects through their interaction with a novel regulatory site on the membrane-bound GABA receptor. Intracellular application of steroids appears to activate no receptor changes (Lambert, Peters, Sturgess, & Hales, 1990).

The potentiation of GABA-related neurotransmission is conceived to be a therapeutically desirable goal, because GABAergic compounds are viewed as potential anticonvulsants (Meldrum, 1975). In fact, sedative steroids often exhibit significant antiepileptic activity in a number of epilepsy models. Progesterone, and especially some of its 5α-reduced metabolites (3α-hydroxy-5β- and 5α-pregnan-20-one), appear to be active in controlling penicillin-induced focal spiking in the cat cerebral cortex (Landgren, Aasly, Backstrom, Dubrovksy, & Danielson, 1987). Surprisingly, pregnanolone was found to be effective against metrazol-, bicuculline-, and pictrotoxin-induced generalized convulsions, but *not* against tonic-clonic seizures elicited by maximal electroshock (Belelli, Bol ger, & Gee, 1989). The hypnotic and antiepileptic effects do not have an obligatory coupling (Belelli et al., 1989) so that the hypnotic potency of a steroid does not guarantee *ipso facto* its anticonvulsant action (File & Simmonds, 1988).

EXCITATORY STEROIDS: EFFECTS OF THE AMIDINE STEROID, RU5135

Ajmone-Marsan (1969) cautioned that, in dealing with focal epilepsy, it is important to maintain a careful distinction between the latent condition of enhanced excitability (vulnerability factor) and overt episodes of stereotypic manifestations of the focus. Despite the proliferation of experimental models, there remains a gap between a variety of laboratory forms of the focus and the focal forms of human epilepsy. There is still little understanding of how the continuous operation of silent, but susceptible neurons would eventually unite into inflamable aggregates generating epileptic spikes. The effects of excitatory steroids seem to aid in the understanding of how this process may be set in motion by a gradual or episodic increase in the level of a naturally occurring ligand, which acts antagonistically to the $GABA_A$ receptor-coupled Cl^- channel. There is an excitatory steroid—pregnenolone sulfate—that, like other 3β-hydroxy-Δ5-steroids, was termed *neurosteroid* (Baulieu & Robel, 1984), now a name for a class of steroids synthesized de novo in the brain. Using fresh crude synaptosomal preparation of the rat forebrain, Majewska and Schwartz (1987) established that pregnenolone sulphate at low micromolar concentrations interacts with $GABA_A$ receptor in a picrotoxin-like fashion. It binds competitively to convulsant, [^{35}S]TBPS recognition site, and inhibits GABA-activated Cl^- transport in synaptoneurosomes. Pregnenalone sulphate injected cerebroventricularly or even I.P. to pentobarbital-anesthetized Fisher-344 rats significantly shortened the sleep time (Majewska, Bluet-Pajot, Robel, & Baulieu, 1989). Another steroid, sulphate of dihydroepiandrosterone, also showed GABA-antagonistic potency (Majewska & Schwartz, 1987). However, [^{3}H]pregnenalone binding was inhibited by dihydroepiandrosterone sulphate, whereas [^{35}S]TBPS was not, thereby suggesting that the two may not interact at the same receptor site.

Unlike pregnenolone sulfate, glucocorticoids and their metabolites also might reduce seizure thresholds by allosterically increasing the affinity of GABA-antagonistic type ligands for TBPS sites. Thus, cortisol, tetrahydrocortisol (3α, 11β, 17,21-tetrahydroxy-5β-pregnan-20-one) and tetrahydrocortisone (3α,17,21-trihydroxy-5β-pregnane-11,20-dione), at nanomolar concentrations, potentiated [^{35}S]TBPS binding at 50% over control values (Majewska, 1987a). Corticosterone, cortisone as well as tetrahydrocorticosterone (3α, 11β,21-trihydroxy-5β-pregnane-20-one) appeared to be much weaker, augmenting [^{35}S]TBPS binding at the level of 20% above control values. By comparison, bicuculline increased [^{35}S]TBPS binding in synaptosomes by 150% above control (Majewska, 1987a). Similar to glucocorticoids and bicuculline, the addition of RU5135 to rat brain P_2 membranes augments specific [^{35}S]TBPS binding by 10%–20% (Squires, Casida, Richardson, & Saederup, 1983).

A synthetic steroid, 3α-hydroxy-16-imino-5β-17aza androstan-11-one (RU5135), described a decade ago (Hunt & Clements-Jewery, 1981) is another example of a compound that could have been misperceived for a sedative with epileptogenic properties. Figure 8.2 shows that it is characterized by an amidine function in ring D and the hydroxyl group in α-configuration. The steroid would not be expected to have hormonal activity in the absence of 3-keto formulation, 4,5-double bond, and hydroxyl function at C-11 and C-17. RU5135 appeared to be a uniquely potent $GABA_A$ receptor antagonist, with an affinity for $GABA_A$ receptor about 500 times greater than a reference GABA-receptor antagonist, bicuculline (Hunt & Clements-Jewery, 1981). Also, RU5135, although a highly potent antagonist at the $GABA_A$ receptor, is a more potent antagonist at the glycine receptor (Curtis & Malik, 1985; Hunt & Clements-Jewery, 1981). Yet, in an exploratory trial in mice, RU5135 showed a depressant-hypnotic action (Boaventura & Boissier, 1978). Based on that effect and my previous experience, I

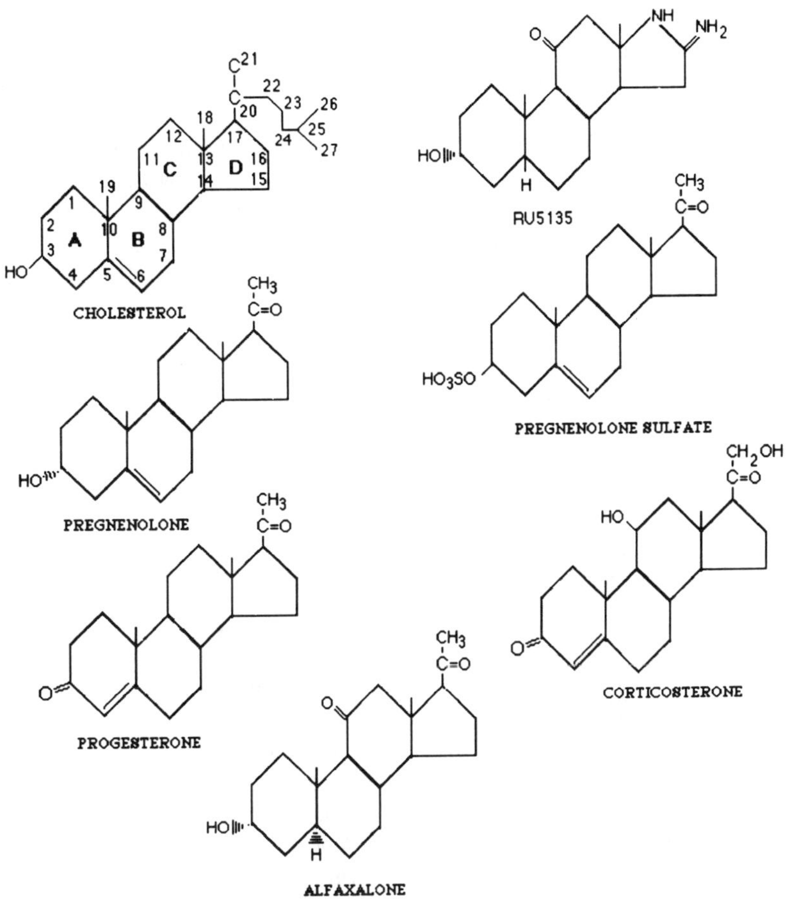

FIG. 8.2. Steroid amidine RU5135 shown in comparison with several other neuroactive steroids mentioned in the text to emphasize structure-activity relationships. The precursor of all adrenocortical steroid hormones, cholesterol, is shown to illustrate the numbering system of individual carbons of the cyclopentanoperhydrophenathren structure. Side chain bonds are represented by dotted lines indicating projection below the place of the ring (α-configuration); solid lines of the side chains denote β-configuration (projection in front of the ring plane).

expected that RU5135 would cause behavioral sedation accompanied by wave-spikes in the EEG, similar to those seen after the systemic administration of another $GABA_A$ antagonist, picrotoxin (Myslobodsky & Valenstein, 1980). However, within a period of 5–30 min, RU5135 administered to waking Wistar rats with implanted electrodes caused reduced motility and ataxic gait, which was followed by and coexisted with a lasting period of epileptic spikes (Myslobodsky & Kofman, 1982). The reduced motility and/or ataxia must have been mistaken by Boaventura and Boissier (1978) for hypnotic effect inasmuch as epileptiform motor manifestations following RU5135 administration are meager (Myslobodsky & Kofman, 1982). Several years later, Myslobodsky, Mintz, Tarrasch and Bar-Ziv (1991) replicated that study, only to show that there was no sign of synchronous waves, let alone wave-spike complexes, in the resting EEG after steroid amidine in both rats and rabbits.

The nature of motor toxicity, heralding, and overlapping with steroid amidine spikes remains uncertain. Systemically administered GABA antagonists may induce a stage reminiscent of behavioral sedation, which antedates behavioral convulsions (Myslobodsky & Valenstein, 1980). This stage is so short-lasting that it often is overlooked. In the latter case, rats would curve or curl up, but this hardly was observed after steroid administration. This effect may be associated with the hypotension and bradiacradia (DeFeudis, 1982). The cardiovascular effects of RU5135 remain to be established.

The Duality of RU5135 Effects and Cortical Injury

The effects caused by RU5135 are intriguing, because these highly stereotyped all-or-none interictal spikes are very similar to interictal discharges caused by topically applied convulsants or other maneuvers associated with neocortical injury. Indeed, brain surgery in small rodents unavoidably is accompanied by brain injury. It has been pointed out that brain injury reduces seizure thresholds (Collier, 1928). More recently, it was noticed that epicortical implants substantially alter brain electrical activity and could ultimately cause brain epileptogenicity (Adler, 1969; Sterman, Shouse, Lucia, Heinrich, & Sarnoff, 1977), thereby leading to hazardous interpretive errors. Does it mean that RU5135 also activates epileptic spikes as a result of cortical damage unwittingly inflicted by surgery? To answer this question, the size of cortical lesion was assessed planimetrically and the dose causing spikes was plotted as a function of its size. Figure 8.3 shows the scatterplot and the regression line drawn through the dose values. A highly significant correlation ($r = .66, p = .001$) was obtained, which confirmed that the hunch was right (Mintz & Myslobodsky, unpublished). The fact that a zero damage by the criteria of light microscopy was still associated with a few low-threshold cases of spiking suggests that the injury might have been more subtle.

These findings were replicated in rabbits, although in the latter animal it was possible to implant an electrode with little, if any, crude signs of cortical lesion. It appeared that injury was still present in the form of the locally breached blood brain barrier (BBB). To reproduce such transient alterations of integrity of the BBB in vivo, a blunt perspex rod (electrode) was implanted over the dura (Jaeger, Aebischer, Winn, Tresco, & Gee, 1991), and the rabbit was submitted to

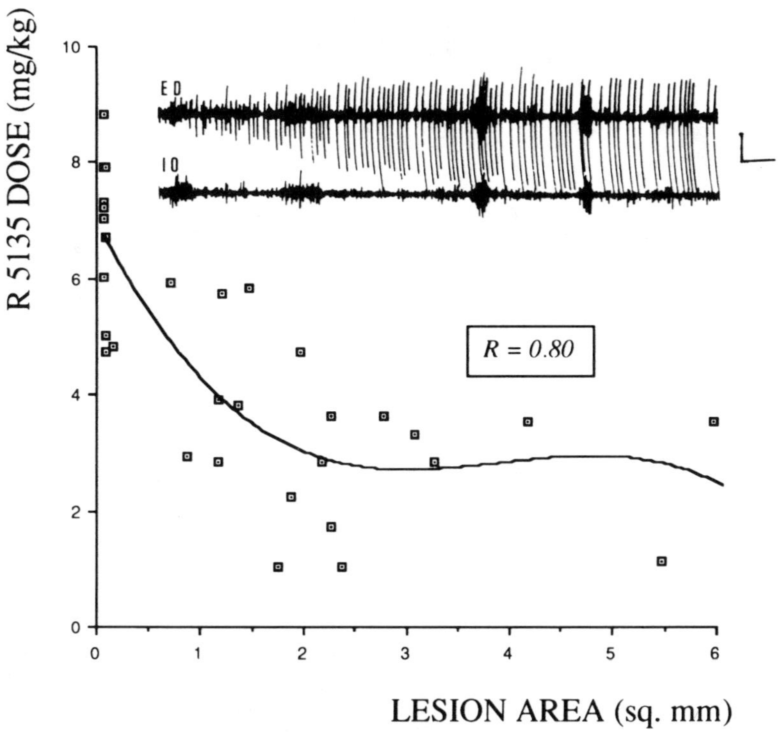

FIG. 8.3. A plot of RU5135 doses eliciting spikes as a function of surgery inflicted cortical injury. Insert shows a fragment of EEG recorded from epicortically implanted silver-ball electrodes (ED) and extradural stainless steel needles placed intraosteally (IO). Waking unrestrained rat.

computed tomography (CT). Normal brain tissue is protected by the BBB from direct penetration of the contrast medium when the latter is administered intravenously. Normally, it takes a dose of 25 ml/50 sec of 50% sodium diatrizoate to disrupt the BBB in a rabbit (Hayman & Hinck, 1988). BBB disruption was assessed by comparing the optical density of the cortex and the brainstem. The CT confirmed the presence of radiodensity increase in the cortical area under the implant (Fig. 8.4). The area of enhanced optic density appeared rather small, within 3–4 mm in diameter, which is in keeping with the minimal size of the cortical field that is believed to be engaged in the generation of penicillin spikes in cats (Goldensohn, Zablow, & Salazar, 1977).

The coincidental appearance of RU5135 neurotoxicity suggests the likelihood of the persistent spilling of excitant neuroactive substances, such as glutamate, into the interstitial space from damaged or depolarized neurons. The event is believed to be the *sine qua non* condition of brain trauma or ischemic lesion

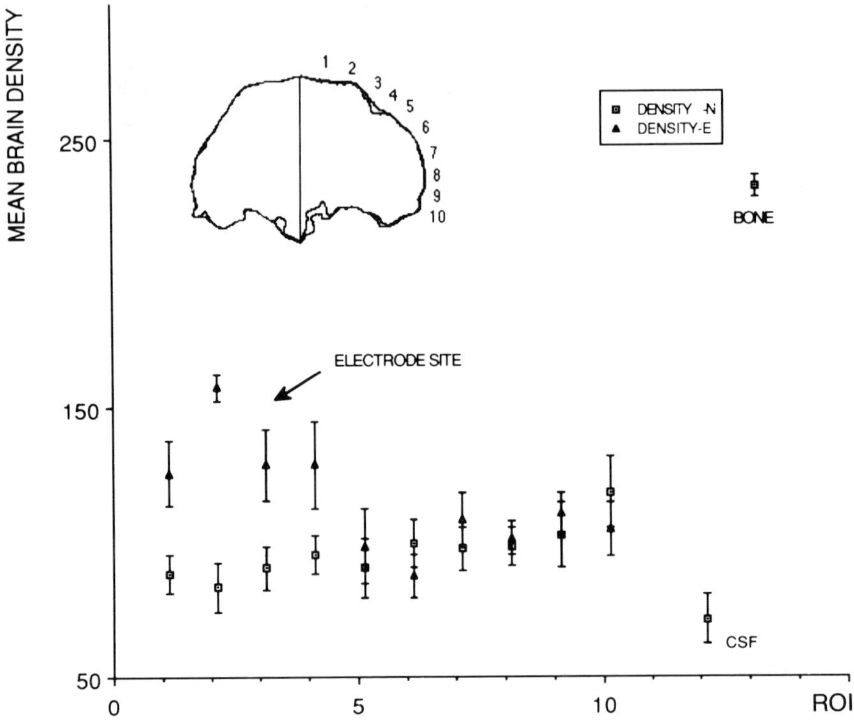

FIG. 8.4. Graph of attenuation values of a selected CT coronal cut of rabbit's head under the electrode before (1) and after (2) 60% Meglumine iothalamate (IOT) administration as a function of a place on the perimeter of the cut. Note increased radiodensity in the area under the electrode. A blunt, 1.5-mm-perspex rod (electrode) was implanted over the dura to sidestep artifacts created by metal electrodes. CT was performed on an Excel 2400 scanner (Elscint, Israel) with a matrix 512 × 512. A rabbit was scanned under Nembutal anesthesia. A sequential set of high-resolution, direct coronal cuts 1.2- and 2.5-mm thick was taken before and after contrast medium. The latter was infused intravenously (IV) in a dose of 1–2 ml/kg over 2–3 min. Readings of HU absorption from a phantom during the period of the study proved stable. The images were digitized and further processed using *Image 1.30* software run on a Mac-2ci image processing station. The size of enhanced area was estimated by assessing the radiodensity of the cortex moving the 2 × 2 region of interest (ROI) along the perimeter of the coronal cut as marked by numbers on the insert. Three rounds of measurements were conducted to form the mean and its standard deviation for statistical comparison on the graph.

associated with a massive NMDA release and the NMDA-induced flux of Ca^{2+} across the membrane. According to current hypotheses, the sustained increase in the intracellular free calcium ($[Ca^{2+}]_i$) initiates a series of reactions that can result in cytoskeletal disruption, neuritic degenetation, and death of excited neurons (Siesjo & Wieloch, 1986). Steroids appear to aggravate glutamate *excitotoxicity.* The glucocorticoid pretreatment prior to kainic acid administration potentiated injury to the hippocampal neurons (Sapolsky, 1986). Hall (1990) drew attention to an important study by Kerr, Campbell, Hao, and Landfield (1989), which showed that corticosteroids augment intracellular free Ca^{2+} concentration in hippocampal neurons. Thus, neurosteroids conceivably may lead to epileptogenicity by adding the enhanced glutamate-mediated excitation to their GABA-antagonistic action. This may contribute to a leaky BBB (Marty, Dusart, & Peschanski, 1991). The development of tissue necrosis and perifocal brain edema adds an additional step to the foregoing cascade, promoting a transient release of short-lived substances—kinins. The latter contribute to secondary brain damage causing a selective opening of the BBB (Baethman et al., 1990), thereby concluding the vicious circle of neurotoxicity.

As soon as we implanted electrodes that did not penetrate the inner table, it appeared that a higher dose of the drug had to be administered to cause spiking under the nontraumatic (intraosteal) electrode (Myslobodsky et al., 1991). Mintz and Myslobodsky (1992), replicated this effect in a group of rats prepared for the analysis of visual evoked potentials (VEP). The pattern of VEP in rats with implanted penetrating and nonpenetrating electrodes proved to be roughly similar. The striking difference in VEP configuration emerged in response to the amidine steroid. At doses of 0.25–0.5 mg/kg, RU5135 appeared to facilitate sensory afterdischarges under intraosteal electrodes, which assumed a form of wave-spike discharges. On the background of higher doses of amidine steroid (up to 3 mg/kg), small doses of metrazol facilitated wave-spike sensory afterdischarges under intraosteal electrodes (Fig. 8.5). The wave-spikes' hypersynchronicity also was seen in the resting EEG derived from noninvasive electrode. However, the triggered spikes under epicortical sites remained unaltered. Apparently, the stage of wave-spike sensory afterdischarges could have been masked in the injured cortex, due to the swift development of triggered focal spikes.

The epileptogenesis may be conceived of as a continuum where wave-spike discharges represent a mild form of pathology, whereas discharges of the focal type (with underlying paroxysmal depolarization) represent its more severe end (Gloor, 1979; Myslobodsky, 1976). The focal and generalized discharges could coexist in the same preparation in reponse to RU5135 because these events represent two different stages of epileptogenesis. The significant and reliable inverse relationship between the degree of damage of the cortical tissue under the recording electrode and the threshold dose of focal spiking suggests that the magnitude of neuronal impairment might determine which epileptogenic re-

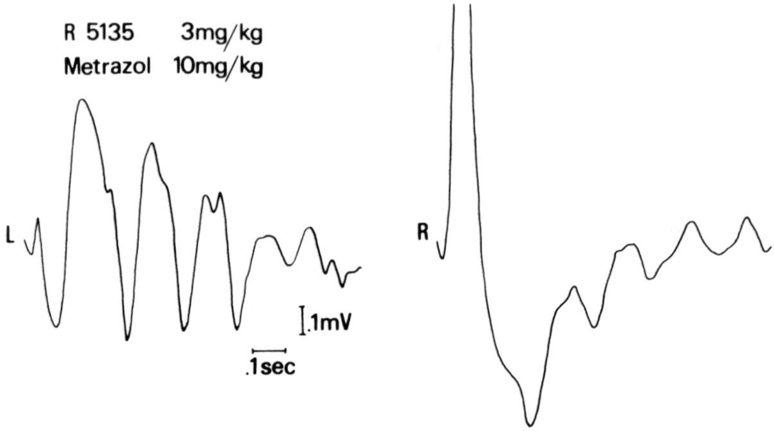

FIG. 8.5. Visual evoked potential (VEP) in a waking rat from intraosteal (L) and epicortical (R) electrodes placed over the visual cortex. Note that after 3 mg/kg (IP) of RU5135 and 10 mg/kg of metrazol, VEP shows normal form with wave-spike shaped sensory afterdischarge under the intraosteal electrode (L). The epicortical electrode records a triggered high-amplitude spike. The rat was connected with low-noise cables and remained freely moving in an electrostatically shielded cage fitted on the sides with mirror panels. Each VEP is an average of 30 tracings to a train of 10 μsec stroboscopic flashes (Grass Model PS22C photostimulator with intensity set at 8 on a 1–16 scale) presented in pseudorandom fashion. Monopolar recording against a reference over the cerebellum. Negativity under the active electrode is upward. Stimulus presentation coincides with the beginning of the average. (Mintz & Myslobodsky, unpublished).

sponse (grand mal or petit mal type) will occur in response to the neuroactive steroid.

Kindled Epilepsy and Steroid-Induced Spikes

The epilepsies frequently arise from or involve the limbic system. The latter has a low seizure threshold, plays a major role in the control of emotions and motivated behaviors, and represents a major feedback and regulatory mechanism of the hypthalamo-pituitary-adrenal axis. It could be expected that RU5135, administered systemically, would activate spikes in the amygdala, which represents an important neurosubstrate for the processing of aversive events into emotionally related behavior (Ben-Ari, 1981) and is a favorite site for kindling epileptic seizures in experimental animals (Goddard, 1987). Yet, it appeared that RU5135-activated spikes failed to codevelop in the amygdala or to be broadcasted to it from the cortical foci within 20–30 min of regular spiking (Kofman, Tarrasch, Mintz & Myslobodsky, 1992).

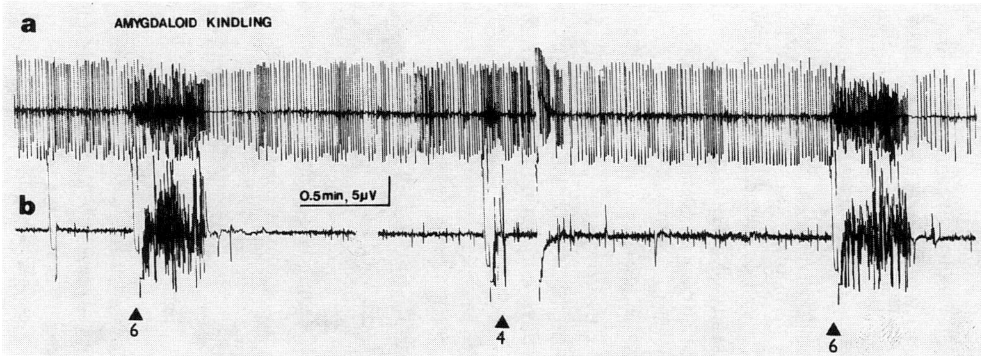

FIG. 8.6. Cortical spiking induced by (a) RU5135 and (b) amygdaloid electrical activity in a rat with kindled epilepsy. A subcortical bipolar electrode consists of two twisted 0.2-mm Teflon-insulated stainless steel wires implanted in the amygdala, 1 mm posterior to bregma, 4.55 mm lateral to midline, and 9 mm below the cortical surface. The amygdaloid kindling was conducted according to the procedure described elsewhere (Myslobodsky & Valenstein, 1980). Triangles denote trains of electrical stimuli delivered to the amydgala, and numbers indicate seizure intensity classified after Racine (1972), adding stage 6 to designate multiple episodes of rearing and falling. Note that cortical spikes do not spread to the amygdala after several generalized seizures, nor do they show a consistent effect on the frequency of cortical spiking.

After kindled seizures are produced, each seizure afterdischarge invariably is followed by interictal spikes (Engel & Ackermann, 1980; Wada, Sato, & Corcoran, 1974). However, in such an enhanced (kindled) state of excitability, amygdaloid neurons were not more responsive to IP administered RU5135 than they were normally (Fig. 8.6). The reason for amygdaloid resistance is not clear. The amygdala must have been traumatized sufficiently by the electrode implant to cause a massive glutamate release. The region of electrode implantation (the basolateral nucleus) contains a high density of benzodiazepine receptors (Young & Kuhar, 1980). After cortisol implantation in the amygdala, rats demonstrated a facilitated extinction of the shuttle-box avoidance response (Bohus, 1968). Increased plasma corticosteroids, observed after amygdaloid stimulation (Brady, 1958), also must add to the effect. That excitotoxic consequences of trauma were obtained in the cortex but not in the amygdala, which has glutamate synapses (Collins, 1984) and responds with a variety of seizure discharges to local injections of KA (Ben-Ari, 1982), might be attributed conceivably to the regionally specific modulation of $GABA_A$ receptor by steroids. Such a possibility was recently demonstrated on the example of regional differences of the allosteric modulation of [^{35}S]TBPS by several 3α-hydroxylated pregnane steroids (Gee & Lann, 1991). Thus, it might be interesting to explore whether the prevalent form of $GABA_A$ receptors in the amygdala have a low affinity to RU5135 compared with the neocortical isoforms.

STEROID-INDUCED SEDATION AND EPILEPTOGENICITY

The resting brain steroid tone represents another factor of the biochemical machinery that channels the focal activity into either wave-spike hypersynchrony or grand mal-type afterdischarges. This suggestion may be illustrated by the effects of progesterone. It was shown to exert a weak potentiating action on the $GABA_A$ receptor. Its 3α-hydroxy-5α and 5β-metabolites are far more potent compounds in this regard: they exert pronounced antiepileptic and hypnotic effects (Wu, Gibbs, & Farb, 1990). 5α-pregnane-3α-ol-20-one shows fluctuations with the ovarian cycle (Ichikawa et al., 1974) and is present in the brain in a concentration about 100 times higher than in plasma (Backstrom, Gee, Lan, Sorensen, & Wahlstrom, 1990). Thus, progesterone and its metabolites could increase potently the GABAergic tone of the brain, thereby normally promoting hypnotic effects. They also are known to cause lasting EEG synchronization in rats, rabbits, and cats (Beyer, Ramirez, Whitmoyer, & Sawyer, 1967; Kubli-Gafrias, Cerventes, & Beyer, 1976; Lincoln, 1969). The special state of mind characterized by reduced concern, relaxation, sleepiness, and bizarre dream-like fantasies, which frequently is experienced by pregnant women (Caplan, 1961; Lewis, 1979), also may be attributed to progesterone potentiation of GABA. The increased resistance to grand mal seizures that is occasionally noticed during pregnancy (Collier, 1928) may be attributed to progesterone as well. The concentration of GABA in the CSF of normal volunteers and patients with no neurological and psychiatric disorders showed a distinct rostrocaudal gradient, more pronounced in females than males. In the former, there was a greater decline in lumbar CSF GABA levels with age. Also, females under 40 years of age showed significantly higher CSF GABA concentrations compared with females older than 40 years of age, thereby suggesting that the foregoing GABA changes are regulated hormonally (Hare et al., 1982).

The same enhanced background GABA tone also is recognized as a favorable one for the activation of wave-spike discharges (Myslobodsky, 1976). In laboratory animals, experimental wave-spike discharges were shown to be facilitated by enhanced GABAergic neurotransmission (Myslobodsky, 1984). In keeping with this, Backstrom et al. (1990) observed, in four of their patients with petit mal, that attacks were more frequent during the luteal phase and less frequent during menstruation. The synchronizing effect of steroids may be a reflection of a normal mechanism that operates in controlling drives and mediating the state of drive reduction that occasionally culminates in epileptogenicity with wave-spike discharges in vulnerable individuals. The synchronous bursting in EEG is associated with a variety of drive-reducing events, such as ingestion of sucrose (in rats) or milk (in cats), escape from painful stimuli, postcoital states, and so on. Collectively, these periods of enhanced synchronicity of brain electrical activity were termed *pleasure waves* (Myslobodsky, 1976). It was suggested that the pleasure waves may serve as precursors of wave-spike discharges in experimental animals and man.

Focal epilepsy is believed to be the expression of an excitatory phenomenon—the paroxysmal depolarization shift. The latter underlies interictal discharges whereas the lasting waves of postsynaptic inhibition (IPSP) set the minimal rate at which depolarization shifts occur (Ajmone-Marsan, 1969). With the reduction of synaptic inhibition (disinhibition), the recruitment of excitatory circuits may gradually increase overall depolarization to the level of cathodic inactivation of the mechanism of spike generation (i.e., a state that ultimately leads to the development of self-sustained afterdischarges) (Ajmone-Marsan, 1969). Although the concept of *disinhibition* as a leading neurophysiological mechanism of reduced seizure thresholds adequately explains the hyperdepolarization events leading to grand mal-type activity (Ajmone-Marsan, 1969; Meldrum, 1975), the same principle can be invoked for the understanding of the origin of wave-spike discharges (Myslobodsky, 1976). Neurophysiologically defined, *wave-spike hypersynchrony* requires two major conditions for its development: (a) a reliable activity of the system of recurrent inhibition, and (b) the excitatory barrage of sufficient intensity. To generalize from Eccles (1965), provided that the inhibitory synaptic action generated by each burst of action potentials is distributed widely in the thalamic neurons, there is no need to postulate any phasic device that causes wave-spike discharges other than rhythmically generated IPSPs and the background excitatory synaptic activity. In keeping with this dictum, the development of wave-spikes could be expected to occur when the balance between sedative and excitatory steroids is shifted and estrogens would continue to remain active at a time of sufficiently high progesterone plasma levels. Estrogens have a more lasting and steady action than progesterone. Therefore, there always will be a time window when the excitatory barrage enhanced by estrogens will be phased by progesterone-augmented waves of postsynaptic inhibition. This situation may be likened to a paroxysmal change in the EEG, which is known to occur in asymptomatic children or infants as a part of arousal response when a child is awakened from any level of sleep (Kellaway, 1979). Thus, absences might predominate in the luteal or progesterone stage of cycle. Alternatively, endogenous GABA antagonists (e.g., sulphated pregnenolone) and/or estrogens (Smith, 1989) would provide sufficient excitatory background to trigger IPSPs, whereas progesterone and its metabolites would facilitate inhibitory postsynaptic action beyond the magnitude required for regulating drives and drive-reduction responses.

The other reason that excitatory synaptic drive is so effective on a background of IPSP–EPSP sequences caused by progesterone may be attributed to the dual nature of the depolarization process. Apart from the tonic mode of discharges of the depolarized membrane, it was established that transient *hyperpolarization* deinactivates a low-threshold voltage-dependent Ca^{2+} current (T-current), which causes a slow, triangular-shaped, depolarizing event (i.e., the low-threshold spike [LTS]) (Suzuki & Rogawski, 1989). The LTS underlies a burst of Na^{+}-dependent action potentials that ride on its crest. Thus, a train of GABA-mediated IPSPs would be a sufficient condition for triggering LTSs (rebound discharges) without the excitatory barrage postulated by Eccles (1965). It remains to be established why and when the frequency of IPSP–EPSP (excitatory postsynaptic potential) sequences is reduced to organize the 3 cps wave-spikes of petit mal epilepsy.

If the process of facilitating GABA-related inhibitory mechanisms were deemphasized, there still would be a way for progesterone to reduce the excitability in the central nervous system. Using voltage-clamped neurons, Wu et al. (1990) showed that progesterone is capable of reversibly antagonizing glycine-induced currents through a site that is distinct from the strychnine and glycine-binding sites. This puzzling effect suggests that progesterone conceivably may cause sedative and antiepileptic effects through glycine-modulated NMDA-receptor functions. The suppression of excitatory epileptogenesis by progesterone is consistent with its attenuation of responses to quisqualate, kainate, and NMDA (Smith, 1990). According to Wu et al. (1990), the range of progesterone concentrations in rat plasma is close to their EC50 values for progesterone to affect glycine-related responses. Therefore, it cannot be ruled out that in vivo progesterone could contribute to EEG synchronization and cause sedative effects both through direct, $GABA_A$-receptor related and indirect (i.e., glycine receptor-mediated) actions.

This scenario is expected to have exemptions because synchronized discharges based on EPSP–IPSP sequences may be a precursor of epileptic discharges (Myslobodsky, 1976), thereby suggesting that sedative steroids may, in certain conditions, show signs of epileptogenicity. A potent sedative steroid, alphaxalone, administered either IV or IP in a dose of 4 mg/kg, paradoxically appeared to potentiate myoclonic seizures in mice with a significant dose-related increase in the duration of the myoclonus. Similar phenomena were noted after the administration of 5-β-alphaxalone and pregnenolone (File & Simmonds, 1988). Although small doses (0.1–0.25 mg/kg) of pregnenolone and its 3α- and 3β-isomers caused synchronous EEG patterns in cats, these steroids also caused focal spiking when given in higher doses (2.5 mg/kg) (Kubli-Gafrias et al., 1976). These effects might be expected, because muscimol, a specific GABA receptor agonist, produces myoclonic jerks in mice in a dose 2 mg/kg (IP) (Menon & Vivonia, 1981).

Based on findings by Smith (1989), one might expect the opposite ratio of the hormonal see-saw, with reduced progesterone and/or increased estrogen level, to contribute to depolarization of neuronal elements and the exacerbation of non-petit mal forms of epilepsy. That female rats may respond with seizures to a dose of picrotoxin, which is subthreshold for male rats (Pericic, Manev, & Lakic, 1985), could be associated with such periods of fluctuations of the GABAergic brain tone. It is known that women with partial epilepsy have two peaks of generalized seizure potentiation; the first is coincident with a reduced progesterone blood level during menstruation, whereas the second follows the preovulatory rise of estrogen. During the luteal phase, the number of seizures is minimal (Backstrom et al., 1990). Clearly, different steroids may have dissimilar effects on these two classes of ictal mechanisms. Also, corticosteroids may act indirectly via numerous participating neurotransmitter systems implicated in epilepsy. As an example, arousal-related suppression of wave-spike discharges could be attributed to either corticoid influence on the biosynthesis of catecholamine (Axelrod, 1974) and/or their impairment of norepinephrine activation through blocking extraneuronal uptake (Iversen, 1971).

STRESS AND EPILEPSY

Emotional stress seldom was claimed to be an important etiological variable in epilepsy. Kraepelin (1904) and Bonhoeffer (1909) indicated that convulsive phenomena are only exceptionally affected by emotional factors. Rather, they felt that emotional upsets could precipitate mood disorders, frenzied motor excitement, and twilight states. The relation of these conditions to the epilepsies seemed to be uncertain and Bonhoeffer (1909) credited Bratz for the distinction he made between *genuine epilepsy* and *reactive attacks*. In part, the problem arises because the concept of *stress* is often elusively abstract when applied to human conditions. It is known that pleasant stimuli evoking amusement are nearly as potent as the unpleasant ones in provoking increased catecholamine excretion; physical properties of stressors are less potent in this respect than is the individual's attitude to the situation (Levi, 1967). The difficulties that are encountered in attempts to define the intensity of stress are too well appreciated to be discussed here. As Yuwiler (1980) put it: "It is not what happens to man that is important but rather what he thinks happens to him" (p. 19).

This notwithstanding, stressful events do change the excitatory/inhibitory balance of the CNS, causing both facilitation and reduction of seizures. Some contradictory reports in this area were illustrated briefly elsewhere (Myslobodsky & Mirsky, 1987). The contribution of neurosteroids in mediating either of these effects of stress is being examined by several groups. Purdy, Moore, Morrow, & Saul (1991) reported that allopregnenolone and allotetrahydroDOC rise in the cerebral cortex to high levels (3–6 ng/ml, 10–20nM) 10 min after swim stress compared with nonstressed male rat (< 1 ng/g). This level of steroids appears to be sufficient to affect GABA-mediated inhibition. All pregnenolone levels peaked in the cortex to the maximal levels of 30–60 min prior to its peak levels in the plasma. This time difference suggests they formed in situ, apparently from progesterone; the latency of the effect is sufficient for the latter to be converted to its metabolites. Unlike allotetrahydroDOC, allopregnenolone still was measurable in the cerebral cortex of adrenalectomized rats (Purdy et al., 1991). The nature of this adaptation is yet to be explored inasmuch as the enhancement of brain GABA tone seems to counter the major adaptive function of stress to recruit all resources for increasing brain excitability. Allopregnenolone, at nanomolar concentrations, appears to potentiate the binding of muscimol and benzodiazepines to the $GABA_A$ receptor and allosterically inhibits the binding of the convulsant TBPS (Majewska, 1990). Observations on voltage-clamped bovine adrenomedullary chromaffin cells in culture showed that allopregnenolone is capable of enhancing GABA responses when administered in the concentration range of 10–30 nM (Lambert et al., 1990).

Steroids elicited during stress may be beneficial because an animal confronted by mortal danger is given a chance to escape rather than develop a panic attack and/or convulsions. As an example, immersion stress administered to the El mice, an inbred mutant strain susceptible to convulsion, caused a complete control of seizures in 38% of animals immediately after stress; the effect was detectable 24 hours thereafter. In 41% of them, seizure reduction was obtained following the immobilization procedure (Mori, Hiramatsu, Kabuto, & Marescau, 1986). Soubrie et al. (1980) showed that swim stress decreased convulsant potency of picrotoxin and pentetrazol and enhanced cortical binding of $[^3H]$flunitrazepam. Devinsky, Emoto, Porter, Theodore, and Nadi (1991) obtained a strong correlation between CSF cortisol level in patients with partial epilepsy and antisocial score of the personality disorders inventory. This effect was attributed to stress-related elevation of glucocorticoids. It would be interesting to see this score compared with seizure data and EEG findings (e.g., "forced normalization").

The above effect of stress may vary in different species, in different strains of rodents (Robertson, 1980), or to different stressors. Also, it may not work well with repeated stressors, which gradually could desensitize GABA receptor-gated Cl^- channel. Weizman et al. (1989) demonstrated this possibility on the example of the in vivo binding of [^{3}H]Ro 15-1788 in conditions of repeated swim stress in mice. It appeared that 7 consecutive days of daily swim session for either 2 or 10 min caused a regionally selective decrease in benzodiazepine receptor occupancy. The effect was especially robust in the cerebral cortex and hippocampus, but also was detected in the midbrain, striatum, and hypothalamus. In parallel with the reduction of [^{3}H]Ro 15-1788 binding, the anticonvulsant clonazepam appeared to be less effective in protecting stressed animals against a challenging dose of pentylenetetrazol. The effect of reduced [^{3}H]Ro 15-1788 binding to hippocampal membranes in vivo was not obtained in adrenalectomized animals, which suggests that peripheral corticosteroids play a role in the regulation of GABA/benzodiazepine receptor synthesis and expression (Weizman, et al., 1990).

The reduction of seizure thresholds in stress may be associated with an increase in the levels of GABA-antagonistic neurosteroid, pregnenolone sulphate (Baulieu et al., 1987). It is not understood why pregnenolone sulphate is released during stress when protective GABAergic neurotransmission also is being enhanced. There are several equally plausible mechanisms that can serve as a foundation for exploring the relationship between pregnenolone sulphate and stress. The first assumes that the neurosteroid may act as endogenous analeptic maintaining the enhanced state of vigilance (Majewska, 1987a). Furthermore, consistent with the effects of flumazenil (Lal, Kumar, & Foster, 1988), it may cause anxiety and thus facilitate exploratory behavior and learning. The second possibility might conceive its release, by analogy with effects of GABA antagonists in rats (Makara & Stark, 1978; Pericic et al., 1985), as a part of the backup system or feedforward circuit, further elevating plasma cortisol level. Another class of explanations may derive from the fact that seizures cause a rapid postictal increase of cortical benzodiazepine receptors (Paul & Skolnick, 1978), so that convulsant properties of pregnenolone sulphate may be essential for the proliferation of GABA receptors that counteract the process of their gradual desensitization. The final scenario is based on the assumption that the brainstem might be the primary target for sulphated pregnenolone, because a neurosteroid with analeptic action conceivably may be useful in the early stages of ontogeny to accelerate pulmonary maturation and antagonize GABA-related anoxia in the neonate.

One might wonder if, in adults, it still is needed primarily in a more mundane capacity to facilitate respiratory functions during emotional and/or physical stress. The increase in ventilation is a common physiological response to acute stress. In anxious individuals, notably with thoracic respiratory pattern, this normal response may evolve into the hyperventilation syndrome (Margarian, 1989). Fetal lungs appear to contain two- to fivefold greater concentration of receptor sites for glucocorticoids than in many other fetal tissues, including the brain (Ballard & Ballard, 1972; Toft & Chytil, 1973). Their role there is ill understood. There is a possibility that steroids may cause ventilatory drive by acting directly on lung parenchyma (Scatrud, Dempsey, & Kaiser, 1978).

Further studies will need to elucidate what determines when excitatory or inhibitory components of steroid action dominate. Among other factors, the type of stress (Drugan et al., 1989), gender, and age (Burgess & Handa, 1991; Early & Leonard, 1977, 1978; McEwen, Brinton, & Sapolsky, 1988; Purdy, Moore, Hagino, Morrow, & Paul, 1991), as well as individual differences in the regulation of pituitary–adrenal functions (McEwen et al., 1988), seem to be relevant to the ways in which the excitatory/inhibitory ratio is being established in the brain. It would be an oversimplification to attribute stress effects solely to neuroactive steroids acting at the GABAergic neurotransmission. Such facilitation may occur consequent to a well-concerted action of norepinephrine at GABA receptors. The GABA-mediated inhibition of Purkinje cells was shown to be potentiated by norepinephrine (Moises, Hoffer, & Woodward, 1980). The proconvulsant effect of muscimol mentioned earlier also requires norepinephrine and serotonin in the production of that response (Menon & Vivonia, 1981). This is an interesting phenomenon in view of the well-recognized role of norepinephrine in stress activation and the possible role glucocorticoids may have in blunting their effects (McEwen et al., 1988).

Psychopathology, Epilepsy, and Stress

Psychopathology is still another problem whose relevance to epilepsy might be significant in the context of the present review. The data on the intersection between the two areas of research are still meager and contradictory. It has long been suggested that frank seizure discharges noticed in the septum and anterior striatum of patients with schizophrenia may characterize actively hallucinating patients (Heath, 1954). The increased firing of epileptogenic septal neurons may cause a significant change of behavior akin to that caused by focal electrical stimulation of the septum. Schizophrenic-like symptoms were described to appear interictally in patients with temporal lobe epilepsy (Slater, Beard, & Glithero, 1963). According to Stevens (1988), atrophic brain changes in limbic structures of schizophrenic patients is an end result of such focal microseizures, which cause excessive loss of neurons. In fact, a number of morphometric studies—some of them conducted in the context of computer assisted tomography (CT) and/or a magnetic resonance imaging (MRI) assessment of the disorder—have been extremely productive in elucidating indices of limbic–prefrontal pathology (Suddath, Christison, Torrey, Casanova, & Weinberger, 1990). The hypothesis of left-hemisphere dysfunction in schizophrenia specifically implicated temporal–hippocampal abnormalities (Flor-Henry, 1976).

In view of the foregoing, I would be more interested in reviewing the effects of early stress, where the AAA (activation, adaptation, and atrophy) syndrome of McEwen et al. (1988) is established more firmly. Similar to schizophrenia, infantile stress in the form of emotional and physical isolation is implicated in epilepsy where parental separation and neglect occasionally are reported as important factors of social background (cf. Taylor, 1972). In laboratory experiments, isolated mice were suggested as a model subject for schizophrenia in the past (DeFeudis, 1984). Isolated animals are highly excitable and known to be excessively aggressive when socially stimulated (DeFeudis, 1984). In contrast, handled (postnatally stressed) animals show resistance to stress in adulthood and reduced susceptibility to seizures elicited by electroconvulsive shock (Levine, 1962). Although an excessive production of glucocorticoids in stress might provide the missing link in the chain of events leading to structural brain damage in psychopathology, the problem of how intrinsic brain vulnerability, infantile stress, and epileptogenic lesion are put together over time hardly has begun to be approached. Weinberger (1987) put forward a few broad speculative suggestions that juxtapose the concepts of brain deficit in schizophrenia in the continuum of aberrant behaviors ranging from attention disorders to Alzheimer's dementia. More recently, in a search for a unifying hypothesis, Feldon and Weiner (1992) restated Sapolsky, Krey, and McEwen's (1986) argument for Alzheimer's dementia to account for *dementia praecox*. The gist of Sapolsky's theory is that stress sets priorities for the organism for a limited period of time. During that time, the previous long-term objectives, motivational demands, and emergencies are overruled as if being subordinated to the major goal of survival. This goal is achieved via glucocorticoids. It has been suspected that, outside this limited emergency, the exposure to glucocorticoids may be harmful unless their action is terminated. Yet, until recently, doubt existed as to the extent to which such a generalized phenomenon may cause selective brain injury. This doubt was dispelled by the studies of McEwen et al. (1988), Sapolsky et al. (1986), and their associates, who emphasized the importance of the length, rather than the intensity, of glucocorticoid effects that determine the susceptibility of hippocampal receptors to down-regulation. Specifically, they have marshaled impressive evidence to suggest that a feedback system that curtails the stress-related tidal wave of exogenous or endogenous glucocorticoids is triggered by activation of both type I and type II corticoid receptors (notably the former), which are abundantly present in the hippocampus. Down-regulation of these receptors, their loss, or genetic deficit might expose hippocampal neurons during repeated episodes of alarm to excessive corticosteroid concentrations, thereby causing irreparable hippocampal damage (McEwen et al., 1988; Sapolsky et al., 1986).

Feldon and Weiner (1992) capitalized on this implication. They proposed that weakened latent inhibition—a phenomenon they believe to underlie disordered attention in schizophrenia—is associated with hippocampal injury, chiefly in nonhandled male rats. In formulating a comprehensive hypothesis on the temporal–limbic dysfunction in schizophrenia, it would be interesting to explore in what way the heterogeneity of hippocampal response to steroids affects the development of aberrant behaviors and whether the latter could be alleviated using antiglucocorticoids (e.g., a glucocorticoid analog RU486) in the neonates. The granule cells of the dentate gyrus actually require glucocorticoids for their normal functioning and appear to lose branches and shrink following adrenalectomy (McEwan et al., 1990). This effect is being reversed to the extent that glucocorticoid replacement appears to prevent neuronal death. In contrast, CA3 neurons are more vulnerable to excessive glucocorticoid levels, but the effect is obtained following a 12-week exposure to glucocorticoids (Sapolsky et al., 1986). This is a long period of stress, considering the life span of a rat.

Assuming that limbic injury in schizophrenia is attributable to excessive glucocorticoids exposure of comparable length, one might question why chronic stress of the postulated duration does not cause other signs of generalized pathology. For example, corticosteroid administrated to young rats during 12 weeks appeared capable of reproducing the aging pattern of neuronal loss in the hippocampus (McEwen et al., 1988), whereas stress-reactive nonstimulated rats appeared to manifest reduced leukocyte count (Levine, 1962). The isomorphic principle of modeling of the disorder requires that hippocampal damage is paralleled by a recognizable picture of hyperadrenocorticism (e.g., Cushing's habitus, growth inhibition, enhancement of trombocyte aggregation, immunosuppression, osteoporosis and signs of muscle atrophy, early arteriosclerosis, retinopathy, delayed development of the BBB, and steroid diabetes, to name a few). The neonatal exposure to glucocorticoids due to emotional and/or physical neglect and isolation is expected to result in the retardation of developmental processes ranging from delayed formation of dendritic spines to EEG slowing and the short stature, designated as the *deprivation dwarfism* syndrome associated with emotional neglect (van Praag, 1979). However, schizophrenic patients often tend to be taller than controls (Pearlson et al., 1989).

Still another question is why excessive glucocorticoids should be postulated to cause schizophrenia and not affective disorders when 5% of patients on exogenous natural and synthetic glucocorticoids develop chiefly confusional and affective symptoms, with euphoria being the most common clinical feature of psychopathology (Johnson, 1981). This is consistent with the hunch that glucocorticoids are, in a sense, endogenous antidepressants (McEwen et al., 1988). Apparently, the concept implicating stress in the catalysis of the psychosis (Weinberger, 1987) and the suggestion that a focal limbic damage is associated with juvenile stress underlying schizophrenia are altogether different. The difference lies in that stress is what happens *to* an individual, whereas the damage is a disease or what happens *in* the brain and/or body.

Asymmetric Brain Injury and Stress

Pre- or perinatal stress is especially harmful to neurons in conjunction with the coincidental injury, hypoxia, infections, and/or opportunistic seizure, which could cause a massive exodus of excitatory amino acids and a loss of Ca^{2+} homeostasis. Human infants are exposed to varying degrees of hypoxia in a number of clinical conditions (e.g., perinatal asphyxia, respiratory arrest, near-miss sudden infant death syndrome, etc.). Because hippocampal corticoid receptors and hippocampal cells are major victims in events initiated or modulated by glucocorticoids (Lowy, 1991; Sapolsky et al., 1986), it might be important to examine why and when a generalized effect of this type should cause injury to a single hemisphere. For example, Ammon's Horn sclerosis, which commonly is found in the brain of epileptics, is frequently unilateral (Falconer, 1971). Given that there is no a priori reason to suspect that hippocampal cells of one hemisphere are able to resist excitatory amino acids neurotoxicity or are better equipped with growth factors than the other hemisphere, the explanation of unilateral foci may be looked for in such factors as the imbalanced neurotransmitter systems, gender-related heterochronicity of the rate of maturation of cerebral hemispheres, stress-related modulation of transmitter asymmetries, brain perfusion imbalances, and so on.

Among more mechanistic concepts, one might recall that McLardy (1969), when experimenting with epilepsy in guinea pigs, attributed the lateralized foci to the postural imbalance of an animal recovering after seizures. He mentioned a tendency for the sclerosis to appear in the underlying, rather than the overlying, hemisphere. To maximize the bilateral symmetry, he alternated the side on which the animal lay postictally during successive seizures. Asymmetric hippocampal lesions in baboons with experimentally induced generalized seizures also occurred on the side the animals were observed lying postictally (Meldrum & Brierly, 1973). It is likely that the underlying side might have been perfused less and the cumulative effect of hypoxia must have caused a massive release of excitatory amino acids, contributing to the lateralized damage. It should be recalled that there is a tendency of head turning in healthy infants (Gesell, 1938). This preference may be frozen in the more persistent motor imbalance (position of comfort) with tilting of the pelvis and lateral curvature of the trunk. In weak and/or preterm babies, this position, along with reduced motility, leads to some degree of skull molding, often in the form of *plagiocephaly* (James, Lloyd-Roberts, & Pilcher, 1959; Robson, 1968). McLardy's (1969) hypothesis is nice in its simplicity, and it might be interesting to explore whether the infants with cranial deformities are at a higher risk for development of unilateral temporal lobe impairment after occasional febrile convulsions.

Apparently, the situation is more complex, because there is firm evidence for interactions among the laterality and gender-dependent risk factors. As an example, although males are more at risk for epilepsy overall, females manifest a greater relative morbidity (cf. Taylor, 1991). This phenomenon may be associated with gender-related differences in the hippocampal response to glucocorticoid exposure (McEwen et al., 1988). For example, the male's greater vulnerability to stress may be seen in an excess of small grown boys among epileptics (Taylor, 1991).

It is uncertain whether the directionality of head turning can be modulated by infantile stimulation. However, such an effect apparently can be modeled in experimental animals (Denenberg, 1981). There are observations that rat pups separated from their mothers and reared in conditions of stress, in the form of artificial feeding, tend to show left-biased eye opening (Smart, Tonkiss, & Massey, 1986). Undisturbed pups manifest no bias, thereby suggesting that eye opening in isolated pups was associated with a preferable pattern of stress-induced lateralization of the brain (Smart et al., 1986). In view of this imbalance, it is of interest that diazepam binding inhibitor (DBI), an endogenous ligand of benzodiazepine receptors, appears to be asymmetrically distributed in the hippocampus (L > R) (Ferrarese et al., 1991).

Seizures and the Circadian Cycle

There is a certain commonality between the machinery of REM sleep and the mechanisms of generalized epileptic attacks of grand mal type (Elazar & Hobson, 1985). Therefore, it is understandable that seizures in some way may substitute for REM (Cohen & Dement, 1966). After electroconvulsive shocks, REM-deprived cats exhibited a reduced compensatory REM rebound (Cohen, Duncan, & Dement, 1967). Likewise, in depressed patients on electroconvulsive therapy, REM sleep was reduced and there was no compensatory REM rebound after the end of therapy (Zarcone, Gulevich, & Dement, 1967). Neuroactive steroids may contribute to the coupling, however imprecise, between epileptic seizures and REM sleep. Glucocorticoids have been recognized to lower seizure thresholds in experimental animals (Woodbury, 1952). The diurnal variation of glucocorticoid levels is a basic resting mode of operation of the pituitary–adrenal axis. The hormonal response to stress varies with the time of day of stress exposure. The major glucocorticoid in humans—cortisol—is secreted daily at a rate of 20 mg, with normal rate of secretion undergoing circadian fluctuation. It reaches a maximum in the second REM epoch (Fehm & Born, 1991). Sectioning the fornix in the rat (Moberg, Scapagnini, de Groot, & Ganong, 1971) or implanting corticosteroids in the hippocampus (Slusher, 1966) eliminates the diurnal variation of circulating corticosteroids, thereby suggesting that the hippocampal–fornix system exerts its inhibition on the cortical secretion via fibers from the fornix. The number of corticosteroid receptors in the hippocampus appears to be crucial for glucocorticoid feedback inhibition (Sapolsky et al., 1986). Estrogens, which are known to increase CNS excitability, would be surmised to act akin to convulsions or ECT in that they should reduce REM-sleep time. Indeed, a reduction of time spent in REM sleep was reported during estrogen-induced behavioral estrous in spayed rats (Yokoyama, Ramirez, & Sawyer, 1966) and guinea pigs (Malven & Sawyer, 1966).

THE SEEDS OF SELF-DESTRUCTION: WHEN DO THEY GERMINATE?

According to an old dictum (Speransky, 1932), a disease intensifies, weakens, or alters normal functions. It does not create these functions de novo. After three more decades of active research, this dictum was reiterated: "Although the phenomena of epilepsy might be thought superficially to represent a hierarchy of bizarre, pathological events, we are confident that epilepsy is really a modification of the normal principles of neuronal operations" (Ward, Jasper, & Pope, 1969, p. 11). As Mayer and Westbrook (1987) appropriately mused, the "brain is loaded with the seeds of its own destruction."

Some neuroactive steroids may seem well suited to act as such seeds. Synthesized peripherally from innocuous precursors, they could reach the brain in quantities sufficient to cause harmful effects. Systemically acting on some of the most vulnerable brain areas, they may cause their damage, and later convulsions, possibly via mechanisms akin to kindling. Assuming that central effects of steroids are a spin-off of their major role in securing some innate biological adaptations, one might be curious why these seeds of self-destruction so seldom germinate and sprout. In other words, what places a limit to steroid epileptogenicity?

One reason is that neuroactive steroids are not stable compounds. They are metabolized and eliminated from the body rapidly. The other reason may be that, among behaviorally active steroids, proconvulsant steroids are probably a minority (Atkinson, Davis, Pratt, Sharpe, & Gomich, 1965); they need to reach high concentrations to cause untoward effects. Still another reason might be that steroids appear to be neurotoxic in the presence of concurrent brain injury. Some neuroactive steroids cannot easily cross the BBB. That may be because a number of steroid metabolites are polar molecules (e.g., dehydroepiandrosterone sulphate) that penetrate the BBB poorly unless administered in high doses and/or appear in the brain in the presence of BBB abnormalities. Marcus, Watson, and Goldman (1966) were the first to show experimentally that cats with intact BBB are highly resistant to conjugated estrogen. By contrast, animals with focally impaired BBB respond with epileptiform discharges to even minute doses of the steroid.

A number of factors may contribute to the increased permeability of the microcirculation in the involved area and malfunctioning of the BBB. For example, focal cortical injury (e.g., ischemic lesions) may underlie epileptiform phenomena known as periodic lateralized epileptiform discharges (PLEDs) (Chatrian, Shaw & Leffman, 1964) by letting in extraencephalic metabolites (possibly steroids?) or environmental neurotoxins in blood plasma, which otherwise are restricted to the brain. Such a possibility is exemplified by a small group of individuals who exhibit idiosyncratic responses following small IV doses of contrast materials injected for cranial computed tomography due to lesions or particular incompleteness of their BBB. Stress, anxiety, and fear seem to predispose to idiosyncratic responses to contrast media (Lalli, 1980). Focal epileptic activity was noticed in conjunction with contrast agents administered to patients with metastatic lesions (Avrahami, Weiss-Peretz, & Cohn, 1987; Scott, 1980). These cases permit one to speculate that there may be a group of patients in whom the BBB cannot keep out blood-born neuroactive steroids or their metabolites, so that that the latter eventually may cause a variety of central symptoms, epilepsy being one of them. If this is a reason of catamenial exacerbation of epilepsy, a leaking BBB easily could be visualized in vivo using CT and/or an MRI.

THERAPEUTIC IMPLICATIONS

The possibility that certain steroids may be useful anticonvulsant compounds is emphasized repeatedly (Belelli et al., 1990; Majewska, 1987b; Paul & Purdy, 1992). However, it is uncertain that this new generation of drugs would be highly focus-selective. The regular practice of antiepileptic medication obeys the principles of the Shotgun-pellet therapy: when a drug is allowed to cross the BBB and reach therapeutic levels in both the focus and in multiple bystander sites, thereby causing undesirable side effects in the same dosage range as that causing seizure protection. The ratio between anticonvulsant and any untoward effect of the drug (e.g., sedative potency) is designated as the *therapeutic index* and represents a useful yardstick by which the size of the therapeutic window is assessed. Steroid-activated spikes appear to be highly resistant to conventional antiepileptic agents, much as interictal spikes in other forms of experimental epilepsy involving tissue damage (Elazar & Blum, 1971; Purpura, Girado, Smith, and Gomez, 1958). Thus, a number of potentially useful antiepileptic compounds cannot be employed unless the problem of poor BBB permeability can be overcome. Among these are some competitive NMDA receptor antagonists that are polar molecules, which, with few exceptions, must be administered in high doses to achieve therapeutic concentrations in the brain (Rogawski et al., 1990). Thus, only drugs with high values of the index are being considered so far in the combat of interictal focal spiking. However, the fact that in focal epilepsy the BBB is often breached locally (Prince, 1972; Purpura et al., 1958) actually may invite using anticonvulsants with restricted passage through the BBB. Remler and Marcussen (1983) advocated the rationale of antiepileptic therapy using drugs that do *not* normally cross the BBB. By virtue of their limited permeability, a more site-specific, focus-directed drug delivery may be achieved.

An alternative approach is to use a compound that selectively improves the ability of injured tissue with little effects on normally functioning areas. Although this requirement might look like an unrealistic goal to find a compound with properties of the "Magic Bullet," such substances may be available. As an example, a deproteinized calf blood extract (Solcoseryl), which contains polypeptides (with a molecular weight under 3,000) amino acids, and nucleic acids conceivably might offer a significant cytoprotection in focal cerebral hypoxic episodes. This agent is distributed in the brain indiscriminately, similar to other organs. But it appears to activate only injured brain tissues by accelerating the recovery of injured mitochondria of cortical cells, notably on the periphery of the cold-inflicted lesion (Ryu, Uemura, Nakajima, Furuya, & Ryu, 1984). A similar preparation, Actovegin, is reported to increase cerebral metabolism depressed by alcohol (Hoyer, Kruger, Oesterreich, & Weinhardt, 1977) and barbiturates (Baethmann & Oettinger, 1977), and to reduce the detrimental effects of a post-ischemic episode to cortical neurons (Hoyer & Betz, 1989).

Still another and more mundane measure of foci excitotoxicity protection may be entertained. Sapolsky (1986) showed that neuronal and glial hippocampal cells are vulnerable to enhanced metabolic demands imposed by neurotoxins (kainic acid and 3-acetylperidine) in the presence of prolonged glucocorticoids exposure. Glucose and, especially, mannose given during glucocorticoid treatment appear to partially protect the hippocampus. From this finding, a practitioner might derive that adding energetic fuel could alleviate an impact of the injury-glucocorticoid synergy. That might mean that proper nutrition, adequate caloric intake, and prevention of opportunistic infections are indicated to a child at risk for epilepsy.

Daily handling of neonatal rats leads to a significant increase in hippocampal glucocorticoid and mineralocorticoid receptors, thereby enhancing their ability to terminate corticosteroid secretion (Sapolsky et al., 1986b). It might be interesting to explore whether similar maneuvers applied to human infants would offer a real therapeutic advantage in elevating immunity to emotional stress and counteracting or minimizing stress-related hippocampal damage in the population at risk for epilepsy. Handling and stimulation, very much similar to that administered to rat pups, appear to be helpful in facilitating growth and cognitive skills of a premature child (Rice, 1977; Solkoff, Weintraub, Yaffe, & Blase, 1969). Surprising as it may seem, even infants that had a hard time after birth have a potential to develop faster. Landauer and Whiting (1964) examined the average stature measurements in 36 societies, some of which used stressors as a routine part of neonatal care-taking practices. These were piercing the skin, molding the head, extreme heat, feeding emetics, swaddling, and so on. It appeared that children in societies that used to inflict neonatal stress were taller by at least 2 inches than their counterparts in more civilized societies. In contrast, postnatal sensory isolation and neglect were recognized as factors contributing to the high incidence of emotional disorders in premature children (Rothschild, 1967). Thus, there is a wide latitude of useful maneuvers, ranging from the sensory stimulation to educational, behavioral, and psychotherapeutic measures, directed at alleviating stress and/or molding individual coping strategies in both early infancy and adulthood when the state of psychological defences can be reflected in levels of adrenal cortical hormones (Mason, 1975).

EPILOGUE

In our concept of brain functions, we often unwittingly lean on models developed in antiquity. Plato distinguished among three segments of the psyche: the *epithumetikon,* a system that governs bodily lusts and appetites; *thumoedes,* a compartment that represents energy and passion; and *logistikon,* or what we designate today as higher cognitive functions, which was believed to preside over the other two. This distinction was still alive centuries later, and these ideas are still of interest in foreshadowing the later models of nervous functioning. Until recently, steroids were believed to participate in altering the synthesis of important proteins, including enzymes that ensure the development and regulation of lower divisions of Plato's psyche. The discovery of neurosteroids and the role of GABA in mediation of their effects have eroded the neurochemical borders of the tripartite psyche. GABA is the most ubiquitous neurotransmitter in the brain, and is especially abundant in the cortex, the likely seat of Plato's *logistikon.* The cortex is also an avid consumer of progesterone. Its concentration there is revealed by no other area, with the exception of the hypothalamus (Bixo, Backstrom, Winbald, Selstam, & Andersson, 1986). There is a 300-fold difference in the cortical level of progesterone between the two phases of the ovarian cycle (Backstrom et al., 1990). How the presence of steroids is translated into the varying patterns of brain excitability remains to be elucidated. Looking at the nature of spikes, wave-spike discharges and self-sustained afterdischarges through a steroid-viewer may help clarify some aspects of steroid interaction with different types of seizures and shed more light on numerous aspects of GABA-steroid effects (sedative, anxiolytic, convulsant, antiepileptic, stress controlling, etc.). Understandably, the story of GABA-steroid interaction is only a small part of the picture currently being grasped. Viewing it from that side is akin to a deliberate surrender to the principle that O'Brien (1989) called the *academic scotomata.* Sir William Hamilton, a 19th-century Scottish philosopher, noticed that when a handful of marbles is thrown on the floor, it is difficult to see at once more than six or seven of them at most without confusion. Such is a sad span of human instantaneous grasp. That is why it remains to be elucidated how many of those neurochemical marbles are implicated in epilepsy and related disorders. Although GABA is uniquely fit to do the job of commutation of the neuronal flow from a number of systems controlling brain reactivity, it hardly does it alone. Only a few possible contributors were mentioned here. This omission is not due to a lack of appreciation of these potential others to the pathophysiology of epilepsy. Simply, very little is known about exact connections of GABA-steroid machinery, with that of endogenous opiates, aspartate-glutamate, catecholaminergic systems, histamine, and prostglandin, which also were implicated in epilepsy. Even less is known of how different components of this broader system interact in vivo when genomic and nongenomic mechanisms cooperate. These may be themes for a different story.

ACKNOWLEDGMENT

I am grateful to Drs. W. Baschong, O. Kofman, S. Pole, R. Purdy, and A. Weizman for critical comments and helpful suggestions on earlier drafts of the chapter. RU5135 was generously donated by Dr. Hunt (RUSSEL).

REFERENCES

Adler, M. W. (1969). Laboratory evaluation of antiepileptic drugs. The use of chronic lesions. *Epilepsia, 10,* 263–280.

Ajmone-Marsan, C. (1969). Acute effects of topical epileptogenic agents. In H. H. Jasper, A. A. Ward, & A. Popc (Eds.), *Basic mechanisms of epilepsies* (pp. 298–319). Boston: Little, Brown.

Atkinson, R. M., Davis, B., Pratt, M. A., Sharpe, H. M., & Tomich, E. G. (1965). Action of some steroids on the central nervous system of the mouse. II. Pharmacology. *Journal of Medicinal Chemistry, 8,* 426–432.

Avrahami, E., Weiss-Peretz, J., & Cohn, D. F. (1987). Focal epileptic activity following intravenous contrast material injection in patients with metastatic brain disease. *Journal of Neurology, Neurosurgery, and Psychiatry, 50,* 221–223.

Axelrod, J. (1974). Regulation of the neurotransmitter norepinephrine. In F. O. Schmitt & F. G. Worden (Eds.), *The Neurosciences. 3d study program* (pp. 863–876). Cambridge, MA: The MIT Press.

Baethmann, A., Schurer, L., Kempski, O., Staub, F., Peters, J., Unterberg, A., Wahl, M., & Maier-Hauff, K. (1990). Brain edema factors. In B. B. Johansson, C. H. Owman, & H. Wildner (Eds.), *Pathophysiology of the blood-brain barrier* (pp. 357–367). Amsterdam: Elsevier.

Backstrom, T., Gee, K. W., Lan, N., Sorensen, M., & Wahlstrom, G. (1990). Steroids in relation to epilepsy and anaesthesia. In D. Chadwick & K. Widdows (Eds.) *Ciba Foundation Symposium 153. Steroids and neuronal activity* (pp. 225–230). Chichester: Wiley.

Baethmann, A., & Oettinger, W. (1977). Effects of a protein-free plasma-hydrolysate (Actovegin) on cerebral blood flow and metabolism. In W. L. Olszewski (Ed.), *12th Congress of European society for surgery research* (p. 200). Basel: Karger.

Ballard, P. L., & Ballard, R. A. (1972). Glucocorticoid receptors and the role of glucocorticoids in fetal lung development. *Proceedings of the National Academy of Sciences of the USA, 69,* 2668–2672.

Baulieu, E.-E., & Robel, P. (1984). Neurosteroids: 3β-hydroxy-Δ5-derivatives in rodent brain. In F. Labrie & L. Proulx (Eds.), *Endocrinology* (pp. 310–315). Amsterdam: Elsevier.

Baulieu, E.-E., Robel, P., Vatier, O., Haug, A., Le Goascpgne, C., & Bourreau, E. (1987). Neurosteroids: Pregnenolone and dehydroepiandrosterone in the rat brain. In K. Fuxe & L. F. Agnati (Eds.), *Receptor–receptor interaction: A new intramembrane integrative mechanism* (pp. 89–104). Basingstoke: Macmillan.

Beach, F. A. (1948). *Hormones and behavior.* New York: P. B. Hoeber.

Belelli, D., Bolger, M. B., & Gee, K. W. (1989). Anticonvulsant profile of the progesterone metabolite 5α-pregnan-3α-ol-20-one. *European Journal of Pharmacology, 166,* 325–329.

Belelli, D., Lan, N. C., & Gee, K. W. (1990). Anticonvulsant steroids and the GABA/benzodiazepine receptor-cloride ionophore complex. *Neurosciences and Biobehavioral Reviews, 14,* 315–322.

Ben-Ari, Y. (1981). *The amygdaloid complex: INSERM Symposium 20.* Amsterdam: Elsevier.

Ben-Ari, Y. (1982). The role of seizures in kainic acid induced brain damage. In K. Fuxe, P. Roberts, & R. Schwarcz (Eds.), *Excitotoxins* (pp. 184–198). New York: Plenum.

Beyer, C., Ramirez, V. D., Whitmoyer, D. I., & Sawyer, C. H. (1967). Effects of hormones on the electrical activity of the brain in the rat and rabbit. *Experimental Neurology, 18,* 313–326.

Bixo, M., Backstrom, T., Winbald, B., Selstam, G., & Andersson, A. (1986). Comparison between pre- and postovulatory distribution of oestradiol and progesterone in the brain of the PMSG-reated rat. *Acta Physiological Scandinavica, 128,* 241–246.

Boaventura, A. M., & Boissier, J. R. (1978). Efeitos comportamentais de esteroide original com um ciclo amidinico (R5135), Abstracts. *VII Congresso Latinoamericano de Farmacologia.* San Paulo.

Bohus, B. (1968). Pituitary ACTH release and avoidance behavior in rats with cortisol implants in mesencephalic reticular formation and median eminence. *Neuroendocrinology, 3,* 355–365.

Bonhoeffer, K. (1909). Zur frage der exogenen psychosen. *Zentbl. Nervenheilk. Psychiatr., 32,* 499–505.

Brady, J. V. (1958). The paleocortex and behavioral motivation. In H. F. Harlow & C. N. Woolsey (Eds.), *Biological and biochemical basis of behavior* (pp. 193–235). Madison, WI: The University of Wisconsin Press.

Burgess, L. H., & Handa, R. J. (1991). *Estrogen (E) affects glucocorticoid receptor (GR) mediated negative feedback and GR mRNA levels in the rat.* Paper presented at the 21st annual meeting of the Society for Neurosciences, New Orleans, LA.

Caplan, G. (1961). *An approach to community mental health.* New York: Grune & Stratton.

Chatrian, G. E., Shaw, C. M., & Leffman, H. (1964). The significance of periodic lateralized discharges in EEG: An electroencephalographic, clinical and pathological study. *Electroencephalography and Clinical Neurophysiology, 17,* 117–193.

Cohen, H. B., & Dement, W. C. (1966). Sleep: Suppression of rapid eye movement phase in cat after electroconvulsive shock. *Science, 154,* 396–398.

Cohen, H. B., Duncan, R. F. II, & Dement, W. C. (1967). Sleep: The effect of electroconvulsive shock in cats deprived of REM sleep. *Science, 156,* 1646–1648.

Collier, J. (1928). *Three lectures on epilepsy.* London: The Lancet.

Collins, C. G. S. (1984). Amino acid transmitter candidates in various regions of the primary olfactory cortex follwing bulbectomy. *Brain Research, 296,* 145–147.

Curtis, D. R., & Malik, R. (1985). Glycine antagonism by RU 5135. *European Journal of Pharmacology, 110,* 383–384.

DeFeudis, F. V. (1982). GABA—an inhibitory neurotransmitter that is involved in cardiovascular control. *Pharmacological Research Communications, 14,* 567–575.

DeFeudis, F. V. (1984). GABA and endocrine regulation-relation to neurologic–psychiatric disorders. *Neurochemistry International, 6,* 1–26.

del Rio, M. R.(1981). γ-Aminobutyric acid system in rat oviduct. *Journal of Biological Chemistry, 256,* 9816–9819.

Denenberg, V. H. (1981). Hemispheric laterality in animals and the effects of early experience. *Behavioral and Brain Sciences, 4,* 1–49.

Devinsky, O., Emoto, S., Porter, R. J., Theodore, W. H., & Nadi, N. S. (1991). Cerebrospinal fluid biochemical corelates of behavior in partial epilepsy. *Journal of Epilepsy, 4,* 81–85.

Drugan, R. C., Deutsch, S. I., Weizman, A., Weizman, R., Vocci, F. J., Crawley, J. N., Skolnick, P., & Paul, S. M. (1989). Molecular mechanisms of stress and anxiety: Alterations in the benzodiazepine/GABA receptor complex. In H. Weiner, I. Floria, R. Murison, & D. Hellhammer (Eds.), *Frontiers of stress research* (pp. 148–158). Toronto: Hans Huber.

Early, C. J., & Leonard, B. E. (1977). The effect of testosterone and cyproterone acetate on the concentration of γ-aminobutyric acid in brain areas of aggressive and non-aggressive mice. *Pharmacology Biochemistry and Behavior, 6,* 409–413.

Early, C. J., & Leonard, B. E. (1978). GABA and gonadal hormones. *Brain Research, 15,* 27–34.

Eccles, J. C. (1965). Inhibition in the thalamic and cortical neurons and its role in phasing neuronal discharges. *Epilepsia, 6,* 89–115.

Elazar, Z., & Blum, B. (1971). Effects of drugs on interictal spies and after-discharges in experimental epilepsy. *Archives of International Pharmacodynamics and Therapy, 189,* 310–318.

Elazar, Z., & Hobson, A. (1985). Neuronal excitability control in health and disease: A neurophysiological comparison of REM sleep and epilepsy. *Progress in Neurobiology, 25,* 141–188.

Engel, J., & Ackermann, R. F. (1980). Interictal EEG spikes correlate with decreased, rather than increased, epileptogenicity in amygdaloid kindled rats. *Brain Research, 190,* 543–548.

Erdo, S. L. (1983). High-affinity, sodium-dependent γ-aminobutyric acid uptake by slices of rat ovary. *Journal of Neurochemistry, 40,* 582–584.

Falconer, M. A. (1971). Genetic and related aetiological factors in temporal lobe epilepsy. A review. *Epilepsia, 12,* 13–31.

Fehm, H. L., Clausing, J., Kern, W., Pietrowsky, R., & Born, J. (1991). Sleep-associated augmentation and synchronization of luteinizing hormone pulses in adult men. *Neuroendocrinology, 54,* 192–195.

Feldon, J., & Weiner, I. (1992). From animal model of an attentional deficit toward new insights into the pathophysiology of schizophrenia. *Journal of Psychiatry Research, 26,* 345–366.

Ferrarese, C., Mennini, T., Pecora, N., Pierpaoli, C., Frigo, M., Mazorati, C., Gobbi, M., Bizzi, A., Godegoni, A., Garattini, S., & Frattola, L. (1991). Diazepam binding inhibitor (DBI) increases after acute stress in rats. *Neuropharmacology, 30,* 1445–1452.

File, S. E., & Simmonds, M. S. (1988). Myoclonic seizures in the mouse induced by alphaxalone and related steroid anaesthetics. *Journal of Pharmacy and Pharmacology, 40,* 57–59.

Flor-Henry, P. (1976). Lateralized temporal–limbic dysfunction and psychopathology. *Annals of the New York Academy of Sciences, 280,* 777–795.

Gee, K. W. (1988). Steroid modulation of GABA/benzodiazepine receptor-linked chloride ionophore. *Molecular Neurobiology, 2,* 291–317.

Gee, K. W., & Lan, N. C. (1991). γ-Aminobutyric acid A receptor complexes in rat frontal cortex and seizure cord show differential responses to steroid modulation. *Molecular Pharmacology, 40,* 995–999.

Gesell, A. (1938). The tonic neck reflex in the human infant. *Journal of Pediatrics, 13,* 455–464.

Gloor, P. (1979). Generalized epilepsy with spike-and-wave discharge: A reinterpretation of its electrographic and clinical manifestations. *Epilepsia, 20,* 571–588.

Goddard, G. V. (1987). Development of epileptic seizures through brain stimulation of low intensity. *Nature, 214,* 1020.

Goldensohn, E. S., Zablow, L., & Salazar, A. (1977). The penicillin focus: I. Distribution of potential at the cortical surface. *Electroencephalography and Clinical Neurophysiology, 42,* 480–492.

Good, C., & Walker, G. (1984). The hip and molded baby syndrome. *Journal of Bone and Joint Surgery, 66,* 491–492.

Hall, E. D. (1990). Steroids and neuronal destruction or stabilization. In D. Chadwick & K. Widdows (Eds.), *Ciba Foundation Symposium 153. Steroids and neuronal activity* (pp. 206–214). Chichester: Wiley.

Hare, T. A., Wood, J. H., Manyam, B. V., Gerner, R. H., Ballenger, J. C., & Post, R. M. (1982). Central nervous system γ-aminobutyric acid activity in man. *Archives of Neurology, 39,* 247–249.

Harrison, N. L., Majewska, M. D., Harrington, J. W., & Baker, J. L. (1987). Structure-activity relationships for steroid interaction with the γ-aminobutyric $acid_A$ receptor complex. *Journal of Pharmacology and Experimental Therapy, 214,* 346–353.

Harrison, N. L., & Simmonds, M. A. (1984). Modulation of the GABA receptor complex by steroid anaesthetic. *Brain Research, 323,* 287–292.

Hayman, L. A., & Hinck, V. C. (1988). Central nervous system angiography: Contrast media. *Neuroradiology and Radiology of Head and Neck,* 3.

Heuser, G., Ling, G. M., & Buchwald, N. A. (1965). Sedation and seizures as dose-dependent effects of steroids. *Archives of Neurology, 13,* 195–203.

Heath, R. G. (1954). *Studies of schizophrenia.* Cambridge, MA: Harvard University Press.

Hoyer, S., & Betz, K. (1989). Elimination of the delayed postischemic energy deficit in cerebral cortex and hippocampus of aged rats with a dried, deproteinized blood extract (Actovegin). *Archives of Gerontology and Geriatry, 9,* 191–192.

Hoyer, S., Kruger, G., Oesterreich, K., & Weinhardt, F. (1977). Effects of drugs on cerebral blood flow and oxydative metabolism in patients with dementia. In J. S. Meyer, H. Lechner, & M. Reivich (Eds.), *Cerebral vascular disease* (pp. 25–28). Amsterdam: Excerpta Medica.

Hunt, P., & Clements-Jewery, S. (1981). A steroid derivative, R5135, antagonizes the GABA/benzodiazepine receptor interaction. *Neuropharmacology, 20,* 351–361.

Iversen, L. L. (1971). Role of transmitter uptake mechanisms in synaptic neurotransmission. *British Journal of Pharmacology, 41,* 571–579.

James, J. I. P., Lloyd-Roberts, G. C., & Pilcher, M. F. (1959). Infantile structural scoliosis. *Journal of Bone and Joint Surgery, 47B,* 719–735.

Jaeger, C. B., Aebischer, P., Winn, S. R., Tresco, P. A., & Gree, L. A. (1991). *Vascular remodeling adjacent to brain implants of empty and PC12 cell-loaded polymer capules.* Paper presented at 21st annual meeting of the Society for Neurosciences, New Orleans, LA.

Johnson, D. A. W. (1981). Drug-induced psychiatric symptoms. *Drugs, 22,* 57–69.

Kawakami, M., & Sawyer, C. H. (1975). Effects of sex hormones and antifertility steroids on brain thresholds in the rabbit. *Endocrinology, 80,* 857–971.

Kendall, D. A., McEwen, B. S., & Enna, S. J. (1982). The influence of ACTH and corticosterone on [^{3}H]GABA receptor binding in rat brain. *Brain Research, 236,* 365–374.

Kerr, D. S., Campbell, L. W., Hao, S.-Y., & Landfield, P. W. (1989). Corticosteroid modulation of hippocampal potentials: Increased effect with aging. *Science, 245,* 1505–1509.

Kofman, O., Tarrasch, R., Mintz, M., & Myslobodsky, M. (1992). Steroid derivative RU5135 fails to precipitate spikes in amygdala-kindled rats. *Brain Research Bulletin, 29,* 511–514.

Kraepelin, E. (1904). Vergleichende psychiatrie. *Zenttrallblatt fur Nervenheilk. und Psychiatrie, 27,* 433–437.

Kubli-Gafrias, C., Cerventes, M., & Beyer, C. (1976). Changes in multiunit activity and EEG induced by the administration of natural progestins and to flaxedil immobilized cats. *Brain Research, 114,* 71–81.

Lal, H., Kumar, B., & Foster, M. (1988). Enhancement of learning and memory in mice by benzodiazepine antagonist. *FASEB Journal, 2,* 2707–2711.

Lalli, A. F. (1980). Contrast media reactions: Data analysis and hypothesis. *Radiology, 134,* 1–12.

Lambert, J. L., Peters, J. A., Sturgess, N. C., & Hales, T. G. (1990). Steroid modulation of the $GABA_A$ receptor complex: Electrophysiological studies. In D. Chadwick & K. Widdows (Eds.), *Ciba Foundation Symposium 153. Steroids and neuronal activity* (pp. 56–71). Chichester: Wiley.

Landauer, T. K., & Whiting, J. W. M. (1964). Infantile stimulation and adult stature of human males. *American Anthropology, 66,* 1007–1028.

Landgren, S., Aasly, J., Backstrom, T., Dubrovsky, B., & Danielson, E. (1987). The effect of progesterone and its metabolites on the interictal epileptiform discharges in cat's cortex. *Acta Physiological Scandinavica, 131,* 33–42.

Leonard, B. E. (1974). The effect of two synthetic ACTH analogues on the metabolism of biogenic amines in the rat brain. *Archives of International Pharmacodynamics and Therapy, 207,* 242–253.

Levi, L. (1967). Sympatho-adrenomedullary responses to emotional stimuli: Methodologic, physiologic and pathologic considerations. In E. Bajusz (Ed.), *Introduction to clinical endocrinology* (pp. 78–105). Basel: Karger.

Levine, S. (1962). Psychophysical effects of infantile stimulation. In E. L. Bliss (Ed.), *Roots of behavior.* New York: Harper & Bros.

Lewis, E. (1979). Inhibition of mourning by pregnancy: Psychopathology and management. *British Medical Journal, 2,* 27–30.

Lincoln, D. W. (1969). Effects of progesterone on the electrical activity of the forebrain. *Journal of Endocrinology, 45,* 585–596.

Lowy, M. T. (1991). *Kainic acid-induced decrease in hippocampal corticosteroid receptors.* Paper presented at the 21st annual meeting of the Society for Neurosciences, New Orleans, LA.

Magarian, G. J. (1989). Chronic hyperventilation syndrom. In H. Weiner, I. Floria, R. Murison, & D. Hellhammer (Eds.), *Frontiers of stress research* (pp. 336–343). Toronto: Hans Huber.

Majewska, M. D. (1987a). Antagonist-type interaction of glucocorticoids with the GABA receptor-coupled chloride channel. *Brain Research, 418,* 377–382.

Majewska, M. D. (1987b). Steroids and brain activity. Essential dialogue between body and mind. *Biochemical Pharmacology, 36,* 3781–3788.

Majewska, M. D. (1990). Steroid regulation of the $GABA_A$ receptor: Ligand binding, chloride transport and behavior. In D. Chadwick & K. Widdows (Eds.), *Ciba Foundation Symposium 153. Steroids and neuronal activity* (pp. 83–106). Chichester: Wiley.

Majewska, M. D., Bluet-Pajot, M. T., Robel, P., & Baulieu, E. E. (1989). Pregnenolone-sulfate antagonizes barbiturate-induced hypnosis. *Pharmacology, Biochemistry and Behavior, 33,* 701–703.

Majewska, M. D., Harrison, N. L., Swartz, R. D., Baker, J. L., & Paul, S. M. (1986). Steroid hormone metabolites and barbiturate-like modulators of the GABA-receptor. *Science, 232,* 1004–1007.

Majewska, M. D., & Schwartz, D. (1987). Pregnenolone-sulfate: An endogenous antagonist of the γ-aminobutyric acid receptor complex in brain? *Brain Research, 404,* 355–360.

Makara, G. B., & Stark, E. (1978). Role of GABA in the hypothalamic control of the pituitary gland. In S. Garattini, J. F. Pujol, & R. Samanin (Eds.), *Interactions between putative neurotransmitters in the brain* (pp. 263–283). New York: Raven Press.

Malven, P. V., & Sawyer, C. H. (1966). Sleeping patterns in female guinea pigs: Effects of sex hormones. *Experimental Neurology, 15,* 229–239.

Marcus, E. M., Watson, C. W., & Goldman, P. L. (1966). Effects of steroids on cerebral electrical activity. *Archives of Neurology, 15,* 521–532.

Marty, S., Dusart, I., & Peschanski, M. (1991). *Changes in the blood-brain barrier to macromolecules after an excitotoxic lesions in the CNS.* Paper presented at the 21st annual meeting of the Society for Neurosciences, New Orleans, LA.

Mason, J. W. (1975). Clinical psychophysiology: Psychoendocrine mechanisms. In: Reiser, M. (Ed.), American Handbook of Psychiatry, v. IV, (pp. 553–582). New York: Basic Books.

Maus, M., Premont, J., & Glowinski, J. (1990). *In vitro* effects of 17β-oestradiol on the sensitivity of receptors coupled to adenylate cyclase on striatal neurons in primary culture. In D. Chadwick & K. Widdows (Eds.), *Ciba Foundation Symposium 153. Steroids and neuronal activity* (pp. 145–153). Chichester: Wiley.

Mayer, M. L., & Westbrook, G. L. (1987). Cellular mechanisms underlying excitotoxicity. *Trends in Neurosciences, 10,* 59–61.

McEwen, B. S., Brinton, R. E., & Sapolsky, R. (1988). Glucocorticoid receptors and behavior: Implications for stress response. In P. Chrousos, D. L. Loriaux, & P. W. Gold (Eds.), *Mechanisms of physical and emotional stress* (pp. 35–45). New York: Plenum Press.

McEwen, B. S., Coirini, H., & Schumacher, M. (1990). Steroid effects on neuronal activity: When is the genome involved? In D. Chadwick & K. Widdows (Eds.), *Ciba Foundation Symposium 153. Steroids and neuronal activity* (pp. 3–12). Chichester: Wiley.

McEwen, B. S., Denef, C. J., Gerlach, J. L., & Plapinger, L. (1974). Chemical studies of the brain at a steroid hormone target tissue. In F. O. Schmitt & F. G. Worden (Eds.), *The Neurosciences. 3rd study program* (pp. 599–620). Cambridge, MA: The MIT Press.

McLardy, T. (1969). Ammonshorn pathology and epileptic dyscontrol. *Nature, 22,* 877–878.

Meldrum, B. S. (1975). Epilepsy and γ-amino butyric acid-mediated inhibition. *International Review of Neurobiology, 17,* 1–36.

Meldrum, B. S., & Brierly, J. B. (1973). Prolonged epileptic seizures in primates. *Archives of Neurology, 28,* 10–17.

Menon, M. K., & Vivonia, C. A. (1981). Muscimol-induced myoclonic jerks in mice. *Neuropharmacology, 20,* 441–444.

Mintz, M., & Myslobodsky, M. S. (1992). Dual effect of a steroid derivative (RU5135) on VEP in rats. Paper presented at the *EPIC X meeting*. Eger, Hungary.

Miller, D. (1992). Caveats and hazards of assessment. Stress and neurotoxicity. In R. L. Isaacson & K. F. Jensen (Eds.), *The vulnerable brain and environmental risks, Vol. 1: Malnutrition and hazard assessment* (pp. 239–266). New York: Plenum Press.

Moberg, G. P., Scapagnini, U., de Groot, J., & Ganong, W. F. (1971). Effects of sectioning the fornix on diurnal fluctuation and plasma corticosterone levels in the rat. *Neuroendocrinology, 7,* 11–15.

Moises, H. C., Hoffer, B. J., & Woodward, D. J. (1980). GABA facilitation by noradrenaline shows supersensitivity in cerebellum after 6-hydroxydopamine. *Naunyn-Schmiedeberg's Archives of Pharmacology, 315,* 35–46.

Mori, A., Hiramatsu, M., Kabuto, H., & Marescau, B. (1986). Effects of emotional stress on E1-mouse convulsions, and their biochemical background. *Neurochemical Research, 11,* 37–45.

Myslobodsky, M. (1976). *Petit mal epilepsy. A search for precursors of petit mal activity.* New York: Academic Press.

Myslobodsky, M. (1984). Petit mal epilepsy: Too much or too little GABA? In R. Fariello, P. L. Morselli, K. G. Lloyd, L. F. Quesney, & J. Engel. (Eds.), *Neurotransmitters, seizures, and epilepsy* (pp. 337–346). New York: Raven Press.

Myslobodsky, M. S. (1988). Metabolic encephalopathies and petit mal epilepsy. In M. S. Myslobodsky & A. F. Mirsky (Eds.), *Elements of petit mal epilepsy.* New York: Lang.

Myslobodsky, M. S., & Kofman, O. (1982). A steroid derivative (R5135) activates long-lasting non-convulsant spiking in rats. *Neuropharmacology, 22,* 157–164.

Myslobodsky, M. S., Mintz, M., Tarrasch, R., & Bar-Ziv, J. (1991). A steroid derivative (RU 5135) exhibits epileptogenicity in the presence of deficient blood-brain barrier. *Pharmacology, Biochemistry and Behavior, 38,* 327–331.

Myslobodsky, M. S., & Mirsky, A. F. (Eds.). (1987). *Elements of petit mal epilepsy.* New York: Lang.

Myslobodsky, M., & Valenstein, E. (1980). Amygdaloid kindling and the GABA system. *Epilepsia, 21,* 163–175.

Newmark, M. E., & Penry, J. K. (1979). *Photosensitive epilepsy: A review.* New York: Raven Press.

Newmark, M. E., & Penry, J. K. (1980). Catamenial epilepsy: A review. *Epilepsia, 21,* 281–300.

O'Brien, M. D. (1989). Academic hemianopia and the treatment of cerebrovascular disease. In A. Hartmann & W. Kuschinsky (Eds.), *Cerebral ischemia and calcium* (pp. 3–6). Berlin: Springer-Verlag.

Paul, S. M., & Purdy, R. H. (1992). Neuroactive steroids. *FASEB Journal, 6,* 2311–2322.

Paul, S. M., & Skolnick, P. (1978). Rapid changes in brain benzodiazepine receptor after experimental seizures. *Science, 202,* 982–893.

Pearlson, G. D., Kim, W. S., Kuboe, K. L., Moberg, P. J., Jayaram, G., Bascom, M. J., & Chase, G. A. (1989). Ventricle-brain ratio, computed tomographic density and brain area in 50 schizophrenics. *Archives of General Psychiatry, 46,* 690–697.

Pericic, D., Manev, H., & Lakic, N. (1985). Sex differences in the response of rats to drugs affecting GABAergic transmission. *Life Sciences, 36,* 541–547.

Pfaff, D. W. (1989). Features of hormone-driven defined neural circuit for a mammalian behavior. *Annals of the New York Academy of Sciences, 563,* 131–147.

Prince, D. (1972). Topical convulsant metals and metabolic antagonists. In D. P. Purpura et al. (Eds.), *Experimental models of epilepsy: A manual for laboratory workers* (pp. 51–84). New York: Raven Press.

Purdy, R. H., Moore, P. H., Jr., Hagino, N., Morrow, A. L., & Paul, S. M. (1991). *$GABA_A$ receptor-active neurosteroids in the rat brain.* Paper presented at the 21st annual meeting of the Society for Neurosciences, New Orleans, LA.

Purdy, R. H., Moore, P. H., Jr., Morrow, A. L., & Paul, S. M. (1991). Stress-induced elevations of γ-aminobutyric acid type A receptor-active steroids in the rat brain. *Proceedings of the National Academy of Sciences of the USA, 88,* 4553–4557.

Purpura, D. P., Girado, M., Smith, T. G., Jr., & Gomez, J. A. (1958). Effects of systematically administered amino and guanidino acids on spontaneous and evoked cortical activity in regions of blood brain area destruction. *Electroencephalography and Clinical Neurophysiology, 10,* 1287–1288.

Remler, M. P., & Marcussen, W. H. (1983). A GABA-EEG test of the blood-brain barrier near epileptic foci. *Applied Neurophysiology, 46,* 276–285.

Rice, R. D. (1977). Neuropsychological development in premature infants following stimulation. *Developmental Psychology, 13,* 69–76.

Robertson, H. A. (1980). The benzodiazepine receptor: The pharmacology of emotions. *Le Journal Canadien des Sciences Neurologiques, 7,* 243–245.

Robson, P. (1968). Persistent head turning in the early months: Some effects in the early years. *Developmental, Medical and Child Neurology, 10,* 82–92.

Rogawski, M. A., Hershkowitz, N., Politi, D. M., Suzuki, S., Thurkauf, A., & Yamaguchi, S. (1990). Novel research strategies for antiepileptic therapy. In B. S. Meldrum & M. Williams (Eds.), *Current and future trends in anticonvulsant, anxiety, and stroke therapy* (pp. 91–111). New York: Wiley-Liss.

Rosciszewska, D., Buntner, B., Guz, I., & Zawisza, L. (1986). Ovarian hormones, anticonvulsant drugs and seizures during menstrual cycle in women with epilepsy. *Journal of Neurology, Neurosurgery & Psychiatry, 49,* 47–71.

Rothschild, B. F. (1967). Incubator isolation as a possible contributing factor to the high incidence of emotional disturbance among prematurely born persons. *Journal of Genetic Psychology, 110,* 287–304.

Ryu, H., Uemura, K., Nakajima, S., Furuya, T., & Ryu, K. (1984). Effects of solcoseryl on experimental cerebral injury: morphological studies of cerebral mitochondria. *Cytoprotection and Cytobiology, 1,* 109–107.

Sadasivudu, B., Rao, T. I., & Murthy, C. R. (1977). Metabolic effects of hydrocorticosterone in mouse brain. *Neurochemistry Research, 2,* 221–222.

Sapolsky, R. (1986a). Glucocorticoid toxicity in the hippocampus: Temporal aspects of synergy with kainic acid. *Neuroendocrinology, 43,* 440–444.

Sapolsky, R. (1986b). Glucocorticoid toxicity in the hippocampus: Reversal by supplementation with brain fuels. *Journal of Neurosciences, 6,* 2240–2244.

Sapolsky, R. M., Krey, L. C., & McEwen, B. S. (1986). The neuroendocrinology of stress and aging: The glucocorticoid cascade hypothesis. *Endocrine Reviews, 7,* 284–301.

Scatrud, J. B., Dempsey, J. A., & Kaiser, D. G. (1978). Ventilatory response to medroxyprogesterone acetate in normal subjects: Time course and mechanisms. *Journal of Applied Physiology, 44,* 939–944.

Schofield, P. R., Shivers, B. D., & Seeburg, P. H. (1990). The role of receptor subtypes diversity in the CNS. *Trends in Neurosciences, 13,* 8–11.

Scott, W. T. (1980). Seizures: A reaction to contrast media for computed tomography of the brain. *Radiology, 137,* 359–361.

Selye, H. (1941). The anesthetic effect of steroid hormones. *Proceedings of the Society for Experimental Biology and Medicine, 46,* 116–121.

Siesjo, B. K., & Wieloch, T. (1986). Epileptic brain damage: Pathophysiology and neurochemical pathology. In A. V. Delgado-Escueta, A. A. Ward, D. M. Woodbury, & R. J. Porter (Eds.), *Advances in neurology* (vol. 44, pp. 813–847). New York: Raven Press.

Slater, E., Beard, A., & Glithero, E. (1963). The schizophrenia-like psychoses of epilepsy. *British Journal of Psychiatry, 109,* 95–150.

Slusher, M. A. (1966). Effects of cortisol implants in the brainstem and ventral hippocampus on diurnal corticosterone levels. *Experimental Brain Research, 1,* 184–194.

Smart, J. L., Tonkiss, J., & Massey, R. F. (1986). A phenomenon: Left-biased asymmetrical eye-opening in artificially reared rat pups. *Developmental Brain Research, 28,* 134–136.

Smith, S. S. (1989). Estrogen administration increases neuronal responses to excitatory amino acids as a long-term effect. *Brain Research, 503,* 354–357.

Smith, S. S. (1991). Progesterone administration attenuates excitatory amino acid responses of cerebellar Purkinje cells. *Neurosciences, 42,* 302–320.

Solkoff, N., Weintraub, D., Yaffe, S., & Blase, B. (1969). Effects of handling on the subsequent development of premature infants. *Developmental Psychology, 1,* 765–769.

Soubrie, P., Thiebot, M. H., Jebert, A., Montastruc, J. L., Hery, F., & Hamon, M. (1980). Decreased convulsant potency of picrotoxin and pentetrazol and enhanced ^{3}H-flunitrazepam cortical binding following stressful manipulations in rats. *Brain Research, 189,* 505–517.

Speransky, A. D. (1932). *Epileptic fit. Experimental analysis of the neocortical mechanisms.* Moscow: Medgiz. (in Russian)

Squires, R. F., Casida, J. E., Richardson, M., & Saederup, E. (1983). [^{35}S]t-butyl bicyclophosphorothionate binds with high affinity to brain specific sites coupled to γ-aminobutyric acid-A recognition sites. *Molecular Pharmacology, 23,* 326–336.

Sterman, M. B., Shouse, M. N., Lucia, M. C., Heinrich, R. L., & Sarnoff, S. K. (1977). Effects of anesthesia and cranial electrode implantation on seizure susceptibility in the cat. *Experimental Neurology, 57,* 158–166.

Stevens, J. R. (1988). Epilepsy, psychosis and schizophrenia. *Schizophrenia Research, 1,* 79–89.

Suddath, R. L., Christison, G. W., Torrey, E. F., Casanova, M. F., & Weinberger, D. R. (1990). Anatomical abnormalities in the brains of monozygotic twins discordant for schizophrenia. *New England Journal of Medicine, 322,* 789–794.

Suzuki, S., & Rogawski, M. (1989). T-type calcium channels mediate the transition between tonic and phasic firing in thalamic neurons. *Proceedings of the National Academy of Sciences of USA, 86,* 7228–7232.

Taylor, D. C. (1972). Mental state and temporal lobe epilepsy. A collective account of 100 patients treated surgically. *Epilepsia, 13,* 727–765.

Taylor, D. C. (1991). Developmental and behavioral differences between males and females with special reference to epilepsy. In M. Trimble (Ed.), *Women in epilepsy.* Chichester: Wiley.

Timiras, P. S. (1969). Role of hormones in development of seizures. In H. H. Jasper, A. A. Ward, & A. Pope (Eds.), *Basic mechanism of epilepsies* (pp. 727–736). Boston: Little, Brown.

Toft, D., & Chytil, F. (1973). Receptors for glucocorticoids in lung tissue. *Archives of Biochemistry & Biophysics, 157,* 464–469.

van Praag, H. M. (1979). Psychopsychiatry: Can psychosocial factors cause psychotic disorders? *Comprehensive Psychiatry, 32,* 357–365.

Wada, J. A., Sato, M., & Corcoran, M. E. (1974). Persistent seizure susceptibility and recurrent spontaneous seizures in kindled cats. *Epilepsia, 15,* 465–478.

Ward, A. A., Jasper, H. H., & Pope, A. (1969). Clinical and experimental challenges in the epilepsies. In H. H. Jasper, A. A. Ward, & A. Pope (Eds.), *Basic mechanism of epilepsies* (pp. 1–12). Boston: Little, Brown.

Weinberger, D. R. (1987). Implications of normal brain development for pathogenesis of schizophrenia. *Archives of General Psychiatry, 44,* 660–669.

Weizman, A., Weizman, R., Kook, K. A., Vocci, F., Deutsch, S. I., & Paul, S. M. (1989). Repeated swim stress alters brain benzodiazepine receptors measured *in vivo. Journal of Pharmacology and Experimental Therapeutics, 249,* 701–707.

Weizman, A., Weizman, R., Kook, K. A., Vocci, F., Deutsch, S. I., & Paul, S. M. (1990). Adrenalectomy prevents the stress-induced decrease *in vivo* [^{3}H] Ro15-1788 binding to $GABA_A$ receptors. *Brain Research, 519,* 347–350.

Woodbury, D. M. (1952). Effect of adrenocortical steroids and adrenocorticotropic hormone on electroshock seizure threshold. *Journal of Pharmacology and Experimental Therapeutics, 105,* 27–36.

Woolley, D. E., & Timiras, P. S. (1962a). The gonad-brain relationship: Effects of female sex hormones on electroshock convulsions in the rat. *Endocrinology, 70,* 196–203.

Woolley, D. E., & Timiras, P. S. (1962b). Estrous and circadian periodicity and electroshock convulsions in rats. *American Journal of Physiology, 202,* 379–382.

Wu, F.-S., Gibbs, T. T., & Farb, D. H. (1990). Inverse modulation of γ-Aminobutyric acid- and glycine-induced currents by progesterone. *Molecular Pharmacology, 37,* 597–602.

Yokoyama, A., Ramirez, V. D., & Sawyer, C. H. (1966). Sleep and wakefulness in female rats under various hormonal and physiological conditions. *General & Comparative Endocrinology, 7,* 10–17.

Young, S. W. III., & Kuhar, M. J. (1980). Radiohystochemical localization of benzodiazepine receptors in rat brain. *Journal of Pharmacology and Experimental Therapy, 212,* 337–340.

Yuwiler, A. (1980). Three paradigms for studies in schizophrenia. In C. Baxter & T. Melnechuk (Eds.), *Progress in schizophrenia research* (pp. 1–26). New York: Raven Press.

Zarcone, V., Gulevich, G., & Dement, W. C. (1967). Sleep and electroconvulsive therapy. *Archives of General Psychiatry, 16,* 567–578.

9 Behavior of Epileptic Patients After Magnetic Stimulation

P. A. Anninos
N. Tsagas
Democrition University of Thrace and Polytechnic School, Alexandroupolis and Xanthi, Greece

The term *epilepsy* refers to a paroxysmal and transitory disturbance of brain electrical functions that develops suddenly, ceases spontaneously, and exhibits a conspicuous tendency to recur. Although in its most typical form it is characterized by the sudden onset of loss of consciousness, which may or may not be associated with tonic spasms and clonic contractions of the muscles, many varieties of epileptic seizures have been described, with their distinctive features depending on differences in the site of origin, extent of cerebral involvement, and nature of the disturbance of function (Adams & Victor, 1985; Dreifuss, 1989).

Epileptic seizure is accompanied by changes in the electrical potentials of the brain and has been described as "paroxysmal cerebral dysrhythmia" (Gibbs, Gibbs, & Lennox, 1937). In the case of a generalized seizure, it may be triggered by spread from a cortical focus or originate from deep cerebral structures. The generalization of the clinical and electrical manifestations are thought to depend on activation of deep, centrally located mechanisms including the midbrain reticular formation and its diencephalic extension, the intralaminar, and nonspecific thalamic projection systems (Adams & Victor, 1985).

In general, partial seizures are those in which the first clinical and electroencephalographic changes indicate initial activation of a system of neurons limited to part of one cerebral hemisphere (Dreifuss, 1989). A partial seizure primarily is classified by whether consciousness is impaired during the attack. Hence, when consciousness is not impaired, the seizure is classified as a simple partial seizure. When consciousness is impaired, the seizure is classified as a complex partial seizure. Impairment of consciousness may be the first clinical sign, or simple partial seizures may evolve into complex partial seizures. Complex partial seizures frequently have bilateral hemispheric involvement, and their elaboration includes elements of the limbic system (i.e., temporal and frontal lobes). Complex partial seizures are not peculiar to any period of life, but show an increased incidence in adolescence and adult years.

In most cases of seizure disorders, abnormal neuronal discharges are associated with electroencephalographic (EEG) changes, although in certain unquestionable attacks of epilepsy, conventional EEG recordings are normal. Localization of these abnormal electrical discharges are critical for documentation and potential therapeutic modalities.

Due to the limitations of the scalp EEG recordings, the interictal EEG is nondiagnostic in many patients with proved seizures (Gastaut & Tassinari, 1975). In cases where EEG recordings have been negative, the use of more invasive methods, such as electrocorticography (ECoG) and stereoelectroencephalography (SEEG), have facilitated the identification of seizure activity (Spencer, 1981; Sutherling & Barth, 1990; Wieser & Elger, 1987). These interventions are associated with a certain degree of risk and expense, and are labor- and time-intensive. Moreover, selection of patients for intracranial electrode implantation assumes that a given seizure disorder is focal, but nonlocalized seizures are found in 18%–20% of patients evaluated by intracranial recordings (Spencer, 1981). This is especially true in patients with frontal lobe epilepsy (Sutherling & Barth, 1990). Furthermore, metabolic imaging techniques, such as positron emission tomography (PET) and single photon emission computed tomography (SPECT), which indicate a focal area in terms of a region of hypometabolism or alterations in cerebral blood flow, have failed to prove reliable in localizing epileptic foci (Engel, 1987; Wieser & Elger, 1987). Hence, considering that approximately 50,000–100,000 persons in the United States are therapy resistant, and hence candidates for epilepsy surgery (Rose, Smith, & Sato, 1987), there is great interest in the development of noninvasive methods that can assist in accurate localization and measurements of the brain's electrical activity.

Measurement of the brain's magnetic activity, with the use of the magnetoencephalogram (MEG), has been reported to permit higher spatial resolution than can be achieved with electric potential measurements of the EEG (Elger et al., 1989; Rose et al., 1987). In addition, the MEG may be superior to the EEG in spatial localization of current sources, because the scalp and the skull are transparent to the associated magnetic fields, whereas they distort the volume currents measured by the EEG (Rose et al., 1987). This implies that for localizing presumed epileptic foci in the depths of the cerebrum, the magnetic counterpart of the EEG, the MEG, might be superior to conventional surface EEG recordings (Elger et al., 1989).

In fact, the MEG has been considered to be potentially more effective in the three-dimensional localization of focal neuronal events (Rose et al., 1987), with an ability to localize a source in the human brain to about 2 or 3 mm (Barth, Beatty, Broffman, & Sutherling, 1986; Kaufman & Williamson, 1982; Rose, Ducla-Soares, Sato, & Kufka, 1988; Weinberg, Brickett, Coolsma, & Baff,

TABLE 9.1
Comparison of EEG and MEG

EEG	*MEG*
Scalp potential differences	Extracranial magnetic field
Tissues and fluids interference	No interference
Sensitive to dipoles in all directions	Sensitive to tangentially oriented dipoles
Maximal signal in cortical gyri	Maximal signal in cortical sulci
Localization to about 20 mm	Localization to about 2–3 mm

1986). In contrast, the EEG was reported to have an accuracy of 20 mm (Smith, Sidman, & Flanigin, 1985). However, a recent study using implanted sources in the human brain failed to confirm the superiority of the MEG over the EEG in terms of depth localization of a focal source (Cohen et al., 1990). In this study, the MEG average localization accuracy was found to be 8 mm, whereas the EEG accuracy was 10 mm.

There are several principal differences between the EEG and the MEG (Rose & Ducla-Soares, 1990) (see Table 9.1). The EEG uses electrodes applied to the scalp with conductive paste, and it measures scalp potential differences. It is sensitive to dipoles oriented in any direction. For the routine EEG, electrodes are spaced evenly around the head, and recording of the signal is done over the entire head at one time. The MEG uses a magnetometer that is positioned close to the head surface, and it measures extracranial magnetic fields. It is primarily sensitive to tangentially oriented dipoles generated by the activity of the cortical pyramidal cells (Nunez, 1990).

The cerebral cortex, like any other electric generator, produces a magnetic field that, although very weak, can be recorded by the MEG (Rose et al., 1987). Unlike the EEG, the MEG is not subject to interferences from the tissues and fluids lying between the cortex and the scalp. The spontaneous magnetic fields produced by the cerebral neuronal activity are about one billionth of the strength of the earth's magnetic field and arise from ion movements produced by changes in the electrical potential of neuronal cell membranes (Rose et al., 1987). Changes in the membrane potential, which usually begin in the dendrite, are followed by compensatory ionic movements throughout the neuronal cell body, creating a current dipole. The MEG is thought to record the activity of the cortical pyramidal cells, which are oriented perpendicular to the brain surface, where many such neurons are aligned parallel to one another (Rose et al., 1987). In contrast, cortical neurons, which are oriented perpendicular to the scalp surface and produce dipoles oriented radially, do not contribute to the component of the extracranial magnetic field perpendicular to the scalp. Neurons with intermittent orientation produce dipoles with both tangetial and radial components. Hence, the orientation of the current dipole is a critical factor affecting the measurement of magnetic fields outside the head (Rose et al., 1987). Because the principal generator of the MEG lies in the layer of pyramidal cells and the MEG is produced exclusively by a flow of electric current tangential to the skull surface, it appears that the signal will originate maximally from the cerebral sulci (where the pyramidal cells are more favorably oriented) and only minimally from the surface of the gyri where their orientation is less favorable.

The magnetic fields associated with an epileptic event are approximately 1 picotesla (pT) and are measured with a superconducting detection coil coupled to a superconducting quantum interference device (SQUID) (Rose et al., 1987). Since the introduction of the SQUID magnetic field sensors, attempts have been made to localize epileptic foci (Cohen et al., 1990; Rose et al., 1987; Sutherling et al., 1987; Sutherling, Crandall, Cahan, & Barth, 1988). It has been known for some time that internal neuronal activity is associated with the generation of magnetic activity (Burr & Northorp, 1939), which can pass virtually undistorted through the highly resistant and low conductive human skull. Using the SQUID, it became possible to measure magnetic fields of the order of 2×10^{-8} G from the brain, which corresponds to brain activities for the alpha frequencies (8–12 Hz) (Anninos, Anogianakis, Lehnertz, Pantev, & Hoke, 1987). Barth, Sutherling, Engel, and Beatty (1982, 1984) mapped the magnetic field distribution after averaging a sufficient number of interictal spikes triggered by the EEG in patients with focal epilepsy. Sato, Rose, and Porter (1985) computed field maps from manually selected individual spikes in a patient with partial complex seizures and reportedly detected a dipolar source in the right temporal area.

It has been argued previously (Elger et al., 1989) that a single dipole model is not appropriate for the conceptualization of seizure activity because (a) an epileptic focus generates different types of seizure activity, the occurrence of which is unpredictable; (b) the brain area generating a single epileptic discharge is varying, and different neuronal populations may contribute to a single epileptic pattern, most of them with a *similar* field potential; (c) the synchronized action potentials of epileptic neurons discharging with high frequency give rise to synchronized projected synaptic activity, resulting in a number of new current dipoles; and (d) the interictal activity is known to be of localizing value only in a limited number of patients with seizure disorders.

Given these difficulties, we have proposed an alternate approach utilizing the MEG for the evaluation of patients with seizure disorders (Elger et al., 1989). Instead of studying the surface distribution of the time domain MEG, our method was based on investigating the surface distribution of frequency domain aspects of the interictal MEG. We propose that the surface distribution of spectral energy in specified frequency bands would exhibit patterns that are specific for specified locations or epileptic foci (Anninos et al., 1987; Elger et al., 1989). Furthermore, we postulated that these patterns would not be detected in normal subjects, and that correlations of a specified pattern with the location of epileptic foci would enable us to establish an atlas of typical cortical projections of interictal seizure activity. This could be used in planning the strategy for presurgical evaluation of patients with seizure disorders (Elger et al., 1989).

In addition to mapping epileptic foci for the presurgical evaluation of patients with seizure disorders, we also were interested in applying magnetic fields back to the brain to attenuate seizure activity (Anninos et al., 1987). This proposal seemed justified in view of the observations in animals, which showed that administration of low-frequency magnetic fields altered electrical activity in the brain and thus influenced the frequency or severity of seizures (Ossenkopp & Cain, 1988). Specifically, it has been shown that exposure of rats to intense acoustic stimulation, which induces epileptiform brain activity, together with exposure to 2- or 3-Hz modulated electromagnetic fields, depresses the paroxysmal brain electrical activity associated with audiogenic seizures (Antimonii & Salamov, 1980). Furthermore, exposure to 50- or 60-Hz magnetic fields has been reported to inhibit the lethal effects of pentylenetetrazol (PTZ)-induced seizures in rats (Ossenkopp, Cain, & Smith, 1985). More recently, Ossenkopp and Cain (1988) reported an inhibitory effect of low-intensity 60-Hz magnetic field exposure on electrically kindled seizures in rats and humans. In addition, changes in the geomagnetic fields have been linked to the incidence of epileptic seizures (Keshaven, Gangadhar, Gautman, Ajit, & Kapur, 1981; Rajaram & Mitra, 1981; Venkatraman, 1976). In brief, these findings indicated a relationship between ambient magnetic field activity and the occurrence of epilepsy. Furthermore, they suggest that application of magnetic field may attenuate seizure activity in epileptic patients.

To test our prediction empirically, we investigated the effects of magnetic stimulation in epileptic patients with partial seizures. Most of these patients had been resistant to conventional antiepileptic therapy. After mapping the presumed epileptic foci, we applied a single magnetic stimulation of the same intensity and frequency to those recorded with the MEG back to the brain and observed a significant attenuation in the frequency and severity of seizure over an observation period lasting from 10 to 14 months.

MATERIALS AND METHODS

The patients were referred to our laboratory in Alexandroupolis, Greece, by a practicing neurologist. Informed consent for the study was obtained from all patients prior to the procedures. Patients had been diagnosed by a specialist neurologist to have partial seizures in accordance with the classification of the Commission on Classification and Technology of the International League Against Epilepsy (1981). All patients had normal serum biochemical studies as well as a normal CT scan. In all cases, mapping of the seizure foci, as well as magnetic stimulation, were performed during the interictal state. None of the patients experienced side effects during or after the procedure.

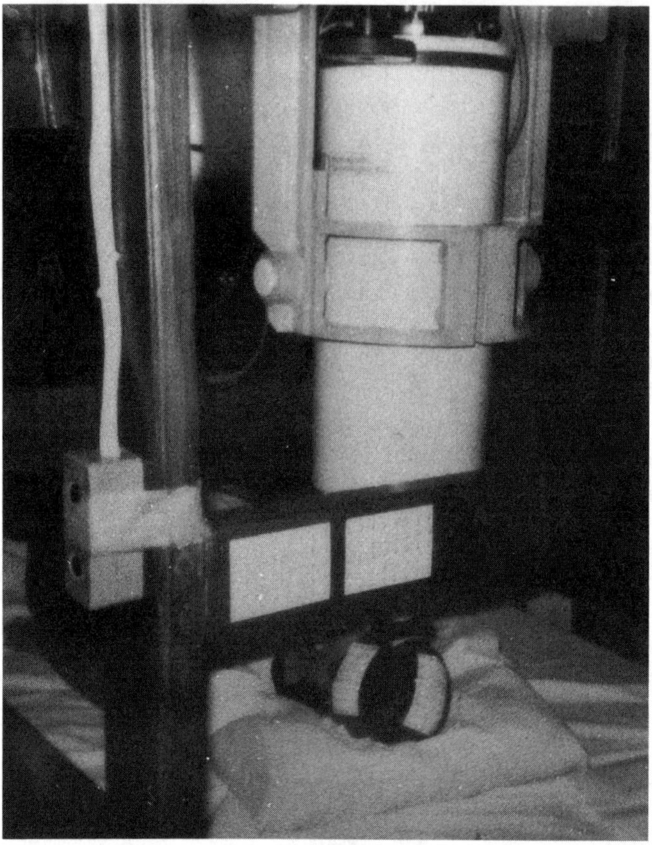

FIG. 9.1. The SQUID and the patient lying on a wooden bed during the MEG measurements.

The method used for the recording of magnetic activity has been described in detail elsewhere (Anninos et al., 1987; Elger et al., 1989). In brief, we used a SQUID second-order gradiometer (D.C. SQUID model 601 of the Biomagnetic Technologies). In an electrically shielded room in our laboratory (Fig. 9.1), the noise level in the SQUID environment was of the order of 30–50 $fT/\sqrt{Hz}$.

During the procedure, the patient lay down on a wooden bed with his head resting on a special cushion filled with air. After positioning the SQUID 3 mm above each particular point on the scalp using an optic system, the patient was asked to relax and close his eyes to avoid artifacts from eye flickering and to enhance the alpha rhythms.

To establish the actual differences between the environmental noise level and the power contained in the MEG spectrum, we proceeded to average all the MEG spectra recorded during an experimental session and compared them with the noise level determined during the same experiment. In particular, at some point during each experimental session, the SQUID probe was placed 30 cm away from the scalp of the patient, and 32 records of 1-sec duration each were taken, keeping all other experimental conditions unchanged. Comparison of the two averaged spectra showed substantial values for the signal to noise ratio (see Fig. 9.2).

The MEG measurements consisted of data recorded from the scalp of the patients at specified points as defined by a recording reference system. This reference system, which is based on the International 10–20 Electrode Placement System (Jasper, 1958), uses any one of the standard EEG recording positions as its origin (Anninos et al., 1987). In this study, we used the P3, P4, T3, T4, F3, and F4 recording positions. The reference system was devised to retrieve maximal information from a specified area of the skull, given that the gradiometer coil is theoretically equally sensitive to all magnetic flux lines perpendicular to a circular area of the brain. In our case, this circle has been an affective diameter of 2.36 cm (i.e., the diameter of the SQUID sensor coil). Around the origin a rectangular 32-point matrix was used (four rows × eight columns, equidistantly spaced in a 4.5 cm × 10.5 cm rectangular) for positioning of the SQUID (Anninos et al., 1987).

The MEG was recorded from each cerebral hemisphere at each of the 32

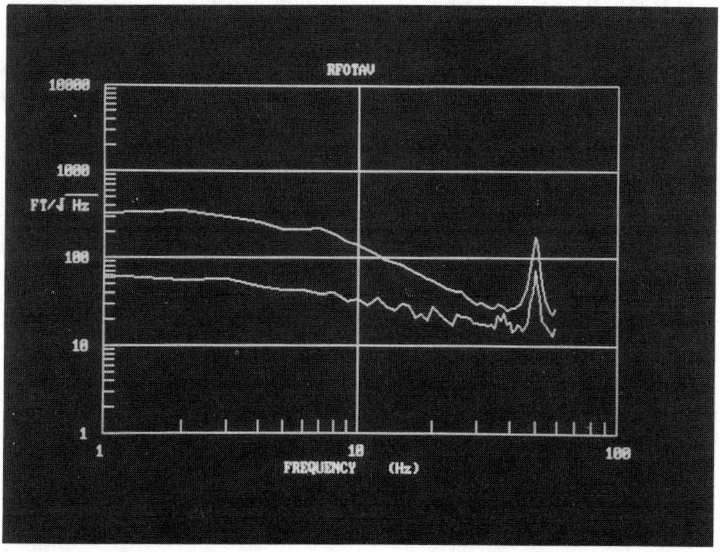

FIG. 9.2. Comparison between the power spectrum of the environmental noise level and the power spectrum of the average of all MEG spectra recorded during an experimental session.

matrix points on the scalp for 32 consecutive epochs. Each epoch was 1,000 ms in duration and was digitized with a sampling frequency of 250 Hz (frequency resolution of the power spectrum being 1 Hz). The MEG signal was band-pass filtered with cut-off frequencies of 0.1 Hz and 60 Hz. The MEG records were digitized with an analog-to-digital converter and stored in an IBM-PC computer for off-line Fourier statistical analysis.

MEG measurements were recorded from both the left and right temporal areas and, in some instances, from the frontal and occipital regions. Thus, 64 or 128 positions were collected. For each subject, the spatial distribution of specified band frequencies of the MEG power spectrum over an extensive area of the scalp ($10.5 \text{ cm} \times 4.5 \text{ cm} = = 47.25 \text{ cm}^2$) was calculated. These were expressed with the use of computer-generated graphics in terms of the total average of ISO–Spectral Amplitude (ISO–SA) distribution on the surface of the scanned areas over the scalp utilizing the frequency bands of 2–7 Hz, 8–13 Hz, and 14–25 Hz, respectively, in the MEG. These maps were useful in obtaining clearly defined areas of high spectral density in the 2–7 Hz band frequency. In addition, the ISO-SA maps helped provide clear identification of the point coordinates on the scalp where the MEG power spectrum emitted for the 2–7 Hz frequency, and its maximal power as well as its maximal magnetic field intensity.

The isocontour lines corresponding to equal spectral amplitudes for each frequency band were calculated providing two-dimensional graphic representations. Different shades in these ISO–SA maps represent different spectral amplitudes (in $\text{fT}/\sqrt{\text{Hz}}$) for the same band frequency. In our graphic illustrations (*vide infra*), the large symbol "+" represents the reference point for the left and right hemisphere for easy identification of the coordinates of the functional focal points. In the same illustration, the small "+" symbol represents the relative positions of the 32 matrix points with respect to the reference points.

Mapping the spectral power distribution over a surface, in the case where the measurements are independently recorded for each position (as in our case, where a single channel SQUID is used), requires the recorded MEG activity to remain invariant in time (Anninos et al., 1987). To ensure that in the course of our recordings the MEG activity was not influenced by long-term variations, we proceeded to repeat the recordings at various positions at different times. Figure 9.3 demonstrates that there was very little difference in the power spectrum between records as much as 60 minutes apart during the experiments. This is also evident in the ISO–SA maps seen in Figs. 9.4 and 9.5, respectively, which were obtained previously from a patient after measuring the same region (Elger et al., 1989). Thus, in our view, the stability of MEG measurements in epileptic patients justified the usage of a one-channel SQUID.

In terms of the MEG activity, we proposed a functional definition of the presumed epileptic foci. A *focus* was defined as a circumscribed cerebral area where, in the band of 2–7 Hz MEG frequencies, it exhibited its maximal power spectral value and the most dense concentration of ISO–SA contour lines (*vide*

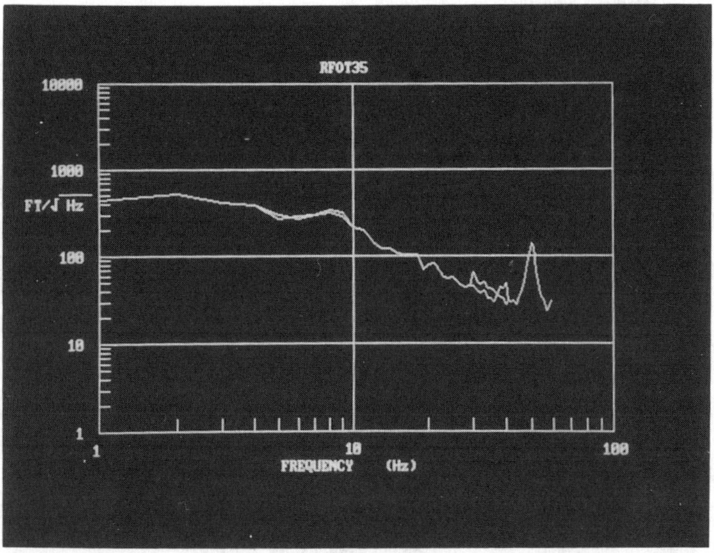

FIG. 9.3. The power spectra obtained by recording the activity with the SQUID at a particular position at different times. The power spectrum remained unchanged during multiple recordings taken as much as 60 min apart.

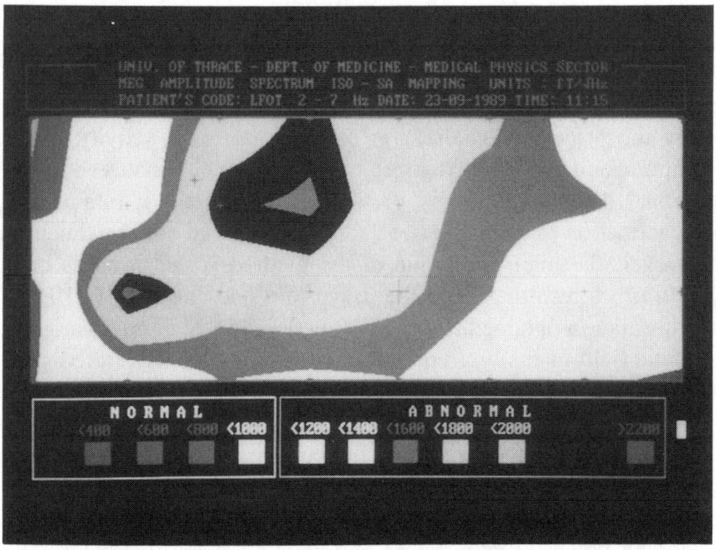

FIG. 9.4. ISO–SA map of the left temporal region for the 2–7 Hz band frequency measured on September 23, 1989.

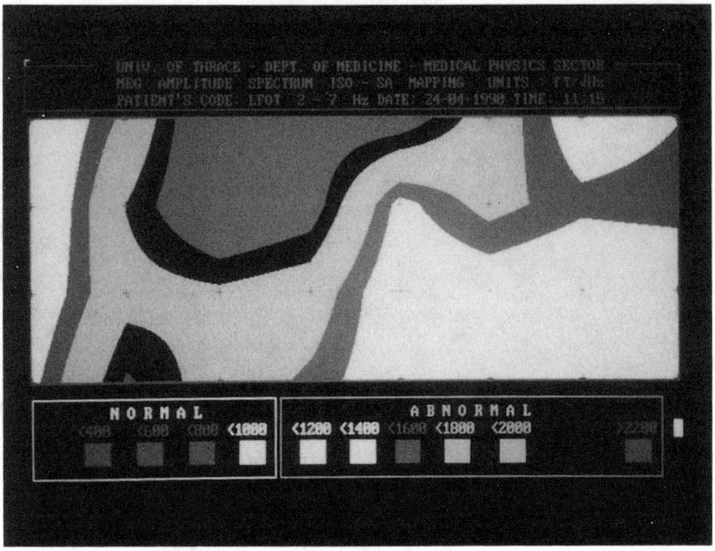

FIG. 9.5. ISO-SA map of the left temporal region of the patient described in Fig. 9.4. It shows the ISO–SA map for the 2–7 Hz band frequency measured on April 24, 1990.

infra) (Anninos et al., 1987). As a corollary to the previously described functional definition of a focus (Anninos et al., 1986), we proposed that when a focus is identified in both hemispheres, the one that is characterized by the highest dense concentration of the ISO–SA lines in its morphology should be considered the dominant one. We consider this method to be simple, because it represents pictorially the projected localization of maximal brain activity. By its nature (i.e., temporal and spatial averaging), the procedure eliminates short-term abnormal neuronal discharges in any cortical area, whereas it retains long-lasting localized activation phenomena (i.e., random interictal abnormal neuronal activity). However, the main limitation of the method is that it relies on long data acquisition times resulting from the usage of a one-channel SQUID.

The information obtained from each functional focal point regarding the emitted magnetic field intensity, frequency, and coordinates was stored subsequently in a special integrated circuit, which was used to energize an electronic device (Fig. 9.6), the principles of which are summarized in Appendix A. The latter was used to emit back a wave of magnetic field of the same intensity and frequency to the previously defined functional focal points (see Figs. 9.7 and 9.8). Figures 9.9 and 9.10 demonstrate the wave forms before and after magnetic treatment. The corresponding power spectra before and after magnetic treatment are shown in Figs. 9.11 and 9.12. The coils of the device were applied for several minutes (1–30 min) to each functional point on the patient's scalp, and resulted in cancella-

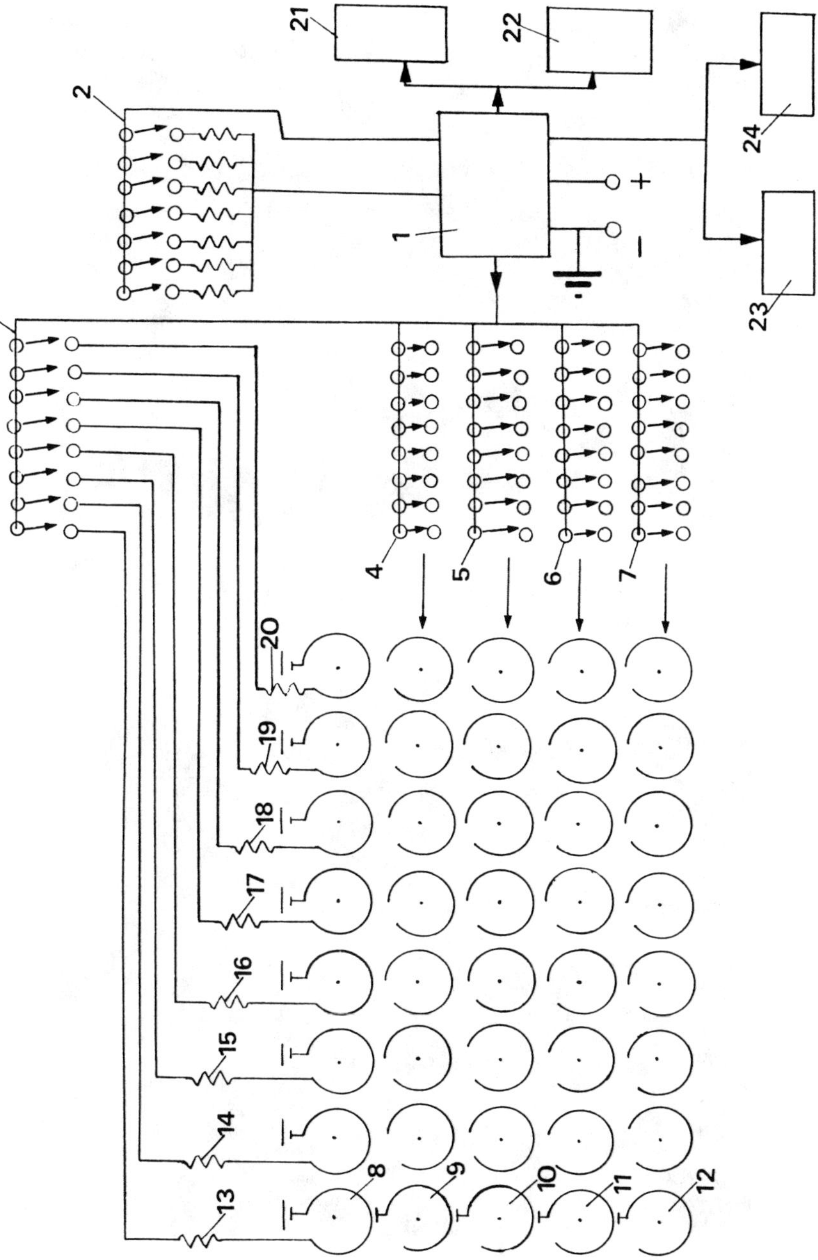

FIG. 9.6. General principles of the electronic device (see Appendix).

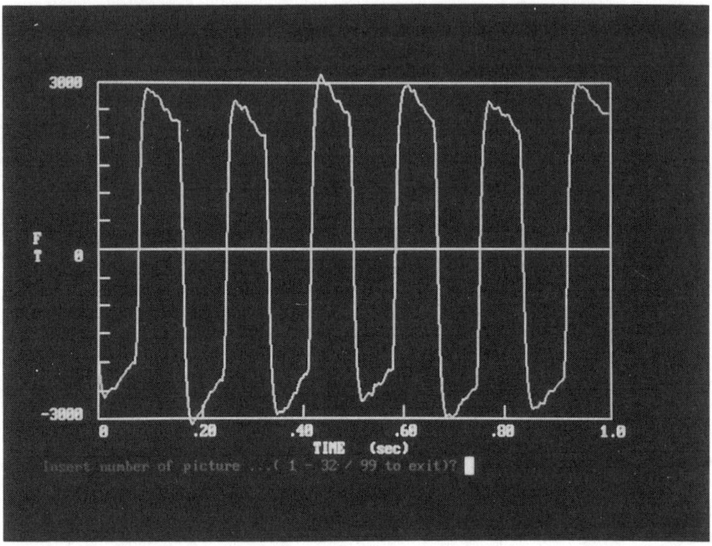

FIG. 9.7. The wave form of the magnetic field emitted from a particular coil of the electronic device.

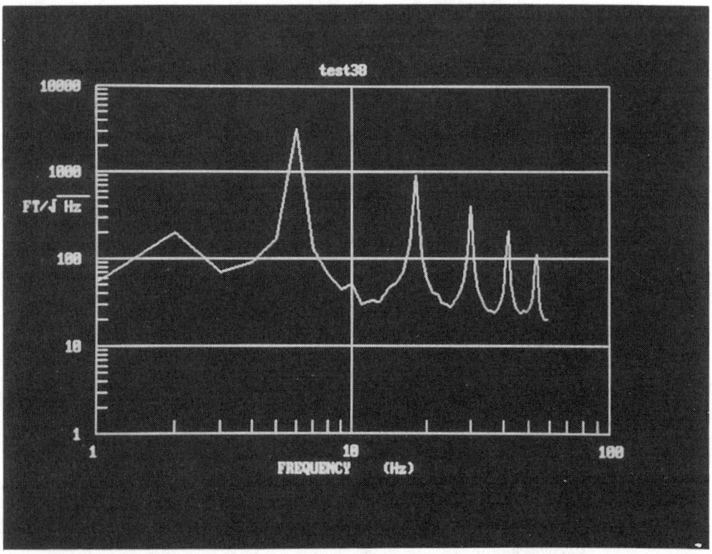

FIG. 9.8. The power spectrum of the wave form illustrated in Fig. 9.7. It shows the power amplitude and its frequency emitted from the electronic device.

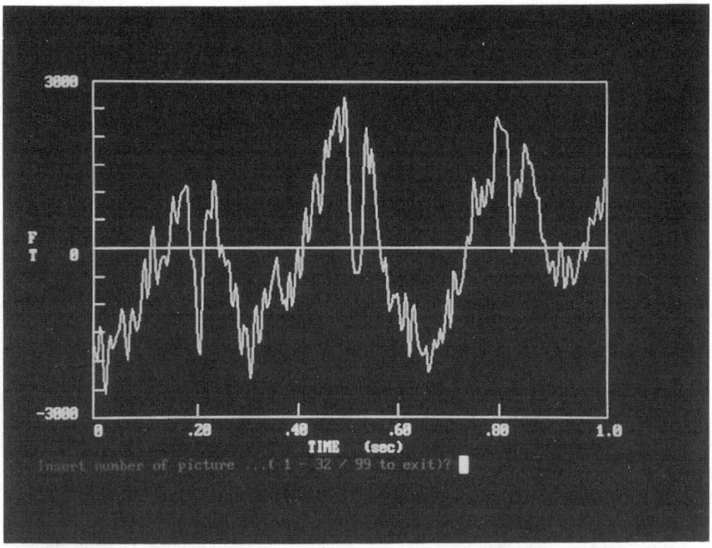

FIG. 9.9. The wave form for one of the identified focal points in the left temporal hemisphere of an epileptic patient.

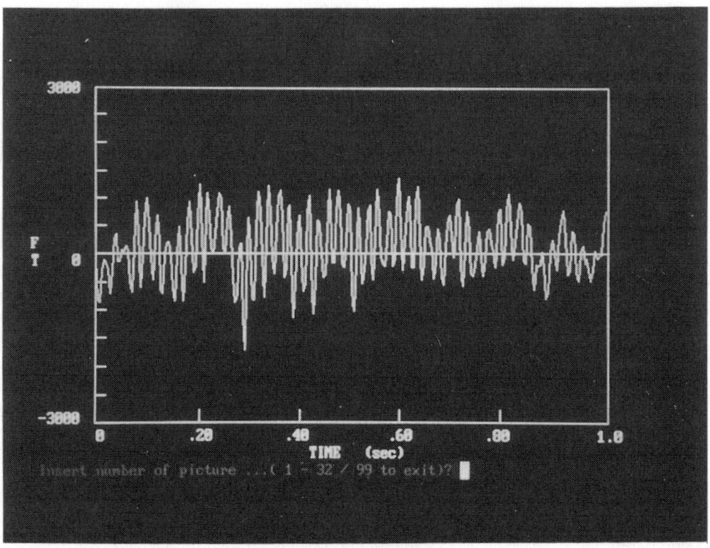

FIG. 9.10. The wave form after magnetic treatment.

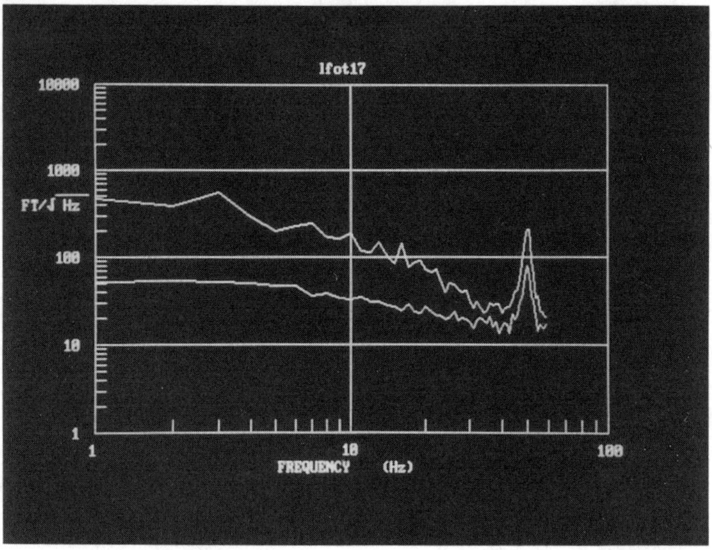

FIG. 9.11. The power spectrum for the wave form of the patient described in Fig. 9.9.

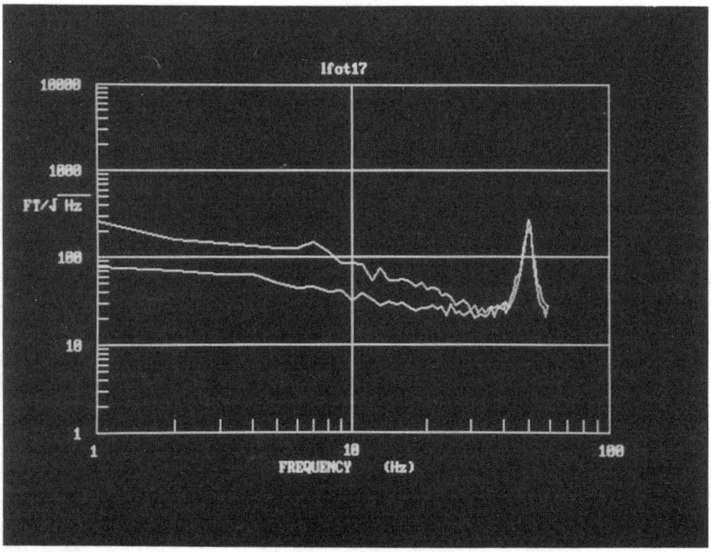

FIG. 9.12. The power spectrum after magnetic treatment.

tion if the magnetic power emitted from the effected brain region returned to a value of $< 1{,}000\ \mathrm{fT}/\sqrt{\mathrm{Hz}}$, a power that is considered to be within the normal limits.

Each coil of the electronic device had a diameter of 1 cm and, depending on the current of the circular coil and its turns, the magnetic field emitted from this coil to a distance of X cm from its center is given by the following equation from elementary physics: $B = uNIS/2\pi X^3$ where $u = 4 \times 10^{-7}$ weber/AM. Thus, for $I = 0.3 \times 10^{-6}$A, N = 6 turns, S = ..$(0.01\ \mathrm{m})^2$, and X = 3 mm, the B ~ 12.6 pico-tesla (pT).

RESULTS

The results of the MEG recordings for a particular patient before and after magnetic smoothing with the electronic device are presented in Figs. 9.13 and 9.14, respectively. Figure 9.13 demonstrates the ISO-SA map of the left temporal area in the interictal state. As can be seen, the maximal total average emitted power in the 2–7 Hz band frequency is $< 1{,}400\ \mathrm{fT}/\sqrt{\mathrm{Hz}}$.

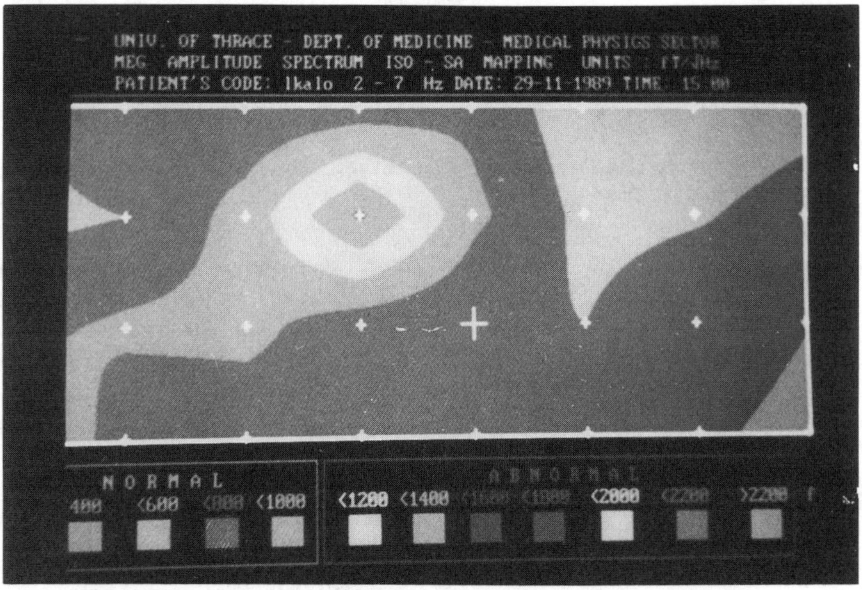

FIG. 9.13. ISO–SA map of the left temporal hemisphere during the interictal state before magnetic smoothing. As can be seen, the maximal total average emitted power in the 2–7 Hz band frequency is $< 1{,}400\ \mathrm{fT}\sqrt{\mathrm{Hz}}$.

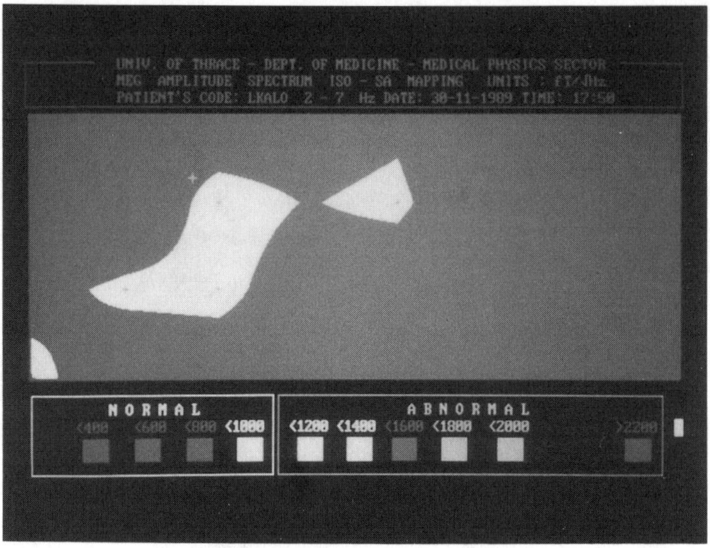

FIG. 9.14. ISO–SA map of the left temporal hemisphere after magnetic smoothing. As can be seen, the maximal total average emitted power in the 2–7 Hz band frequency is < 1,000 fT/$\sqrt{\text{Ha}}$.

The ISO–SA map of the patient after magnetic smoothing is presented in Fig. 9.14. The maximal total average emitted power in the 2–7 Hz band frequency is reduced to < 1,000 fT/$\sqrt{\text{Hz}}$.

Thus, our findings demonstrate that, by using the ISO–SA mapping technique, we were able to map and localize the presumed projections of interictal epileptic foci. Prior to magnetic smoothing with the electronic device, the ISO–SA maps of the epileptic foci showed dense concentrations of ISO-SA contour lines in the 2–7 Hz band frequency. Following magnetic stimulation of the same intensity and frequency back to the functional focal points of the brain, all patients demonstrated a reduction in the total average emitted power. As described below, this procedure was associated with normal psychological behaviour and with attenuation in the frequency and severity of the patients' seizures.

DISCUSSION

Using the ISO–SA maps in normal subjects, we found that the ISO–SA maps in the 2–7 Hz band frequency do not show dense concentrations of ISO–SA contour lines (Figs. 9.15 and 9.16) and, additionally, appear to change with time, thus indicating unstable brain activity (Elger et al., 1989; Lehnertz et al., 1989). In contrast, the ISO-SA maps of epileptic patients showed dense concentrations

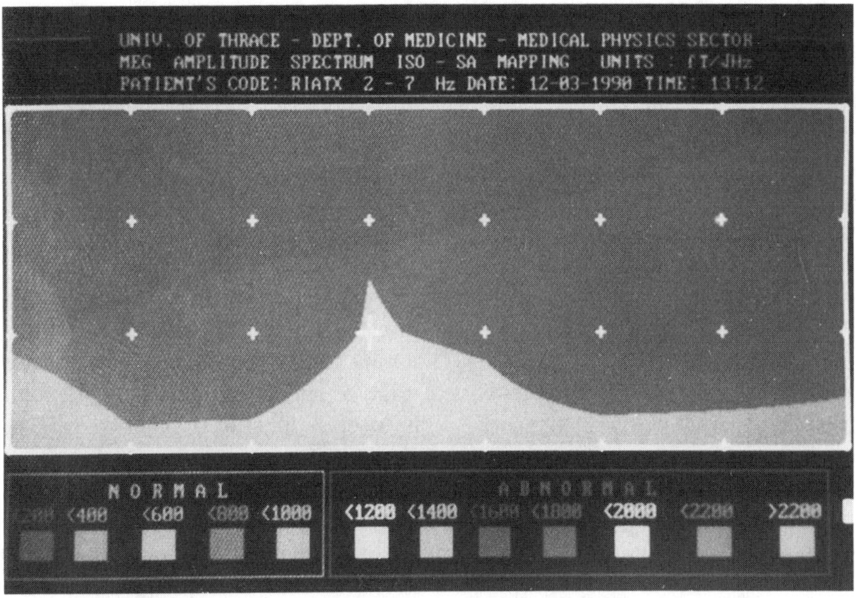

FIG. 9.15. ISO–SA map from a normal subject. The total average emitted power in the 2–7 Hz band frequency measured on August 2, 1989, is < 600 fT/$\sqrt{\text{Hz}}$.

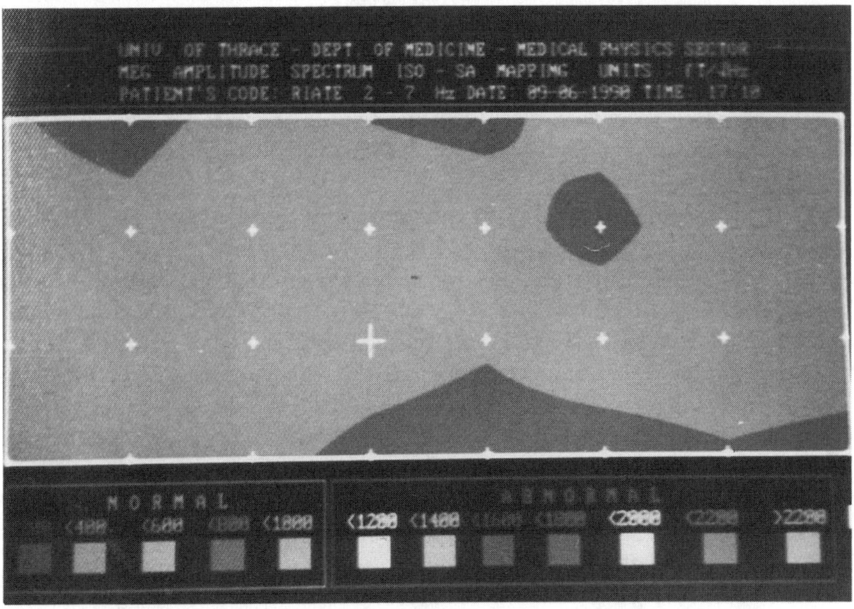

FIG. 9.16. ISO–SA map from the subject shown in Fig. 9.15 measured 1 month later. The change in the ISO–SA map with time is suggestive of unstable cerebral activity.

of ISO-SA contour lines in the same band frequency range. Characteristically, the patterns of epileptic patients appeared to be invariant with time, and repeated measurements showed them to occur over the same area of the brain (Figs. 9.4 and 9.5). Thus, the stability of MEG measurements in epileptic patients justified, in our experience, the application of a one-channel SQUID for the identification of epileptic foci.

Because epileptic foci emit coherent magnetic activity, we proceeded, following the identification of presumed foci of seizure activity, to influence these foci with the use of a specific electronic device. The coils of this device were constructed to emit back magnetic fields of the same intensity and frequency to those emitted from the brain to each functional point of epileptic foci. The application of such coherent varying magnetic fields to each functional point of seizure activity resulted in reduction (i.e., cancellation) of the maximum total average emitted power from these areas. We believe that this effect was related directly to the attenuation of the patients' seizure activity and also to their normal behavior.

However, we caution that we are unable to assert with total validity that we have identified the presence, as well as the position, of the epileptic foci. In a previous study (Elger et al., 1989), we found that the localization of presumed epileptic foci, as determined by conventional EEG recordings, coincided with the location of the accumulation of spectral energy in the ISO–SA maps in a large proportion of patients. Furthermore, that application of magnetic fields, which have similar characteristics to those emitted from the foci of abnormal neuronal activity, resulted in reduction in the average emitted power and coincided with the clinical attenuation of the patients' seizure activity clearly supports the efficacy of our procedure. Finally, the findings in animals—that the magnetic field inhibits seizure activity (Ossenkopp & Cain, 1988)—are in accordance with our clinical observations.

With regard to the position of the presumed epileptic focus, our data clearly demonstrate the perpendicular projection of the foci on the scalp. Thus, we assume that the magnetic stimulation placed above these points intersected with these points. Furthermore, we are aware that the fields of our dipoles had a fixed geometry and could not be adjusted. Furthermore, we contend that a single orientation of the SQUID cannot detect magnetic fields in every direction emanating from a spherical source, and that individual wave characteristics, amplitudes, and phases cannot be determined from power spectra averaged across broad frequency bands. In fact, Fig. 9.9 shows arrhythmic activity, and our treatment device produces an approximate sine wave oscillator. However, it is evident from Fig. 9.11 that the spectral distribution of the arrhythmic activity showed a dominant frequency. Our device was set to this dominant frequency and emitted this frequency back to the presumed foci of seizure activity. Therefore, it appears that the emission of the dominant frequency was sufficient to exhibit therapeutic, as well as behavioral, good response in our patients.

Despite these limitations, we are confident that this method is useful in identifying cerebral areas reflecting foci of seizure activity, and that our technique provides a novel method that is effective in suppressing seizure activity.

We wish to emphasize that all our patients exhibited frequent tonic–clonic seizures over a prolonged period of time, and that two of these patients obtained insufficient response from the administration of anticonvulsants despite showing good compliance with antiepileptic medication, as evidenced by therapeutic plasma anticonvulsant levels. Although the patients continued to take antiepileptic medication, magnetic stimulation appeared to have potentiated the anticonvulsant efficacy of these drugs. Moreover, in one patient, phenytoin was discontinued with no change in seizure frequency.

Although our patients have been followed for a period of only 10–14 months, we tentatively conclude that magnetic stimulation could be considered an effective adjunctive procedure in the management of a subgroup of patients with partial seizures who fail to benefit from conventional pharmacologic treatment. Clearly, a much larger sample of patients and a longer period of observation are required before more firm conclusions can be drawn concerning the efficacy of the procedure in the treatment of partial seizures.

APPENDIX: GENERAL PRINCIPLES OF THE ELECTRONIC DEVICE

The device consists of a generator of alternating low voltage, which can produce low frequencies from 2 Hz to 7 Hz (1); a switch of selecting frequencies (2); switches of selecting coils (3–7); one group of similar coils properly arranged in rows (8–12) or more similar groups (21–24); and resistances (13–20) that connect the coils of the first row (8) with the switch of selecting coils (3) and similar resistances that connect all the other coils of the rows (9–12) with the switches (4–7) and similarly for the other groups of coils. The coils are 1 cm in diameter. They are enclosed between two parallel plane surfaces in such a way that the axis of the coils is situated perpendicular to these surfaces, which are located parallel to the projection of the epileptic focus on the skull.

REFERENCES

Adams, R. D., & Victor, M. (1985). *Principles of neurology.* New York: McGraw-Hill.

Anninos, P. A., Anogianakis, G., Lehnertz, K., Pantev, C. H., & Hoke, M. (1987). Biomagnetic measurements using SQUID. *International Journal of Neuroscience, 37,* 149–168.

Anninos, P. A., Kokkinidis, M., Hoke, M., Pantev. C. H., Lehnertz, K., & Lütkenhoner, B. (1986). MEG measurements with SQUID as a diagnostic tool for epileptic patients. *Brain Research Bulletin, 16,* 549–551.

Antimonii, G. D., & Salamov, R. A. (1980). Action of a modulated electromagnetic field on experimentally evoked epileptiform brain activity in rats. *Bulletin of Experimental Biology and Medicine, 89,* 145–148.

Barth, D. S., Beatty, J., Broffman, J., & Sutherling, W. (1985). Magnetic localization of a dipolar current source implanted in a sphere and a human cranium. *Electroencephalography and Clinical Neurophysiology, 63,* 260–273.

Barth, D. S., Sutherling, W., Engel, J., & Beatty, J. (1982). Neuromagnetic localization of epileptiform spike activity in the human brain. *Science, 218,* 891–894.

Barth, D. S., Sutherling, W., Engel, J., & Beatty, J. (1984). Neuromagnetic evidence of spatially distributed sources underlying epileptiform spikes in the human brain. *Science, 223,* 293–296.

Burr, H. S., & Northorp, F. (1939). Evidence for the existence of an electrodynamic field in living organisms. *National Academy of Science, 25,* 284–288.

Cohen, D., Cuffin, N., Yunokuchi, K., Maniewski, R., Purcell, C., Cosgrove, G. R., Ives, J., Kennedy, J. G., & Schomer, D. L. (1990). MEG versus EEG localization test using implanted sources in the human brain. *Annals of Neurology, 28,* 811–817.

Dreifuss, F. E. (1989). Classification of epileptic seizures and the epilepsies. *Pediatric Clinics of North America, 36,* 265–279.

Elger, C. E., Hoke, M., Lehnertz, K., Pantev, C., Lütkenhoner, B., Anninos, P. A., & Anogianakis, G. (1989). Mapping of MEG amplitudes spectra: Its significance for the diagnosis of focal epilepsy. In K. Mauer (Ed.), *Topographic brain mapping of EEG and evoked potentials* (pp. 565–570). Berlin: Springer Verlag.

Engel, J. (1987). *Surgical treatment of the epilepsies.* New York: Raven Press.

Gastaut, H., & Tassinari, C. A. (1988). The ictal and interictal EEG in different types of epilepsy. In A. Remond (Ed.), *Handbook of electroencephalography and clinical neurophysiology* (vol. 13, pp. 3–6, 47–64). Amsterdam: Elsevier.

Gibbs, F. A., Gibbs, E. L., & Lennox, W. G. (1937). Epilepsy: A paroxysmal cerebral dysrhythmia. *Brain, 60,* 317–342.

Jasper, H. H. (1958). The ten-twenty electrode system of the International Federation. *Electroencephalography and Clinical Neurophysiology, 10,* 367–380.

Kaufman, L., & Williamson, S. J. (1982). Magnetic location of cortical activity. In I. Bodis-Wollner (Ed.), Evoked potentials. *Annals of the New York Academy of Science, 388,* pp. 197–213.

Keshavan, M. S., Gangadhar, B. N., Gautman, R. U., Ajit, V. B., & Kapur, R. L. (1981). Convulsive threshold in humans and rats and magnetic field changes: Observations during total solar eclipse. *Neuroscience Letters, 22,* 205–208.

Lehnertz, K., Elger, C. E., Hoke, M., Pantev, C., Lütkenhoner, B., Anninos, P. A., & Anogianakis, G. (1989). Two-dimensional spectral analysis of MEG data in epileptic patients. *Advances in epileptology* (Vol. 17). New York: Raven Press.

Nunez, P. L. (1990). Localization of brain activity with electroencephalography. In S. Sato (Ed.), *Magnetoencephalography* (vol. 54, pp. 39–65). New York: Raven Press.

Ossenkopp, K. P., & Cain, D. P. (1988). Inhibitory effects of acute exposure to low-intensity 60-Hz magnetic fields on electrically kindled seizures in rats. *Brain Research, 442,* 255–260.

Ossenkopp, K. P., Cain, D. P., & Smith, S. (1985). Low intensity 60-Hz magnetic fields and epilepsy reduced incidence of lethal pentylenetetrazol induced seizures in rats pre-exposed to magnetic fields. *Society for Neuroscience, 11,* 1280.

Rajaram, M., & Mitra, S. (1981). Correlation between convulsive seizure and geomagnetic activity. *Neuroscience Letters, 24,* 187–191.

Rose, D. F., & Ducla-Soares, E. (1990). Comparison of electroencephalography and magnetoencephalography. In: S. Sato (Ed.). *Magnetoencephalography.* New York: Raven Press, vol. 54, pp. 33–37.

Rose, D. F., Ducla-Soares, E., Sato, S., & Kufka, C. V. (1988). MEG measurement of a subdural dipole in a patient. *Epilepsia, 5,* 656.

Rose, D. F., Smith, P. D., & Sato, S. (1987). Magnetoencephalography and epilepsy research. *Science, 238,* 329–335.

Sato, S., Rose, D., & Porter, R. (1985). Single magnetic spike mapping. In H. Weinberg, G. Stroink, & T. Katila (Eds.), *Biomagnetism: Applications and theory* (pp. 261–263). New York: Pergamon Press.

Smith, D. B., Sidman, R. D., & Flanigin, H. (1985). A reliable method for localizing deep intracranial sources of the EEG. *Neurology, 35,* 1702–1707.

Spencer, S. S. (1981). Depth electroencephalography in selection of refractory epilepsy for surgery. *Annals of Neurology, 9,* 207–214.

Sutherling, W. W., & Barth, D. S. (1990). Magnetoencephalography in clinical epilepsy studies. The UCLA experience. In S. Sato (Ed.), *Magnetoencephalography* (vol. 54, pp. 231–245). New York: Raven Press.

Sutherling, W. W., Crandall, P. H., Cahan, L. D., & Barth, D. S. (1988). The magnetic field of epileptic spikes agrees with intracranial localizations in complex partial epilepsy. *Neurology, 38,* 778–786.

Sutherling, W. W., Crandall, P. H., Engel, J., Darcey, T. M., Cahan, L. D., & Barth, D. S. (1987). The magnetic field of complex partial seizures agrees with intracranial localizations. *Annals of Neurology, 21,* 548–558.

Venkatraman, K. (1976). Epilepsy and solar activity—a hypothesis. *Neurology, 24,* 1–5.

Weinberg, H., Brickett, P., Coolsma, F., & Baff, M. (1986). Magnetic localization of intracranial dipoles: Stimulation with a physical model. *Electroencephalography and Clinical Neurophysiology, 64,* 159–170.

Wieser, H. G., & Elger, C. E. (1987). *Presurgical evaluation of epileptics*. Berlin: Springer-Verlag.

10 Role of the Community Agency in the Comprehensive Treatment of the Epilepsies

Reina Berner
The Epilepsy Institute, New York

RAISON D'ETRE FOR A COMMUNITY AGENCY

Experientially, we have developed services to address the core issue: a sudden lack of control caused by a seizure, experienced by both the person experiencing the episode medically and the onlooker. The treatment approach encompassed by the Epilepsy Institute has a two-prong approach (i.e., strengthening the individual/family unit to cope with seizure events and the reactions this elicits in them, and helping the others deal with these events).

The following common situations and subsequent feelings, faced daily by people with epilepsy and their families, can be addressed and remedied through varying modalities of interventions (e.g., counseling, therapy, and education).

EXPERIENCING A SEIZURE

Because control is regarded at a premium in our society, the person with epilepsy episodically and involuntarily faces a loss of this (i.e., seizures). However, not only is the person having the seizure momentarily out of control, vulnerable, and helpless, but onlookers share these feelings. As we seek to avoid such feelings, we often blame and shun the person who has caused this discomfort. The feedback given to people with epilepsy, the mirroring they often receive, is of disgust for an event that is beyond their control. It is not surprising that feelings of shame often are deeply rooted and entrenched over centuries of stigmatization (Dell, 1986).

DEALING WITH MEDICAL CARE

Manifestations of lack of control and self-mastery extend to the need for daily medications and reliance on physicians—to depend on these outside sources for one's perceived quality of life (Schneider & Conrad, 1986). Unfortunately, these authority figures are usually unable to provide any significant comfort because cause and effect are often missing from this diagnosis. The cause usually cannot be determined; seizure control cannot be predicted or guaranteed. We often cannot explain why a seizure occurs at one time on medication and not another; which medications will be most effective and at which dosages; and if seizure frequency will change at different stages of life and for whom. These endless unknowns can cause anxiety as well as feelings of inadequacy in family members. Parents often do not know what questions to ask, and sometimes do not fully understand the answers provided. They must make judgment calls constantly and often do not receive the medical information or emotional support needed for such a process. Obviously, these feelings can be transmitted to the child with epilepsy. Adults with recent onset often experience the same feelings in trying to restructure their lives. The way one learns to cope with this anxiety will directly affect one's sense of control.

LABELING/IDENTIFICATION

Epilepsy generally is avoided by society. There has been an effort among some professionals to change the word *epilepsy* to *seizure disorder.* Although these terms at times can be used interchangeably, no other group with a medical label denoting symptoms, not cause (e.g., cancer, diabetes), appears to be trying to effect a change in nomenclature. The extent of this aversion and its effect on individuals and parents, who are told never to use the word *epilepsy,* only serve to reinforce stigma and shame. Simultaneously, the word *epileptic* still is utilized widely to designate a person with epilepsy. However, this word denotes only a seizure event and not necessarily that a person is involved in this process.

SELF-PERCEPTIONS

With all these taboos, readily obtaining information on this condition can become an arduous undertaking (Temkin, 1971). People with epilepsy often know little about the condition, reflecting the misunderstandings of society at large. This includes the unawareness that transient feelings of intense terror or fear may be from seizure activity. These feelings are negated by others, because they are not triggered mutually by an external stimulus that can be identified. One can begin to question the validity of one's perceptions and secretly harbor the feeling of being crazy. This can hamper a person from describing such symptoms to physicians or from seeking services from mental health practitioners. Sadly, many of these professionals would not necessarily know that these could be manifestations of epilepsy. It also can serve to limit a person socially for fear of exposure, reinforcing shame, secrecy, and fear.

The inability to readily identify another person with epilepsy creates additional burdens. It rests with the diagnosed person whether to tell someone and at which point in a relationship. Often, people with epilepsy do not realize what information other people need to know about this condition. This invisibility also limits contact between people with epilepsy, so that a mutual sharing of experiences cannot take place. People with epilepsy and their family members often feel, and are, alone. Many others are hesitant to raise the issue of epilepsy, because they have been advised not to do so.

COMPLYING WITH DENIAL

Because society seeks to deny this condition, can people with epilepsy and their families easily seek psychological assistance? Does this collude with the general belief that people with epilepsy are crazy? Does this defy the authorities who have advised them not to discuss “it”? These conditions set up barriers to seeking services, as does the reality that there is generally a lack of such services—a collusion by professionals and consumers, creating a cycle from which few can deviate. One must try to pass regardless of the emotional toll this can take.

Shame and denial are feelings that can be dealt with, freeing up a person and allowing him or her to cope more effectively. Unfortunately, services to deal with these issues are not provided routinely where people are diagnosed or treated, nor is it our experience that the majority of people are provided with educational materials and/or informed of services. Often, it is not even recognized that this can be a difficult diagnosis to cope with, and that some supportive assistance might be needed. This kind of acknowledgment from an authority figure would give a portion of this population the freedom to seek outside help, and not necessarily perceive it as another flaw or deficit.

HISTORY OF AGENCY

In 1967, the agency was incorporated as a 501(c)3 not-for-profit agency, focusing on the provision of educational presentations, and information and referral services. This beginning effort afforded the opportunity to ascertain and document needs. After several years, it became clear that these efforts alone could not change nor significantly alter the impact of epilepsy on one’s life. Results from the information and referral services validated that persons with epilepsy and their families generally could not obtain the same services from generic providers, especially in the areas of psychosocial interventions, vocational assessment, counseling, and training.

At this juncture, time-limited grants were awarded by The New York State Developmental Disabilities Council to develop program models of direct services. This included a counseling service staffed by clinical social workers, psychologists, and psychiatrists. These professionals provided: individual, marital, family, group counseling/therapy; psychiatric evaluations and chemotherapy, as needed; and psychological and aptitude batteries. This program element was granted certification in 1976 as a unique and needed outpatient treatment facility to a traditionally underserved population by the New York State Department of Mental Hygiene, which, at that time, had some responsibility for service delivery to people with epilepsy. The clinic is now certified by the New York State Office of Mental Retardation and Developmental Disabilities (NYS OMRDD). To obtain local governmental funding, application was made to the New York City Department of Mental Health, Mental Retardation and Alcoholism Services (NYC DMH, MR & AS). Initially, funding was minimal; but over the years, this has increased. However, the clinic rate remains at half of that for the identical service provided at a mental health agency. An annual average of 550 individuals and families is seen for over 6,200 direct client sessions.

Another grant was utilized to establish a Work Activities Center. It was the agency's contention that people with epilepsy should not be relegated to their homes once they finished their public education, because they have seizures. It believed that a majority of the persons served would be capable of training for and obtaining employment.

The participants in this 5-day-per-week program routinely had been rejected by New York State Vocational and Educational Services to Individuals with Disabilities (NYS VESID, a.k.a. Office of Vocational Rehabilitation), which has as part of its mandate the sponsorship of eligible candidates with disabilities for vocational training and related programs. Some who had been granted VESID sponsorship previously had been terminated from programs where one could obtain a skill leading to competitive employment because of their seizure activity.

The persons enrolled in the Work Activities Center readily proved our hypothesis. Some went directly into competitive employment through the agency's job placement service; some proceeded to vocational training programs, which would now accept them; and a minority, for one reason or another, could not realistically engage in activities toward and/or in actual competitive employment. This service, as well as vocational assessment, counseling, and job placement, became funded partially by NYS VESID. Unfortunately, after several years, the low rate of reimbursement for this labor-intensive service made it impossible for the program to continue. However, a vocational component was always sustained. Currently, through the auspices of NYC DMH, MR & AS, the following services are maintained: career and vocational assessment and counseling, and job placement services.

The information and referral service is well utilized, as are educational materials. Annually, over 15,000 requests are handled nationally. The issues most frequently raised dictate the content of our educational materials and advocacy stances. These latter efforts include, but are not limited to, negotiating with schools, employers, and unions and/or seeking legal remedies when necessary; and advocating for or against proposed legislation as it could pertain to the quality of life of those persons whom the agency represents. Partial funding for these services over the years derived from NYS DDPC, NYC Department of MH, MR & AS, and NYS OMRDD. Currently, they barely are funded.

Epilepsy appears to be volleyed between governmental agencies, with its ultimate designation seeming quite arbitrary at times. Governmental funding has been nominal over the years, with the current exception of the NYC Department of MH, MR & AS. Raising private dollars is an even greater challenge.

AGENCY MODEL

Because epilepsy can affect every aspect of one's life, numerous programs should be developed to address the many issues. However, one also must look at available governmental funding streams. As epilepsy rarely fits neatly into most of these, some flexibility and creativity are needed. Due to funding constraints and/or institutional politics, there are certain identified areas for which the agency does not provide services.

Programs primarily address the intrapsychic and environmental factors that affect people with epilepsy, through psychosocial/psychological exploration and interventions, as well as vocational and employment options. The medical picture is addressed and, wherever necessary, remedied as much as possible.

By having daily contact with people with epilepsy, the agency is acutely aware of and subjected to the issues and treatment that they encounter. The major feat for professionals is to learn how to cope with the myriad issues that can arise, and be able to offer effective strategies. One needs a highly skilled multidisciplinary staff composed of clinical social workers, psychiatrists, psychologists, vocational rehabilitators, and nurses. Professional staff not only must be skilled in their respective disciplines with a sound grasp of intrapsychic and environmental factors, but also must be able to learn and integrate the medical, psychosocial, familial, vocational, and legal aspects of the epilepsies. *Medical* not only implies basic knowledge of epilepsy, diagnostic procedures, seizure types, surgical interventions, medications, and potential side effects, but also interactions between medications; not only interactions between anticonvulsants if there should be any, but also between anticonvulsants and other classes of medications. Psychiatrists not only must have diagnostic and, preferably, psychoanalytic training, but also knowledge and skill in psychopharmacology. Vocational aspects not only imply knowledge about different vocations, careers, and labor trends, but whether a person's seizure type(s), frequency, times of occurrence, and manifestation(s) will influence choices based on abilities and interests. Clinical social workers and psychologists require psychological sophistication to sort through numerous theories of personality/behavior, which often utilize small and/or skewed samples and/or offer no actual differences from those seen in studies of the general population. Frequently, these often exclude the external influences a person with epilepsy and their family members experience daily; these grossly generalize about this population, attributing everything to the condition of having epilepsy, thus effectively negating the individual.

This has led to the usage of several modalities, which, although obviously not inclusive of all, provides the basics available to the general population. These include individual, marital, family, and group counseling/therapy (which utilize an eclectic approach); educational, vocational, and career counseling; job placement assistance; prescribing of psychoactive medications; short-term educational/information workshops; support groups; referral for reevaluation of neurological care; and advocacy.

Educational and advocacy efforts stem from our constituents and complement direct care services. These include responding to phone and written inquiries; producing up-to-date printed materials on various aspects related to the epilepsies; the development of the *American Epilepsy Digest* (formerly the *New York Journal of Epilepsy*), which contains articles on psychosocial and employment issues, legislative and legal remedies, various treatment approaches, first-person accounts, and books of interest; conducting conferences for employers, physicians (CME credits), educators, and health-related professionals; and disseminating up-to-date information, via professionally conducted consumer workshops. For consumers, it can mean learning more about themselves and available options. Feeling empowered helps individuals become partners in their health care and their lives. For the others, it hopefully clarifies some myths and helps sensitize them.

Advocacy and legal remedies are needed to enforce laws to protect the civil liberties of people with epilepsy. It is clear that society's view of epilepsy as shameful has led to a full cycle of denial on every stratum. Because epilepsy does not exist, people do not need services. Laws supposedly designed to protect this group seldom are enforced even by the very helping professionals who ostensibly should want this accomplished. Thus, tremendous effort may be placed on one person's situation, as doubtlessly many others are experiencing the same. When people see that there are those who acknowledge and recognize them as worthy and worth fighting for, it sets a tone not only for that particular person, but for others who, hopefully, will then be spared that kind of discriminatory treatment. It can force systems to reevaluate and reformulate policies concerning people with epilepsy.

While listening to people, one learns of recurrent incidents, although sometimes of an anecdotal nature, that need to be addressed. The Institute took an early stance on the issue of generic switching of anticonvulsant products when many of its clients began to experience breakthrough seizures. Although some sources criticized the Institute for this, it was vindicated by scientific documentation several years later. The point is not necessarily to be right, but to listen and raise questions when relevant. It listened to people who spoke about "seizure alert dogs" (i.e., dogs with the alleged ability to detect seizures before a person is aware of them). This is something that even the most modern technology cannot do. It listened because 50% of people with epilepsy cannot become seizure-free on available anticonvulsants. It realized how such dogs could improve the quality of a person's life *now*—not in 10, 20, or 100 years. Many sources have chided the Institute, but it tenaciously held to exploring this phenomenon until monies to pilot such a study could be obtained.

By listening to enough people, the Institute has learned not to discount environmental factors as potential precipitants for seizures. Surely, it does not have the resources or manpower to explore all these issues, but listening and learning, rather than negating the person with epilepsy and their family members, produces profound growth for all concerned parties.

THERAPEUTIC PROGRAM

Anyone who has epilepsy and/or a family member is eligible to apply for assistance. Within the first three sessions (i.e., the initial assessment), historical and current information is gathered. Besides identifying data, this includes:

1. The person's reason(s)/perception(s) for seeking assistance and source of referral.
2. Ages when developmental milestones were achieved; general medical, neurological, and psychological care received; nature of treatment(s); and medication(s) prescribed past and present.
3. Composition and description of family of origin and nuclear family.
4. Educational, vocational, and work experiences.
5. Social relationships, athletic activities, hobbies and interests, and usage of alcohol and other substances.
6. Mental status.

Although the components of this assessment are quite consistent with those used for the general population, there is an emphasis on obtaining a very complete medical and neurological history. The medical history might reveal: other conditions, that could impact the individual/family physically, intellectually, and/or psychically; the potential interactions of medications, if prescribed, with anticonvulsants; and/or if psychoactive medications are indicated. The neurological history includes: cause if known; age at onset of seizures; age when diagnosed; description of seizure type(s); frequency, past and present; duration of seizures; nature of postictal recovery phase; and current medication(s), those previously prescribed, and any periods of time when medications were not utilized.

The reasons for these questions are manifold. Two of the primary ones, beside social and vocational implications, are that most people, regardless of racial, ethnic, educational, or economic factors, do not know which type(s) of seizures they have, nor do they receive adequate neurological care.

Generally, people are only familiar with grand mal (tonic–clonic) and petit mal (absence). Petit mal is often offered, when in fact the person has some form of partial seizures. This confusion is essentially due to a lack of information.

Depending on the information provided, a referral for a second opinion, preferably from an epileptologist, might be needed. Income does not stand in the way of this. If a person cannot afford private care, the Institute has established rapport with selected seizure clinics that will accept referrals regardless of designated catchment areas. The Institute is fortunate to have these relationships, and that there are epileptologists in this geographical area from whom to select.

However, seeking a second opinion can become a treatment issue, because the individual/parent might feel criticized for having utilized what they had thought was the best care available and/or might have a long-term relationship with the treating physician in question.

During this process, those seeking assistance are informed of the following agency procedures:

1. Because all care must be coordinated, releases for information must be signed.
2. Within six sessions, an evaluation with an agency psychiatrist must be completed.
3. Minors and/or adults who live with their parents and/or live separately, but are financially supported by their parents are seen with their parents during this assessment phase.
4. If a person is a substance abuser, an appropriate program to deal with this issue must be entered within a designated period of time.

Upon completion of these sessions, the information obtained from the person(s) applying, or the lack of it (usually a diagnostic indicator), is presented to the full interdisciplinary team to develop recommendations and treatment strategies tailored for each individual/family. This, in turn, is presented to the applicant(s) to see if it is acceptable. If it is, the treatment process commences.

Treatment recommendations may include any one or a combination of the following services: individual, marital, family, or group therapy (therapeutic techniques are dependent on the needs/abilities of each client to utilize different approaches); the prescribing of psychoactive agents; psychological testing; aptitude testing; vocational counseling; job placement assistance; medical and/or neurological referral(s); and advocacy in cases of alleged discrimination.

The primary therapist is responsible for conducting treatment sessions as well as coordinating all internal and external services provided to an individual, and initiating referrals for any other form of assistance that the person might require and/or benefit from. Clients who could benefit from a group experience are matched carefully to other group members based on functioning level, not the fact that they have epilepsy. This is not a homogeneous population, thus considerations for joining a group involve a careful selection process. A potential group member is invited to participate for three sessions, at which time the client and

TABLE 10.1
At Intake Assessment

Variable	*Percent*	*Variable*	*Percent*
Gender		Educational Level (*cont*)	
Female	45	10–12th grade dropout	24
Male	55	High school graduate	33
Age		Business school graduate	6
0–5	1	Some college	10
6–12	3	College graduate	13
13–18	11	Source of Referral	
19–25	20	Self	37
26–36	39	Relatives/friends	25
37–47	18	Other agency	13
48–58	6	Hospital/doctor	18
59–69	1	School	4
70+	1	Unknown	3
Race		Reported Seizure Types	
White	49	Generalized	57
Black	28	Partial	15
Hispanic	22	Partial & generalized	28
Asian	1	Reported Seizure Frequency	
Living Situation		Daily	9
Alone	23	Weekly	16
Family of origin	46	Monthly	35
Spouse and/or children	24	2–3 months	14
Friends	7	4–6 months	15
Marital Status		Yearly	10
Single	67	Controlled 1 year	1
Married	14	Sources of Income	
Separated	8	Governmental disability and welfare subsidies	37
Divorced	9		
Widowed	2	Relatives	24
Educational Level		Employed	33
Completed ninth grade	14	Unemployment benefits	6

TABLE 10.2
At Termination

Variable	*Percent*
Average Time Seen	
Not proceed after assessment period	36
1–3 months	14
4–6 months	15
7–12 months	18
13–18 months	13
19–24 months	2
25–36 months	2
Reported Changes in Anticonvulsant Medication	
Yes	56
No	44

group leader review whether this is a beneficial match. Clinical progress is reviewed at least quarterly, or sooner if, for some reason(s), the treatment plan has to be revised (see Tables 10.1 and 10.2).

Of those people specifically seeking employment, 85% are successfully able to engage in this process and be placed. Follow-up services are offered after placement, and, for some, highly recommended. For various factors, the remaining 15%, will not be able to engage in competitive employment.

Although it is the Institute's clinical opinion that a sizable population developed improved coping mechanisms, thus reducing and/or eliminating presenting symptoms of anxiety and/or depression, they have not administered scales to measure this at intake and termination.

Unfortunately, as of this date, the Institute has not correlated which persons involved in clinical treatment have moved from being unemployed to becoming involved in school/and or jobs and/or for those who were employed at onset who gained promotions and/or moved to better jobs in other companies. Although much of this information is available, a computerized database would need to be established to retrieve such information. This also could produce a profile of which people seeking assistance sustain this process.

OUTCOME OF ACTIVITIES—CASE EXAMPLES

Case 1: Ms. R

Identifying Information. Ms. R is a 28-year-old college educated, employed, Caucasian female. She shares an apartment with a friend and plans to marry her fiancé in June.

Reason for Contact. Ms. R requested an immediate appointment following a flurry of seizures that had been observed by her fiancé during Christmas vacation. She expressed confusion, as 2 years ago she became aware of episodic, rapid changes in her breathing. After contact with an internist, she was referred to a psychiatrist. Diagnosed as having panic attacks, she was placed on an antidepressant medication and was seen twice weekly for psychotherapy. As the episodes continued, Ms. R was prescribed larger and larger dosages of the antidepressant medication. However, during this most recent episode, people were present who could describe the entire event. She called her psychiatrist. In his absence, the covering psychiatrist suggested that the problem appeared to be neurological and referred her to a neurologist. Diagnosed with complex partial seizures, an anticonvulsant medication was initiated and Ms. R discontinued the other. She wondered what was actually true—which professional to trust. She questioned whether it was epilepsy or a symptom of something else, because she believed that one had to be born with this condition. Whatever "it" was, she questioned how it would progress, because she feared mental deterioration and death.

Ms. R's fiancé accompanied her to the initial session. He described Ms. R as an independent, social, and calm individual, as opposed to how she currently was presenting herself.

Medical/Neurological/Psychological. Ms. R is aware of no major medical condition in herself or family of origin. The only instance of psychological care was started after she had become aware of the episodic, rapid breathing episodes.

The neurologist initially consulted had diagnosed complex partial seizures and prescribed an anticonvulsant medication. Seizure episodes still occurred. The dosage of the medication prescribed was minimal and it was suspected that a therapeutic level had not been achieved.

Family. Ms. R was raised in a suburban, middle-class area, the youngest of four children. Her siblings are college educated, married, and residing with their own families. Ms. R moved to this city after graduating from college, and has been employed here ever since. Family dynamics were not of concern to her, and reportedly these were explored in her prior therapy. She has contact and visits with all family members.

Education and Work Experience. Since college, Ms. R had been employed at two different companies. She has worked at her current position for the past 4 years with good evaluations. However, she had planned to look for another job with more potential prior to receiving her current diagnosis.

Social Relationships. She reported numerous friendships, and had known her fiancé for 2 years prior to engagement. She acknowledged that she was spending less time with her friends due to preoccupation with her health.

Plans had been made to marry in June, but Ms. R now questioned if she should proceed with this. Her fiancé understood epilepsy, because his mother, a physician, explained it to him. He did not perceive epilepsy as a reason to interfere with their marriage date. He was open about his feeling for and toward Ms. R.

However, Ms. R saw her medical condition as a potential problem, and felt it was unfair. She became engaged before the diagnosis of epilepsy was confirmed. She now questioned whether there was an underlying disease process going on, and, if not, would seizures interfere with her ability to work, have children, or drive (a move to a suburban area was planned in the near future). She did not want to become a burden. Her fears of epilepsy reflected those commonly held by society.

She could not quite understand her fiancé's easy acceptance of her condition, nor his apparent lack of sensitivity to what she was experiencing. She had not disclosed her condition to any coworkers or friends.

Her fear of episodic losses of control decreased her willingness to socialize. When she had to do so, she felt as if she were becoming boring, because her overriding concern interfered with her ability to relate spontaneously and participate freely in conversations and/or activities.

She reportedly was a social drinker, but now feared drinking alcohol, despite learning that this was not prohibited. She was afraid to do anything that she believed could possibly precipitate a seizure, although she was unsure of how to handle this situation socially. She also expressed fear of losing her job.

Ms. R had participated in athletics all her life. She had discontinued all such activities, as well as driving.

Mental Status. Ms. R is a neatly groomed, slender woman. She is relevant and coherent. Affect is appropriate to content with features of anxiety and depression. She expressed feelings of hopelessness and inability to cope. She reported that, at times, she could not concentrate at work, had racing thoughts, and had difficulty with sleeping and a decreased appetite.

Treatment Recommendations. Ms. R's treatment recommendations included the following:

1. Referral to an epileptologist.
2. Consideration of antianxiety medication for short-term usage.
3. Individual sessions to address the myriad issues disrupting Ms. R's life and educate her about epilepsy as well as explore her attitudes toward this diagnosis.
4. Consider group therapy sessions as Ms. R stabilizes emotionally to reduce feelings of being unique in her experiences and to learn effective coping mechanisms.

Outcome. Ms. R accepted the referral for neurological reevaluation. Tumor and/or other disease processes were ruled out. Anticonvulsant dosage was too low and gradually was raised. When she eventually became seizure-free, she continued for a period to worry and to expect another seizure to occur. This concern became less prominent with time. She also experienced periodic difficulty with word finding when at higher levels of medication. She accepted this as a trade-off for being seizure-free. Although this raised some of her prior fears about deterioration, she was able to put these into a more realistic perspective. Much later, when anticonvulsant medication was decreased, the problem with word finding was resolved.

A benzodiazepine was prescribed, but Ms. R resisted taking it. Her episodic racing thoughts probably were due to seizure activity. However, her anxious state was impacting negatively on her ability to concentrate, sleep, and eat. She decided to utilize the medication on a short-term basis—only when these symptoms interfered significantly with her ability to concentrate on her work.

Individually, she was able to overcome the fears of mental deterioration and death: what she erroneously thought she might do during a seizure that would be hurtful to others, and conversely what could happen to her during one. She feared how other people would perceive her once they knew her diagnosis: would she be able to keep her job, strive toward a promotion, or ever be hired by a different company?

After having seizures at work, on the street, in stores, and on the subway with no negative outcomes, these experiences, combined with her inner strength, enabled her to discuss her epilepsy openly. As well, she resumed swimming and proceeded with the marriage she initially had postponed.

Beyond resuming her former life, she developed a sensitivity and empathy toward others whom society perceives as different. To conquer her fear of having a damaged child and/or being unable to take care of an infant, she volunteered at a hospital on the children's floor. Battling concerns of having a seizure while left alone with these youngsters, she developed relationships with several, especially, as chance would have it, a child with refractory seizures who had been left there by his mother. When she became pregnant, her anticonvulsant medication was reduced as far as possible. She fought her belief, despite contrary information, that if anything was wrong with the infant, it only could be her fault. Being caught between an obstetrician and a neurologist was avoided by a referral to one capable of handling this. Again, the thought of having a seizure during labor, an unlikely possibility, and hurting the baby was dealt with successfully. She gave birth to a healthy 8 lb. boy.

Ms. R finally decided to join an appropriate group, because she no longer harbored the feeling that other group members would somehow be strange or weird, as she perhaps had perceived herself to be. Although initially focusing on seizures, which other group members respected and addressed, the focus was on the whole person, not just a seizure event. Later on, she was able to provide the help she had received from others to a new group member who experienced the onset of seizures in his thirties, and could not imagine carrying on with his career, maintaining relationships, developing new ones, or being anything but reclusive. He, too, was surprised to learn that having a seizure in public would not end his world, and that people react in various ways—some of these even quite helpful.

Ms. R completed therapy before the birth of her child. She had postponed looking for another job prior to pregnancy. Although she had gone on interviews and received offers, she did not change positions. However, several months after she returned to her job, she was offered one at a different firm. It not only provided a promotion, but more time to spend with her family. She did not resume driving immediately, but this has now become part of her routine. As previously planned, she and her family have moved to a suburban area.

Case 2: Mr. D

Identifying Information. Mr. D is a 36-year-old college educated, employed Black male. He currently resides with his spouse.

Reason for Contact. Mr. D reports that his wife has become increasingly aware of his having episodes of kicking and convulsive movements during sleep. He has been diagnosed with epilepsy and has started on medication. During this time, he also experienced a seizure at work. He states that he wants to be involved in a group situation to learn more about epilepsy, because he feels he has become more withdrawn, anxious, and depressed since his diagnosis.

Medical/Neurological/Psychological. Mr. D reports one seizure during infancy during a high fever. He reports no major medical illnesses in self or family of origin. He remembers black outs during adolescence that lasted, to his knowledge, for 10–15 sec. He did not fall, but stopped whatever he was doing. He recalls during the past few years waking up episodically with headaches, but being unsure of the cause. Apparently, he did not seek medical care until nocturnal seizures became either more frequent and/or involved.

Family. Mr. D is the third child of six from an intact, middle-class family. All siblings, save one, are college educated. His father is deceased, and his mother resides alone. He reports contact with all family members. Shortly after college graduation, Mr. D obtained employment. He has been married for 6 years.

Education and Work Experience. He has been employed at the same company for 14 years. He is dissatisfied with his current situation, but is undecided as to whether to proceed with any changes.

Social Relationships. He has several friends whom he socializes with in various activities. He denies any close friends in whom he can confide. He knew his wife for several years prior to marriage, and reports marital discord prior to diagnosis.

Mental Status. He presented as neatly dressed and groomed, pleasant, and cooperative throughout the interview. His motor activity was unremarkable, and his speech showed a circumstantial form of thought. His thought content was dominated by appropriate concern for recent diagnosis. He showed no suicidal, assaultive, or psychotic ideation. His fund of knowledge was good, and he was able to serially subtract 7s from 100 accurately. Proverb interpretation was abstract and appropriate. His insight and judgment were good. His mood was mildly depressed, and his affect was constricted.

Treatment Recommendation. Mr. D's treatment recommendation included the following:

1. Individual sessions to address medical aspects of epilepsy, issues of disclosure, employment, and marital concerns.
2. Group sessions to mitigate against tendency to withdraw.

Outcome. Individual sessions were difficult for Mr. D, because seeking assistance was viewed as a sign of weakness. This served to reinforce his feelings of being damaged due to epilepsy.

It was agreed that these sessions would be time limited and would focus on specific areas. Mr. D, once understanding epilepsy, realized the need for medication compliance and for keeping a record of episodes while the neurologist was adjusting dosage. He felt more confident discussing epilepsy with his family of origin once he fully grasped this condition. He eventually requested a transfer at work, which was honored, and rendered a more tolerable employment situation, while he considered longer term objectives.

Group sessions offered Mr. D an easier vehicle to discuss issues of feeling different while growing up, due to blackouts. He acknowledged that other children had perceived him as strange, and he never chose to drive because he knew that something was wrong with him. In hindsight, he realized that this might have interfered with his ability to readily develop relationships and a reluctance to engage in competitive team sports.

He used group sessions not only to work out issues of epilepsy, but eventually to overcome his fear of being recognized—of being seen. He became more assertive in relationships and presented his thoughts in a clearer and more precise manner. He reported improvements both with coworkers and his wife, and was particularly pleased that he was able to develop a more open relationship with a male friend.

Case 3: Ms. J

Identifying Information. Ms. J is a 14-year-old Caucasian female attending high school. She was referred by school personnel because of poor grades and episodic crying spells.

Reason for Contact. Ms. J's parents stated that, over the past year, their daughter had gone from being an "A" student to one barely passing course work. They described her as becoming more defensive and argumentative and believed she would be free of tonic–clonic seizures if she took her medications as prescribed. This had led to family battles.

Although there were substantial family problems, other than Ms. J, it was clear her parents only would engage in several sessions to provide history and learn more about epilepsy. They agreed to be available at some later date if this was requested. Otherwise, they expressed no feelings about epilepsy, except that they did not understand their daughter's current behaviors, which they wished to be corrected.

Medical/Neurological/Psychological. Ms. J has no major medical illnesses. Milestones were reached within average limits. Onset of tonic–clonic seizures was diagnosed at age 12. She acknowledges being frightened at the unpredictable nature of epilepsy.

Family. Ms. J is the youngest of five children from a middle-class family. Her siblings were all students at the high school or college level. She acknowledged feeling unable to compete with her older siblings, and made reference to escalating problems between her parents, on which she would not elaborate.

Education and Work Experience. Ms. J is enrolled in an academic high school and had planned to attend college. She now felt that this would be unlikely, and wondered if her aspirations and career plans would be thwarted due to epilepsy. She expressed confusion over her recent decline in academic performance and her apparent inability to concentrate, although she stated she tried very hard and wanted to succeed. However, her grades continued to fall.

She had worked as a baby-sitter and questioned (as did her parents) whether she should continue.

Social. Ms. J reportedly has lots of friends, but is afraid to have a seizure in front of them, because she fears rejection and humiliation. She also imagines being called "stupid" by peers if a seizure should occur. Thus, she now avoids social activities and is doubtful about dating for the same reasons.

Mental Status. This 14-year-old female looks her stated age. She is well nourished and her hygiene appears excellent. She is neatly and appropriately dressed, and her only noticeable mannerisms are great hesitancy and a voice that is extremely low and difficult to hear. She is friendly and cooperative, and has good eye contact. Her speech, although very low and somewhat difficult to understand at first, is relevant and coherent, with no evidence of any thought disorder. The client appears to be somewhat depressed. She denies any history of auditory hallucination or delusionary thinking. She claims that she sleeps well. The client's affect is appropriate to her stated ideas. Her intelligence appears to be within normal range. Her memory is good for both recent and remote events, and she has relatively good insight and normal amount of judgment.

Treatment Recommendations. Short-term, planned individual sessions were recommended, because it was unlikely Ms. J needed extensive intervention, nor that she could tolerate being the identified patient because she already felt herself to be the family failure. Focus would be on (a) how she perceives herself, (b) issues with medications, (c) factors interfering with school work, (d) role-playing to facilitate discussion of epilepsy with others, and (e) concerns about baby-sitting and her future educational/work options. Her parents were to be seen with Ms. J as needed to discuss recommendations/compromises.

Outcome. When seizure activity was explored fully, it became evident that Ms. J was increasingly experiencing brief seizure episodes. She did not know that these were seizures, had not discussed it with anybody, nor had anyone previously ever asked her these questions. Permission had been granted by parents and Ms. J to speak to her neurologist, hence contact was initiated. Seizure episodes were described, Ms. J was evaluated further, medication was changed, and episodes soon were resolved. Not surprisingly, her school performance quickly corrected itself; however, it was too late in the semester to avoid failing two subjects. Ms. J did not hesitate to enroll in summer school to repeat these courses so that she would be able to graduate on schedule.

As for her medication regime, Ms. J feared being observed taking pills during school hours. She felt she would either be accused of drug abuse or would have to disclose that she had epilepsy. She could be called on to view this behavior and fear of disclosure in terms of how it could later affect her stated school objective, which was a realistic goal.

She learned about epilepsy, to role-play how to tell people about this, and to provide the information they might need to know, but be afraid to ask (i.e., what seizures look like, how frequently they occur, and what they should do if one occurs). She needed to decide which people to tell and when. As her fears of a seizure occurring decreased in importance, Ms. J resumed her social activities, baby-sitting, jobs, and dating.

Case 4: Mr. G

Identifying Information. Mr. G is a 46-year-old, unemployed, widowed Black male, father of three children from a prior marriage.

Reason for Contact. He reportedly was fired several years ago from a good position at a hotel due to a seizure. Since then, he has been unable to get back into the hotel business and has tried a number of different, lower paying jobs. He has not adjusted to these, is currently receiving unemployment benefits, and reports that he cannot make ends meet.

Medical/Neurological. Mr. G states that tonic–clonic seizures were diagnosed when he was 17 years of age. He states he tried to deny this in the past by continuing to drink at social occasions, at times to excess, and not complying with medications. Currently, he is experiencing nocturnal seizures that sometimes make it difficult for him to wake up in a timely manner. With limited financial resources, he acknowledges that he does not maintain adequate medical care.

Family. He is the older child of two from his mother's first marriage, and has two half siblings from her second. He states relationships are maintained with all family members. He married at 18 years of age, and from this union had three children. His wife subsequently divorced him, which still angers him. He remarried at 33 years of age, and apparently was very close to and dependent on his wife. She died 3 years ago, after 10 years of marriage. He sees his children regularly; two are self-supporting, and the youngest is well maintained by mother and her husband.

Education and Work Experience. Mr. G reports dropping out of school at 14 years of age. He states he could not keep up with school work. Over the years, he obtained various jobs in several capacities at hotels, until he achieved a good position. Several years ago, he reports losing such a job due to a seizure. Coupled with his wife's death, he appears to have coped by taking whatever positions he could obtain.

Mental Status. He is a neatly groomed man, and presented no prominent signs or symptoms, despite the restricted and unfulfilled life-style he described. He denied feeling depressed, although he has been lonely since his second wife's death. He has the capability to relate to others. His intellectual functioning seemed to be slightly below average. He was coherent, relevant, and goal directed. There was no evidence of a thought disorder or psychotic symptoms. His mood was neutral and his affect blunted, but appropriate. In trying to elucidate the impact of seizures, the patient has developed an attitude of resignation, viewing epilepsy as something that he has to live with, because of his upbringing and religious beliefs. It appeared that he is performing in life below his capabilities, but does not seem to be aware of it. The main themes of his character organization seemed to be passivity and masochistic acceptance.

Treatment Recommendations. The treatment recommendations for Mr. G include the following:

1. Assistance in obtaining benefits to pay for necessary neurological care.
2. Job placement assistance.
3. Group sessions to assist in presenting for job interviews and obtaining support from others during this period.

Outcome. Although Mr. G received limited medical coverage, he resisted changing physicians. He did state he was complying with current regimen of medication and was adjusted to occurrences of nocturnal seizures.

As a comparable position could not immediately be obtained for him, he continued whatever jobs he could locate, rather than accept governmental financial aid. However, this contributed to a continuous lowering of his self-esteem.

Group sessions provided social contact, as well as the opportunity to meet other people with epilepsy who shared mutual concerns. When an appropriate job was found, he was especially relieved, because this would be the first time an employer knew he had epilepsy. He visibly was freed, and his entire presentation was more spontaneous, alive, and alert.

He has successfully held this job, and one suspects that he will become more attentive to his own health needs.

Case 5: Mr. and Mrs. T

Identifying Information. Mr. and Mrs. T, 42 and 40 years old, respectively, are a married Caucasian couple, and the parents of two children. Both have postgraduate degrees and both hold executive positions.

Reason for Contact. Mr. and Mrs. T called on several occasions before agreeing to an appointment. Concern focused on their 4-year-old son, J, whose seizures had not become fully controlled on medication as had been anticipated. Further, they stated they had been informed that J would "outgrow" the seizures. In the interim, seizure activity continued and dissension about how to handle the numerous and varied situations that were arising had affected the entire family. The older child had stolen a trinket from a store and suddenly had poor school performance; J and his mother were engaging in a power struggle over medication; Mr. T, to avoid the tension at home, spent more and more hours away from the house.

Medical/Neurological/Psychological. For brevity, only information pertaining to J will be presented, although it is customary to ascertain information on all family members and/or residents of a household.

J was a full-term pregnancy and a normal delivery. Milestones were early and parents were hopeful of a bright child. No unusual illnesses or complications were noted. Seizures were noticed about 1 year ago. Mrs. T reported that the second neurological expert they had seen stated that the repeated episodes were "seizure fragments." When more was elicited, it became evident that Mr. and Mrs. T were misinformed as to their son's actual seizure type, and that the type of seizure suspected would not respond well to the medication prescribed, nor would it be outgrown as this couple expected.

Family. Again, J will be the focus of information. Mr. and Mrs. T's expectations for their children appeared to reflect their own capabilities: competency and success in academics, athletics, and social situations. Mr. T relied solely on his wife to meet his needs. Mrs. T's need for perfection fit well with this. However, the stress of J's condition created unexpected, additional stressors. As is often encountered, neither parent could cope easily with the continued episodic, involuntary losses of control. They feared for J's safety and whether he should or would be able to continue in a part-time nursery program; and if they might be away from home in the evenings because a baby-sitter might not really know what to do, and that this beloved child could die. In turn, feelings of inadequacy—of not being sure how to handle each and every situation—left little energy for themselves or their older child.

Education. J was enrolled in a part-time nursery program. He reportedly played well with other children, handled tasks quickly, and was responsive to his teachers' instructions.

Social Relationships. Until recently, J not only played in his nursery school, but with neighborhood children. However, as his parents' concerns and fears grew, this activity decreased proportionately.

Mental Status. So far, J was fine. Mrs. T was becoming increasingly anxious and depressed, and Mr. T was withdrawing emotionally.

Treatment Recommendations. Treatment recommendations for J included the following:

1. Referral to an epileptologist.
2. Short-term marital sessions to help (a) work through reevaluation process and expected outcome, which would be different from the one anticipated; (b) facilitate and normalize the process people undergo when something is "wrong" with one's child (i.e., feelings of denial, anger, loss, grief, and acceptance); and (c) partialize family responsibilities, thereby strengthening their marriage and relationship with their older child.
3. Participation in a parents' group, where situations, as they arose, could be

discussed, coping strategies could be explored, and feelings and frustrations could be ventilated.

Outcome. Mr. and Mrs. T reluctantly agreed to start over again with an epileptologist. J's seizure type did not carry a good prognosis for becoming seizure free on medication, nor for outgrowing them. Intellect was intact.

Sessions did help Mr. and Mrs. T reassess their commitment. They found partializing tasks in a more balanced manner to be helpful. It served as well to reestablish time for parenting both children, and family balance was restored. They did not wish to explore other issues, and this was respected.

Mr. and Mrs. T did as much work on their reactions to having an "imperfect" child as they could at this point. They were informed that, at different developmental stages, concerns and issues might arise. This was normalized, as well as the possibility that assistance might be needed at some future date.

Mr. and Mrs. T periodically attended a parents' group, utilizing the presence of an expertly trained professional to their advantage in modifying their parenting skills to cope with varied situations. They gained from other involved parents, as well as offering help to others.

Case 6: Mr. A

Identifying Information. Mr. A, a 21-year-old Black, single, high school graduate was referred by a social worker from a community agency. Apparently after high school he was referred to VESID and, while in a vocational training program under their sponsorship, was terminated due to a seizure.

Reason for Contact. Mr. A was escorted by his mother for the initial session. Both confirmed that after having attended a vocational training program for 6 months, he was terminated due to seizure activity and told not to return until he had achieved seizure control.

Commonly, *seizure control* and *seizure-free* are used interchangeably, when in fact these are not synonymous. *Seizure control* means the best reduction of seizures with available treatments. *Seizure-free* equates to no seizure activity. Although this interchange is incorrect and confusing, the message was clear: Mr. A was to stay at home until he was seizure-free, at least, as it concerned both the vocational rehabilitation program he had been attending and VESID.

Medical/Neurological/Psychological. According to his mother, Mr. A had encephalitis as an infant and was hospitalized for several weeks. Several months later, seizures began. Mr. A has never been seizure-free on medications. He appeared to have complex partial seizures that, at times, secondarily generalize.

Although from the history it did not appear that Mr. A would ever become seizure-free on medications, current neurological care was not adequate. No other major medical illnesses were reported. Mr. A had never received any form of psychological assistance except for school placement testing.

Family. He is the youngest child of four from a working-class family. Siblings completed high school, and two were living on their own. Mother, when questioned, stated she allows Mr. A to travel independently, assist with household responsibilities, and handle his own money.

Education and Work Experience. Throughout school, Mr. A was placed in special education classes due to mild mental retardation, probably, like epilepsy, a sequelae to encephalitis. He reported enjoying school and having friends. He had been referred by school personnel to VESID for vocational assistance, and was deemed eligible for VESID sponsorship. Reports received from the vocational training program he had attended substantiated that he was considered reliable, dependable, punctual, cooperative, and completed tasks satisfactorily. However, he experienced a seizure and was terminated.

Social Interactions. Reportedly, Mr. A is involved with various family members and family-oriented activities. He also participates in events at a community center.

Mental Status. He is a well-dressed and groomed man who appeared to be his stated age. He made poor eye contact during the interview, and often gave inadequate responses to questions. His speech was very limited and often unclear. Vocabulary was poor, and he used inadequate sentence structure. Mood was depressed and affect was very constricted. Thought content showed no dominant theme other than his interest in vocational training. He showed no psychotic, assaultive, or suicidal ideation. He was fully oriented; recent and remote memory were poor. His fund of knowledge was poor, and he would not attempt the interpretation of proverbs. He was able to perform similarities. He was unable to perform any serial subtractions. Insight was poor and judgment was limited.

Treatment Recommendations. Treatment recommendations for Mr. A included the following:

1. Referral to a specialized epilepsy clinic.
2. Group sessions to further develop interpersonal skills.
3. Individual sessions to support him through neurological reassessment and VESID and vocational process, providing advocacy as needed.

Outcome. Parents agreed to recommendation, and mother escorted him for initial clinic appointment. Several anticonvulsants were tried, and, as expected, Mr. A had improved seizure control, but a poor prognosis for becoming seizure-free.

In group sessions, Mr. A responded to how the group members and leader were affected by certain of his behaviors (e.g., averting eyes, yawning, and apparently not listening at times). He was able, with reminders and cues, to reduce these behaviors, and was able to carry this to outside situations as well.

Mr. A found individual sessions somewhat difficult, because he was reluctant to discuss family issues or feelings. He did respond to support and guidance. He was referred to VESID and, with continuous advocacy, was finally sponsored for a vocational evaluation at an appropriate facility. This accomplished, he was placed in a sheltered workshop ostensibly to continue evaluating work tolerance.

After some time elapsed, Mr. A reported he was on "interrupt status" because one morning he had a seizure on the subway. This event had not stopped Mr. A from continuing his journey and arriving at his program on time. When program staff were contacted, they reported that Mr. A is a good worker and would not say whether it was their determination or that of the VESID counselor to place him on "interrupt status." The VESID counselor was appalled to learn that the Institute would want him to continue his present independent manner of functioning while he was still experiencing seizure activity, and mandated that a neurologist complete another form verifying that it was safe for Mr. A to resume program activity. Fortunately, due to the Institute's relationship with this particular seizure clinic, Mr. A did not have to wait several months for a clinic appointment to obtain this.

Although Mr. A was reinstated at his program, he was being denied vocational training that could potentially lead to competitive employment. As his VESID counselor was also not in favor of this, a meeting was convened. It was agreed to allow Mr. A to become involved with an agency that places people in temporary supervised positions with the goal that he would then be hired.

Mr. A was placed in the housekeeping department of a hospital as his first assignment. After several days of working, he experienced a seizure. He handled himself well, recovering in a few minutes and resuming his duties. The next day he was dismissed. Although Mr. A was given another work assignment in a different company, the experience was devastating. The Institute is still in the midst of negotiating with the agency that handled this initial placement, hospital personnel, and all their funding sources to remedy this obvious example of discrimination.

It is likely that, in the near future, Mr. A will have a job in competitive employment. One suspects that his tendency to withdraw is a survival defense, which has kept him going at a tremendous emotional price.

Case 7: Ms. G

Identifying Information. Ms. G, a 35-year-old, divorced, Hispanic mother of one child, was referred by members of her church.

Reason for Contact. Ms. G was escorted by a church member, due to the frequency of her seizures and concerns about traveling alone. Because her daughter was in school, an appointment had to be arranged according to that schedule, as well as to when someone could escort her.

The nature and frequency of her seizures were severely limiting Ms. G, placing increasing responsibilities on her 11-year-old daughter. She expressed concern about this, as well as becoming increasingly depressed over her situation.

Medical/Neurological/Psychological. Onset of seizures occurred during adolescence, and, although not frequent, she reported being limited socially by her parents. In high school, she became increasingly isolated and depressed, and received short-term counseling. She reported her seizure activity had increased steadily over the past few years. Neurological care appeared inadequate. No other medical conditions and/or illnesses were elicited.

Although Ms. G received some financial support from her ex-husband for their daughter, she had had to apply for public assistance for herself. Thus, she was eligible for ambulette/car service, which would allow her to keep regularly scheduled appointments, because church members could not routinely escort her.

Family. Ms. G is the middle child of three and grew up in a middle-class family in a suburban area. She felt she could never please or be accepted by her mother. Although maintaining phone contact, she experienced her as critical and rejecting. Contacts with siblings also were limited.

Ms. G remembered feeling very sad in high school because her parents would not allow her to participate in any social activities. Nor was she able to drive in an area of limited public transportation. She recalled being treated in a much more restrictive manner than her siblings when they had been her age. She became more and more withdrawn, and eventually school personnel offered her short-term counseling. Her parents did not pursue any other psychological assistance.

She married at 22 years of age and moved to another state. She was unable to work in this area, in large part due to a lack of public transportation. Her husband filed for divorce when their child was 3 years old. Ms. G, without a significant support system, moved back to the city where she had completed her secretarial studies, worked, and knew that public transportation was available.

Education and Work Experience. Graduating from high school, she enrolled in a 2-year secretarial program, which she successfully completed. Working for the same company for several years, she left due to her marriage and relocation. Although she wished to resume employment, she was cognizant that her frequent seizures mitigated against this, and that her skills needed to be updated.

Social Relationships. She reported a diminishing circle of friends from the time her parents restricted her. She had met some people in secretarial school and on her job, but, once she moved away, she lost touch with them.

Likewise, her move back to the city eliminated whatever limited contacts she had established in the previous locale. She found her family of origin too critical, and social contacts primarily consisted of people from her building and church members, whom she viewed as supportive and understanding.

Mental Status. She was neatly groomed and cooperative. Her speech was of normal tone, pitch, and speed. Her mood was anxious and depressed. Her affect was appropriate to thought content. She denied auditory and visual hallucinations. Serial of 7s was fair. Calculations were good. Fund of information was fair. Her abstract ability was good. She admitted to phobias.

Treatment Recommendations. The treatment recommendations for Ms. G included the following:

1. Referral to specialized epilepsy clinic arranging for necessary transportation/escort services.
2. Prescription of antidepressant medication.
3. Group sessions to reduce isolation and strengthen coping mechanisms.
4. Individual sessions to (a) assist her through neurological reevaluation; (b) assess if part-time homemaker is needed to alleviate responsibilities placed on child; (c) encourage her to bring in child to evaluate whether assistance is needed; (d) learn how to handle and interact with family of origin in a more productive way; (e) formulate realistic perceptions of herself and her accomplishments; (f) review marriage, divorce, and any residual feelings that may be impacting on father maintaining contact with daughter.
5. Vocational exploration, when ready, to assess level of skills and options.

Outcome. Referral to specialized epilepsy clinic and transportation arranged. Medications changed and seizure control eventually improved.

An antidepressant was prescribed and accepted. This was coordinated with the treating neurologist. As Ms. G began to successfully resolve several major issues, antidepressant medication was discontinued.

Ms. G was quite active in group sessions, displaying a sense of humor and compassion. She began to perceive herself more objectively, as group members and leader reflected their observations, which differed from those of her family. She left this group, which had impacted profoundly on her life, when she began working. She maintained phone contact with some of the members.

Individually, Ms. G recognized that the responsibilities placed on her daughter were beginning to interfere with school performance and the ability to pursue after-school activities and socialization. Certainly, Ms. G did not want her daughter's experience to replicate her own. Her clear devotion to this child overcame any feelings of inadequacy she had at accepting help from someone else for a short time. Likewise, her feelings of shame for being on public assistance were addressed.

She agreed to bring her daughter to sessions. Individually, to help her child cope with fears of losing her mother because she barely had contact with her father; and periodic joint sessions, to facilitate communication.

Ms. G had a much harder time sorting out her feelings toward her family of origin. She initially found her feelings of rage unacceptable until she fully grasped that contrasting positive and negative feelings can coexist. By getting in touch with her sadness and pain, she could move forward and was able to establish a more satisfactory relationship with her mother.

She acknowledged resentment toward her ex-husband for leaving her, but, beyond that, the resentment extended to his irregular child support payments and erratic phone contacts. Ms. G was helped to role-play situations with her ex-husband so that some friction was reduced. It also was arranged between them that their daughter could spend part of the summer with her father and his family.

As Ms. G stabilized emotionally as well as neurologically, and traveled on her own, she was eager to begin vocational counseling. Through testing, it appeared that her basic skills needed to be upgraded to be ready for competitive employment. She was referred to VESID. Her counselor there agreed to the Institute's recommendations about the site for course work and the skill areas to be addressed. Although this facility was aware that Ms. G had epilepsy, when a seizure finally was observed, she was asked to go home. She was placed on "interrupt status." Negotiations with all involved entities, including the Institute's commitment to do job placement, resulted in Ms. G returning to successfully complete her program.

Ms. G is currently working full time. She has increased her circle of friends, and is engaged to be married. She also is quite proud of her college-bound daughter.

Case 8: Mr. C

Identifying Information. Mr. C is a 23-year-old, single, Hispanic male, residing with his parents, after having dropped out of college 2 years ago.

Reason for Contact. He is seeking advice about finding some direction in his life regarding school, work, and finances. He states that he has difficulty prioritizing his goals and communicating with others.

Medical/Neurological. Mr. C stated that at 19 years of age he was diagnosed with tonic–clonic seizures. He recalled periods of transient lightheadedness and headaches throughout grade school, and wondered in hindsight if these were seizures. He acknowledged having problems concentrating on studies, and dropped out of college shortly after he was diagnosed. When seizure symptoms were explored, Mr. C acknowledged that he has been told that, episodically, he appears to stare off and mumble. He did not identify these behaviors as seizures. He reported no major medical illnesses.

Family. He is the older child of two from his mother's first marriage, and he has three younger half siblings from her second marriage. He reports his mother was abusive toward him throughout childhood, and that this stopped in adolescence when he physically stood up to her. He readily took the opportunity to move away from home by utilizing his high school advisor's suggestion that he attend college. This decision was reportedly not supported by his mother.

Returning to live with his family has been very difficult. He states he wants to move out, is unsure how to proceed with this, and that his mother is opposed to it because of his diagnosis. However, they have frequent fights, and the living situation is tense for all involved.

Education and Work Experience. He reports difficulty with school work, and wonders now if this might have been due to undiagnosed seizures. As well, he has experienced an extremely conflictual home situation. After leaving college and returning to his mother's house, he eventually found a job as a salesman, having worked in this capacity during summer vacations. However, after several months, he lost this job due to stated conflicts with his supervisor.

Social Relationships. Mr. C reports fearing rejection and not readily engaging in relationships, of which he reports a limited number. He believes his failure in athletics has interfered with his relationships with men. He also fears being unable to please women, although he has had two extended relationships. Even in these, however, he felt somewhat withdrawn and unable to express himself.

Mental Status. This is a tall, thin, attractive young man who appears somewhat tense and anxious. He spoke quietly, and is moderately relevant and coherent. His speech was somewhat evasive and tangential. He was able to subtract serial 7s fairly well, but was completely concrete in his attempts to explain proverbs. He showed average intelligence, insight was minimal, and judgment was very questionable.

Treatment Recommendations. The treatment recommendations for Mr. C included the following:

1. Referral to epileptologist.
2. Neuroleptic medication.

3. Individual sessions to work through intense feelings toward mother, which are interfering with current relationships and separation process.
4. Vocational assessment and counseling to formulate areas for client to pursue, while addressing immediate financial concerns. Determine feasibility of job placement.

Outcome. Mr. C agreed to a second neurological consultation after being assisted to obtain medical coverage for this. Complex partial seizures secondarily generalizing were diagnosed and medications altered accordingly. It is doubtful that seizures will be eliminated totally.

Although Mr. C acknowledged an inability to organize his thoughts, he resisted a neuroleptic medication. At first, he attributed this to neurological concerns, but this had been cleared with the treating neurologist. Mr. C eventually realized that a trial period of such medication could help him achieve his stated goals. Instead of viewing the medication negatively, he perceived it as a tool toward this end. He complied and, at a low dosage, became much more focused and goal oriented. He continued on this medication through critical treatment stages.

Individually, Mr. C's inability to communicate stemmed, in great part, from his unresolved rage at his mother. Being cut off emotionally, he was unable to express himself. Because he was able to articulate and deal with this anger, he could perceive more clearly what he wanted. During this process, he moved out of the parental home to a rented room. Eventually, he became involved with a woman whom he subsequently married. He also reported improved relationships with authority figures at work because his anger was no longer displaced.

Through psychological and aptitude testing, it was clear that Mr. C had the ability to complete college studies, as well as engage in various careers not requiring this degree. Because Mr. C needed to separate from his mother first, he agreed to take some courses in computer science while working in a part-time sales job. After he completed these successfully, the Institute was able to obtain a job for him, despite seizure frequency, because Mr. C had learned how to cope and compensate effectively. Once he decided to marry, he chose not to pursue college courses toward his degree.

Case 9: Mr. S

Identifying Information. This 36-year-old, Caucasian male has been married to his second wife for 2 years. He is employed, but dissatisfied with his current position.

Reason for Contact. Mr. S requested a referral to a neurologist, as well as marital and individual sessions. He expressed feeling depressed due to seizure frequency, and a lack of a sense of control, resulting in poor self-esteem and confidence. He hoped that both he and his wife could learn more about epilepsy. Ms. S expressed confusion over complex partial seizures, because she was unaware of these and their manifestation.

Medical/Neurological/Psychological. Mr. S reports German measles at 2 years of age, and encephalitis, for which he was hospitalized for a period of time. He does not know when seizures actually started, except that, at age 9, a teacher recommended he be taken to a doctor. Apparently, his parents complied with this. A diagnosis of epilepsy was made, of which he states he was unaware, and medication was prescribed. According to Mr. S, his parents discontinued this medication after several days.

At 20 years of age, he experienced a tonic–clonic seizure while with friends and was taken to a hospital. Anticonvulsant medication was prescribed, but Mr. S apparently, continuing with his family's denial of his condition, was lax about pursuing neurological care and medication evaluation.

Prior to their marriage, Mr. S's wife suggested that Mr. S engage in individual therapy. Reportedly, he tried this for a short period, but did not feel he obtained anything from it. His wife is involved in her own therapy at this time.

Family. Mr. S is the younger child of two, and from a working-class family. He reported an extremely conflictual relationship between his parents, and that his older sibling excelled academically. His parents often referred to him as "crazy" or "stupid," apparently when complex partial seizures occurred. His mother is deceased, he has had limited contact with his father, and he is unable to engage his sibling in any ongoing kind of relationship.

Education and Work Experience. Mr. S reports some difficulties with school work, starting around the third grade. He never was placed in special classes, but felt that he was slower than the other children. Mr. S remembers periods of blacking out and being told he did strange/weird things. He often was called names and was ostracized by other children. His third-grade teacher tried to get him neurological care and encouraged him in his studies.

He did well athletically, and, although invited to compete in team sports, shied away from these in high school, and instead pursued ones that he could do on his own. He excelled at these and continues his involvement to this day.

Mr. S found part-time work throughout high school and states that, due to fatigue from these jobs, he dropped out in his last year. Shortly afterward, he moved away from his parents' home, holding various positions and engaging in illicit drugs for a period of time.

Eventually, he obtained his GED and attended a community college, which he did not complete. He married, and, after a flurry of tonic–clonic seizures, was advised by a physician to discontinue his then current career choice. Mr. S states his wife became overprotective and fearful; he was at a loss as to what to do, and felt that this led to their eventual separation and divorce.

Mr. S continued with various jobs while obtaining a certificate in another trade. He has pursued that successfully over the years. Recently, he left a job for a much higher paying one, but, due to the shifts involved, he believes he experienced increased seizure activity, lost that position, and has assumed one at a lower salary. He acknowledges difficulty adjusting to the substantial cut in income.

Social Relationships. Mr. S appears to pursue activities that he can do on his own, probably due to family and school experiences. He utilized illicit drugs during late adolescence, possibly as a way of escaping from his situation and as a way of seeking acceptance. Some frightening experiences while on these drugs led him to discontinue usage.

He attributes the failure of his first marriage primarily to his and his wife's reactions to his epilepsy. He is determined to make this second union work successfully. They socialize as a couple; he maintains a high degree of involvement in athletics.

Mr. S seeks to avoid conflict in social relationships and at work, and has difficulty asserting himself. His parents reportedly would argue continuously with no conflict resolution. Additionally, his father would have angry outbursts and physically assault his older sibling and mother. He also seeks to avoid being criticized and ridiculed, as he was during grade school.

Mental Status. He is a very tall, attractive, casually dressed, boyish looking man. His lack of intellectual knowledge about his seizures was striking, probably due to denial and inability to accept them, as well as to his tendency to minimize them. At the same time, he used them to defend himself against all situations, external and internal, which are anxiety provoking for him. His attitude was not that unusual, taking into consideration his parents' reaction to his epilepsy.

On the one hand, his parents displayed total denial that the condition existed by allowing him to avoid taking medication, yet permitting the seizures to manifest; on the other hand, they displayed the need to hide the seizures as something shameful, which said something intrinsically bad about both their son and themselves. Mr. S's seizures became the family secret. Apparently, the situation became even more confusing for him. Although there was a denial of his condition, his parents treated him as if he were a handicapped, special child—someone who was incapable of independent thoughts and actions.

Although not very articulate, he was capable of conveying emotions, not only with words, but with facial expressions and body movements. He was coherent, relevant, logical, and goal oriented. His mood was somewhat depressed, with an underlying anger that he constantly needed to control. His affect was appropriate and full. His insight was partial. He had the capacity to connect past, present, and internal conflicts. His judgment was, in some areas, compromised by his denial of conflict. His concentration and attention span were within normal range. All his cognitive functions were grossly intact.

Treatment Recommendations. The treatment recommendations for Mr. S included the following:

1. Referral to an epileptologist.
2. Time-limited marital sessions to facilitate an understanding of epilepsy and alternative communication patterns.
3. Individual sessions to help Mr. S differentiate from his father, whom he perceives as a business failure, with a passive, inadequate personality marked episodically with angry and assaultive outbursts.
4. Consider group sessions where his denial and shame over epilepsy can be addressed.

Outcome. Mr. S accepted a referral to an epileptologist as per his request. One suspects it was more to please his wife than an actual acknowledgment of his epilepsy. It was questionable, in the beginning phases, how accurately he reported known episodes to the treating neurologist. His desire not to have this condition and to be in control at all times, which seizures worked against, was a recurrent theme. Although anticonvulsant medications were changed appropriately, his compliance with this regimen was questionable at times.

Ms. S grasped different seizure types and appeared to accept that her husband had not been deliberately deceitful about his condition. However, their ways of negotiating issues often resulted in Mr. S assuming a seemingly uninvolved stance. Both of their approaches were explored and ways of modifying them were addressed. Although, of course, not fully resolved, some improvement was reported as well as observable.

Initially, Mr. S had difficulty with individual sessions. He negated exploring issues pertaining to epilepsy, and often was at an impasse with what material to discuss. Increasing contacts with his father, who was becoming more dependent on him, his sense of duty and responsibility toward him triggered many unresolved feelings, which formed the basis for treatment. It became clear that Mr. S's interactions with his supervisor, marked by intimidation and fear, caused Mr. S to block out (i.e., to feel temporarily paralyzed and out of control) the ones with his father. Often he tried to "work around" his supervisor, although this was not always possible. He also expressed difficulty with setting expectations and deadlines with those whom he supervised. This mode of interaction extended to his marital situation as well.

It appeared at times that Mr. S's loyalty to his family of origin prevented him from being and perceiving himself as adequate. As well, this served to avoid any feelings of competition with his father, with whom he identified. This loyalty extended to his feelings about epilepsy. Engaging in treatment allowed him to work through this separation and to begin to identify his own needs and abilities. Eventually, he was able to assert himself with increasingly reduced fears of repercussions. He decided to resume college studies, thus successfully contesting his earlier school failures. At termination, he reported that he and his wife were planning to start a family.

In group sessions, Mr. S's fear of loss of control attributed to seizures encompassed, as well the aggressive and explosive outbursts of his father and his own disinhibiting experiences while using illicit drugs. This acknowledgment provided some perspective for him: that what actually occurred during his seizures could not reasonably be viewed as aggressive or goal directed. However, his identification with his father and his own feelings of rage toward his parents, which he constantly warded off, contributed to this fear. Participating in a group with people who did not need to deny their epilepsy, and through his empathy toward others, he finally developed some for himself. His ability to be multidimensional, accepting and coping with various feelings, bodes well for all areas of his life.

OTHER ISSUES

Other case examples not covered here include postoperative people who are seizure-free and people seeking advocacy assistance. In recent years, more and more people who are postoperative and seizure-free contact the Institute. The main issue for all is the need to restructure their lives without seizures. No matter how happy someone is that their seizures are gone, it is still a loss, necessitating changes in prior ways of coping.

Other people contact the Institute solely for assistance in cases of alleged discrimination, generally in the areas of education, program accessibility, and employment. The latter two are requested most frequently. In some instances, interventions and negotiations with agencies and/or employers and unions have proved successful. Other cases have required legal counsel, either leading to litigation or being settled out of court.

FUTURE

The Epilepsy Institute has upheld its mission of providing high-quality, comprehensive services to a traditionally underserved population. It has been strengthened by this, yet remains flexible enough to explore new approaches and incorporate those which prove successful. Its unique program models have been recognized by various professional and governmental entities. Its resources are expended to enable people with epilepsy and significant others to fulfill their goals for an improved quality of life. If additional funds could be realized, expansion in the following areas would be fruitful as well:

- Establish additional clinics that are geographically accessible to public transportation whenever feasible, and located within reasonable commuting distances.
- Maintain a maximal professional staff so that all those requesting aid could be served. This also would permit more easily the training of interns from various disciplines. Because training interns is labor intensive by supervisory personnel, an experienced staff is needed for this. The obvious benefit is that more professionals would be knowledgeable about epilepsy and treatment interventions.
- Develop and maintain a computerized database. Various factors could then be correlated more easily to treatment outcomes. This database also could serve to document needs for other services, improving outreach and educational programs, as well as serving as a resource for potential candidates for research studies.
- Expand current clinical psychosocial programs to include and integrate the approaches of hypnosis, breathing/relaxation exercises, and biofeedback services.
- Continue the study designed and implemented by the Epilepsy Institute to scientifically document the phenomenon that certain dogs allegedly are able to "seizure alert" (i.e., to warn a person of an impending seizure). Establish a training program teaching dogs to seizure alert and match them with appropriate candidates. Conduct research on selected variables as to how such dogs improve quality of life (i.e., increased socialization, reduction in family tension and anxiety, increased involvement in community resources, and effect on seizure frequency).

REFERENCES

Dell, J. L. (1986). Social dimensions of epilepsy; Stigma and response. In S. Whitman & B. P. Hermann (Eds.), *Psychopathology in epilepsy: Social dimensions.* New York: Oxford University Press.

Schneider, J. W., & Conrad, P. (1986). Information, and the control of epilepsy: A patient's perspective. In S. Whitman & B. P. Hermann (Eds.), *Psychopathology in epilepsy: Social dimensions.* New York: Oxford University Press.

Temkin, O. (1971). *The falling sickness: A history of epilepsy from the Greeks to the beginnings of modern neurology* (2nd rev. ed.). Baltimore, MD: The Johns Hopkins University Press.

11 Influence of Psychosocial Factors on Seizure Occurrence

Y. Løyning
H. Bjørnæs
P. G. Larsson
S. Areng
R. Aronsen
A. Bragason
R. Kloster and
R. Lossius
The National Center for Epilepsy, Sandvika, Norway

Probably all manifestations of epileptogenic neuronal activity (i.e., overt seizures, "subclinical" seizures, and subclinical activity apparent only in the EEG) have negative consequences of somatic, psychological, and/or social character. Hence, the ultimate goal of epilepsy treatment should be to eliminate all these manifestations. However, most of the present antiepileptic therapies have their main effect on seizures and, hence, are directed against this manifestation.

Apart from antiepileptic drugs, many factors in the patients' internal and external environment are known to influence the epileptogenic manifestations, increasing as well as decreasing them. To institute the most effective and least harmful treatment for seizures, their provoking and inhibiting factors should be analyzed and dealt with effectively.

A comprehensive service center for difficult cases with epilepsy, like our National Center for Epilepsy in Sandvika, Norway, should be proficient in analyzing all factors influencing epileptogenic manifestations and familiar with all treatments known to reduce them. However, as far as we know, most centers of this kind, like ours, have hitherto performed a rather limited analysis of seizure influencing factors and used mostly antiepileptic drug treatment and partly surgical treatment in their daily work. Regarding seizures, analysis of influencing factors of various nature, particularly the psychosocial ones, and antiepileptic psychosocial treatment, like behavioral treatment, undoubtedly are underutilized, despite the increasing evidence of influence and usefulness (Dahl, Brorson, & Melin, 1992; Goldstein, 1990).

Realizing that, for a few selected patients who have seizures obviously provoked by psychosocial factors that seem likely to be reduced by behavioral treatment, we have used the comprehensive interview questionnaire of Dahl

(1988) to reveal these factors as a basis for the treatment Dahl et al. (1992) used with great success. So far, our results are promising enough to continue this approach.

It is necessary to quantify the fraction of patients with an influenceable seizure frequency to plan the future treatment strategies. However, Dahl's (1988) questionnaire is too elaborate and time consuming to fill out for selection or screening of possible candidates for behavioral treatment in our center. For that purpose, elements from the inventories developed by Balaschak and Mostofsky (1981) are more suitable.

METHODS

The Questionnaire

For screening purposes, we have made a less comprehensive questionnaire (Fig. 11.1A) with guidelines for its use (Fig. 11.1B), partly using questions from the inventories of Balaschak and Mostofsky (1981) and from the interview questionnaire of Dahl (1988). Our questionnaire is used to obtain information from the patients and relatives when the history is taken by the doctors and the psychologists on admittance, and from all staff members' observations during the patients' stay in the center. Questions evaluating the patients' possible gain of the seizures, and the compliance and motivation to be seizure-free, are answered later during the stay when the patients are better known.

The interview starts out with open and general questions, proceeding to more specific and exemplifying ones. These screening questions are related to the patients' types of seizures and grouped in the following conditions, known to either influence seizure occurrence or in elements known to be influenceable for further seizure development.

Prodromes/Auras. Does the patient feel in advance when a seizure is coming? Does the patient have any initial seizure phenomena?

High- and low-risk situations for seizure occurrence. In particular, the patient is asked if seizure occurrence is related to social situations, stress, affect, relaxation, changes in arousal and activity, menstruation, the time of the day, the week, the season, the holidays, and so on.

Seizure-provoking factors. The questions specify several factors known to precipitate seizures, such as sleep deprivation, alcohol abuse, physical and mental stress, ovulation, or menstruation.

Self-induced seizures. Can the patient do anything to induce seizures? If so, what?

Factors influencing seizure duration. Can other persons do anything to influence the patient's seizures? If so, what? Can the patient influence seizure duration? If so, how?

Negative and positive consequences of having seizures. What are the negative consequences of having seizures (pain, injuries, rejection, etc.)? How are family members responding to the patient's seizures? Does the patient like/dislike these responses? Does the patient have any gain of having seizures that might reinforce seizure frequency and duration, such as pleasure, concern, care, privileges, less demands, or less conflicts? The evaluation of secondary gain and its subjective importance may be the most difficult part to fill out in the questionnaire, because such mechanisms usually are hidden to the patient and the information must be based on observations by relatives and staff members.

Information Qualifying for Therapy. The interviewer also seeks information of importance for the final selection of a patient for therapy. For instance, it is asked how often the patient tries to influence seizure occurrence and how often these attempts are successful. The patient's ability to cooperate in recording seizures, following instructions, and the motivation for therapy are evaluated by the staff members.

The Patients

Of the patients referred to our center during 1 month, 64 were able to answer the questions in the screening interview or had relatives who could do so, and were given the screening interview in this pilot study.

The mean age of the patients is 28.3 years (range 13–60). Thirty-four were men and 30 were women, and forty-eight answered the questions mainly themselves. Information about 16 patients was obtained from dependents; 15 of these patients were mildly to severely mentally retarded. The parents of the remaining patient wanted to answer for her.

All patients had true epileptic seizures of simple partial, complex partial, primary generalized, or secondary generalized type. Patients with pseudoepileptic seizures were excluded. All patients or their dependents are required to keep seizure calendars before admission. All were on antiepileptic medication monitored by the serum levels. All had their EEGs analyzed and, in some cases, quantified for epileptogenic activity.

RESULTS

The Questionnaire as a Screening Tool

The doctors and psychologists found that completion of the questionnaire took about half an hour, in addition to the ordinary taking of history on admission to

SCREENING INTERVIEW FOR POSSIBILITIES OF INFLUENCING SEIZURE OCCURRENCE

Pat. name________________________born____________dep._____Rec. by:___

If the patient has several types of sz., describe them briefly
Sz.type 1:______________________
Sz.type 2:______________________
Sz.type 3:______________________
Sz.type 4:______________________
Sz.type 5:______________________

Scores
P = info. from Patient
C = --- " ---- Comparents
O = Staff Observation

Interview taken during history

Scores pertain to sz. type no.	specifications/descriptions	influence on sz: reliable/ convincing	probable	possible	doubtful	none
	High risk situations for having sz					
	1. in general					
	2. social situations					
	3. stress (physical/mental)					
	4. changes in arousal (physical/mental)					
	5. affect					
	6. periodicity					
	Low risk situations					
	7. in general					
	8. stable level of activity					
	9. stable level of relaxation					
	10. periodicity					
	Sz triggers					
	11. (describe)					
	Self control possibilities					
	12. pat. able to release sz himself					

Final evaluation	Item					
	if yes, how is this done?					
	Initial phenomenae 13. prodromes					
	14. auras					
	Reactivity during sz 15. no responses to external stimulation					
	16. responds to external stim.					
	Sz duration influenceable by 17. external stimulation					
	18. pat. own behavior					
	if the pat. <u>can</u> infl. sz duration how often is this tried? (approx. % of sz).					
	how often are such trials successful? (approx. % of sz).					
	19. Pat.´s preferences about sz-situation					
	Consequences of sz					
	20. privileges					
	21. attention/care					
	22. avoidance of demands, conflicts					
	23. anxiety reduction					
	24. rejection					
	25. sz annoying or pleasurable (underline)					
	26. family members´ reactions to sz					
	27. pat. likes/dislikes to these reactions					
	28. Supposed motivation for treatment					
	29. Supposed ability for compliance					

FIG. 11.1A. Screening interview for possibilities of influencing seizure occurrence.

Guidelines:

The first part of the interview should be taken as part of the history taken at the admittance. It is important that the patients understand the intention of the questions, so the questions must be adapted to the patients´ intellectual functioning and age. The last part of the questionnaire is best answered when the patient is better known by the team.

The patients should answer as many questions as possible themselves, but for children and mentally retarded patients their relatives/attendants must be consulted when necessary.

<u>Sample questions</u>

1. Do you know of any situation where the possibilities of having szs are greater than usual. Which?
2. Do szs occur more frequent when you are together with other people? In particular situations?
3. What about situations where you are late and have to hurry up, when you are very busy, or when you are otherwise stressed?
4. How is it when you are going to bed or turning out of bed? Or when you suddenly pause and relaxe after heavy physical activity or stress? What about when you start up activities abruptly?
5. Do you more often have szs when you are in affect ? (angry, frightened, irritated, or happy, excited).
6. Are there times of the day, week, month, year when you more often have szs? Other forms of periodicity? Do you have szs in series? Are there any regularities in sz occurrence?
7. Are there situations when you never or more seldom than usual have szs? Which?
8. What when you engage in stable levels of activity?
9. What about stable levels of relaxation/rest/sleep?
10. Are there periods of the day, week, month and year when you more seldom have szs?

11. Do you know of anything that can start/release a sz? What?

12. Can you do anything to release a sz? What? Have you ever done anything that released a sz? What? Do you believe this can start a seizure again if you do the same thing?

Have you ever done anything that prevented a sz? What? Can you do this again?

13. Do you sometimes/always know/feel that you soon will have a sz? What?

14. Do you experience any initial changes, eg. sensations (auras), when you have szs? What?

15 - 16. During a sz, are you able to notice/observe anything in your surroundings? What? Are you able to interact with other people ? How? Can you hear, understand speech/situations? Can you talk/answer?

17. When you have a sz, can other people do anything that influences the duration or strength of the szs? Eg. shorten it, preventing it from developing fully? How? Prolonging it? What?

18. Can you yourself do anything to influence the duration or strength of a sz once it has started? Shorten/prolonging it. What?

Do you always/often try to influence sz duration? Are you always/often successful when trying this?

19. If you could choose, would you like to have more szs, less szs or just the same number you have now? How many szs would you like to have every week? When, were and with whom would you like to have them?

20 - 26. Does the patient have gains from having szs (privileges, attention/care, less demands or conflicts in home/residence/school/working place)? Are any of the significant people reacting by rejecting the pat. because of his szs? Does the pat. experience relief from anxiety after szs? Are szs painful, annoying, peculiar, or pleasurable in any way? How do family members/attendants react to the patient´s szs, and how is the pat. experiencing these reactions?

27. Is the patient motivated for getting better?

28. Will the patient be able to comply/cooperate during treatment?

FIG. 11.1B. Guidelines.

naire, there were few misunderstandings and misinterpretations of the questions and how they should be answered.

Degree of Seizure Influence

Figure 11.2 shows the percent of patients having seizures they believed to be truly or most likely influenced by factors grouped as indicated. Forty-two percent of the patients reported that stress is a high-risk situation for getting seizures; 26% has experienced that change in arousal, mainly relaxation after physical or mental strain, is a high-risk situation; 7.8% is able to provoke seizures in various ways themselves; whereas 14% can influence the duration of seizures.

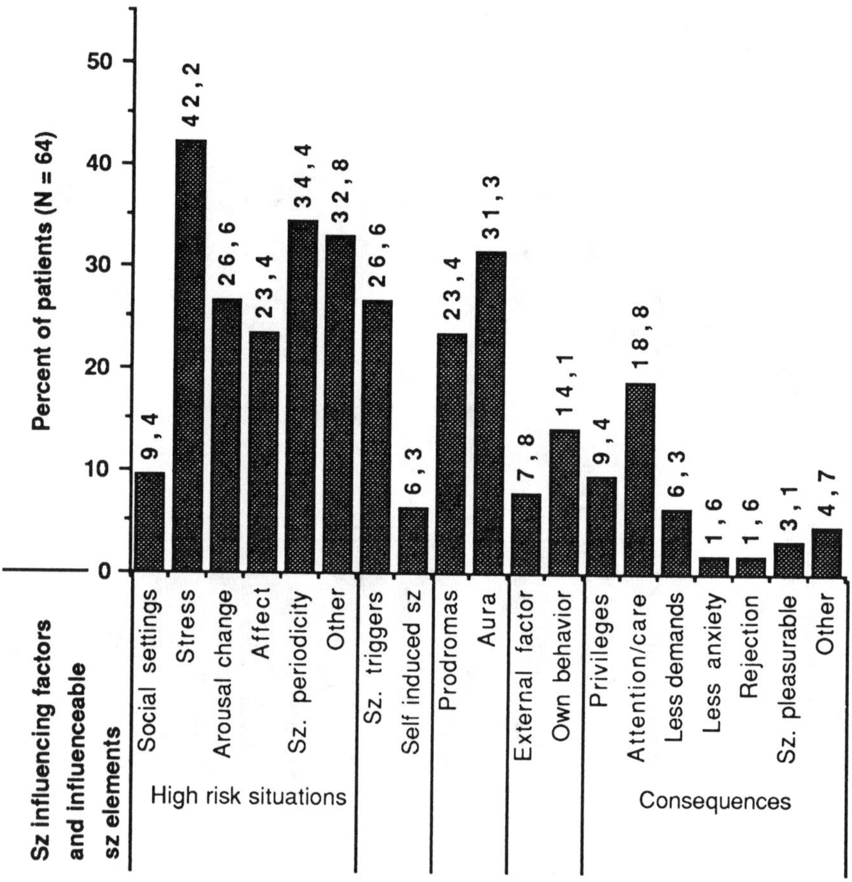

FIG. 11.2. Percent of patients having prodromes, auras, or seizures that they believe to be influenceable by factors grouped as indicated. $N = 64$.

Seizure Consequences

Only 6.3% appeared to have a gain of their seizures in terms of less demands and/or conflicts. Two patients (3.1%) reported that their seizures are pleasurable. One of them, who was under consideration for surgical therapy because her seizures were socially intolerable, had serious concerns about how to manage without seizures.

Suitability for Behavioral Treatment

Patients with several conditions influencing their seizures probably have more possibilities for behavioral therapeutic intervention than patients with few or only one influential condition. Hence, we have arbitrarily grouped patients with three or more influential conditions as best suited for therapy, those having two influencing conditions as promising candidates, those with only one condition as possible candidates, and those without any influential condition as no candidate.

The percentage of patients in these groups are: 35.9% as "best suited candidates," 29.7% as "promising candidates," 17.2% as "possible candidates," and 17.2% as "no candidates." However, this grouping also is chosen for our practical possibilities for intervention, although we realize that a patient with only one, but a very significant, factor might be a particular good candidate. The questions seeking other information qualifying for therapy intend to identify such candidates. Patients considered as good or promising candidates are evenly distributed by age and gender.

Fifteen patients in this pilot study are moderately to severely mentally retarded (estimated IQ < 70). Even among these patients, 5 (33%) meet the criteria qualifying them as good or promising candidates for behavioral treatment of their seizures. However, 4 of them are considered not able to cooperate, nor sufficiently motivated for therapy, rendering only one moderately retarded patient (6.7%) as a seemingly suitable candidate.

Five of the nonretarded patients with ability to cooperate are not considered sufficiently motivated for therapy. Two patients are considered motivated, but are not able to cooperate, and four lack both motivation and cooperability. Thus, when the qualifying evaluations are taken into consideration, 42.2% of the patients seem well suited or promising for therapy, including the mentally retarded ones. There are no significant differences in lack in cooperability and motivation between the genders.

DISCUSSION

The Questionnaire as a Screening Tool

The questionnaire is probably comprehensive enough to catch the majority of patients having seizures influenced by defined psychosocial factors to such a degree that they might be possible candidates for behavioral treatment. Definitely, the questionnaire is not too elaborate and time consuming to fill out during the taking of history on admittance and at an evaluation somewhat later during the stay. Hence, after some adjustments and simplifications, the questionnaire is now being used in a larger study to analyze and quantify the influenceability of the patients' seizures and the suitability for behavioral treatment.

The Results

The screening questionnaire revealed that 82.8% of the patients had influenceable seizures. Of these, 35.9% were well suited, 29.7% promising, and 17.2% possible candidates for behavioral treatment. These figures are certainly much higher than we hitherto have believed on the basis of ordinary history taking on admittance. However, they are somewhat in accordance with information derived from many of the patients being intensively observed during selection for surgical treatment; they are as anticipated after trying out various questionnaires. The ongoing larger study will compare the information formerly derived from ordinary history taking in a control group and those obtained with the actual questionnaire.

There were no significant differences in seizure influenceability related to gender, age, and mental capacity, but the number of children and mentally retarded patients are too small. In the greater ongoing study, children and mentally retarded patients are analyzed separately.

The fraction having specified gain as a consequence of their seizures was less than anticipated from experience. The questionnaire used in the ongoing main study is modified to explore better this gateway to antiepileptic psychotherapy.

The Usefulness of Screening

Identification of patients having seizures influenceable by various factors is of interest, and could be the basis for several treatment strategies. The usefulness for behavioral therapy is to try the therapy; such trials now are being performed on patients selected by the screening method.

Perspectives

If a cost–benefit analysis of behavioral treatment of patients selected by this screening method is favorable, it will have several consequences: (a) the screening method must be perfectionated; (b) this therapeutic approach must be tried out on a larger scale and on drug intractable cases before surgical treatment is performed; (c) the staff must be increased and altered accordingly; (d) the effect must be studied on various types of seizures and also on subclinical seizures and subclinical epileptogenic activity; and (e) the effect also should be studied on patients with both epileptic and pseudoepileptic seizures and pseudoepileptic seizures alone.

General Comments

Goldstein (1990) pointed out, in her review of behavioral epilepsy treatment studies before 1990, the necessity to clarify the specificity of treatment types to types of seizures, epilepsies, and patients. That calls for a relevant characterization of a larger group of potential candidates than is hitherto done. In our opinion, the best description of relevant characteristics is found in the work of Dahl (1988). To perform such a characterization, some kind of screening tool must be developed before trying out different therapeutic approaches. This complex task calls for a multicenter approach. Such a screening tool is what we are developing at our center.

Most of the patients selected for behavioral intervention so far have been drug intractable cases. The treatment has been most successful in the patients evaluated for surgical treatment; one patient unsuccessfully operated is being treated behaviorally with satisfactory results.

When even otherwise intractable patients can be helped by means of behavior therapy, this is proof of its effectiveness. However, it is also possible that these patients are best suited for such therapy; their unresponsiveness to other kinds of treatment is due to their seizures having an important function in the patients' lives, or being under strong negative influence by environmental factors.

Behavioral intervention in difficult epilepsies is so time consuming that it is even difficult to try it out with limited personnel resources. We consider the screening interview as the first step in this selection. The subsequent steps should encompass:

- Evaluation of how incapacitating the seizures are,
- Evaluation of drug resistance, and
- A more comprehensive analysis of treatment relevant factors by means of the expanded interview of Dahl (1988).

Behavioral therapy may be successful in the mentally retarded without motivation and compliance if seizure precipitating or reinforcing factors are detected (Goldstein, 1990).

REFERENCES

Balaschak, B. A., & Mostofsky, D. I. (1981). Seizure disorders. In E. Mash & L. Terdal (Eds.), *Behavioral assessment of childhood disorders* (pp. 601–637). New York: Guilford.

Dahl, J. (1988). Behavior therapy in the treatment of epilepsy: An application of applied relaxation. *Scandinavian J. of Behaviour Therapy,* 17, 139–153.

Dahl, J., Brorson L.-O., & Melin, L. (1992). Effects of a broad-spectrum behavioral medicine treatment program on children with refractory epileptic seizures: An 8-year follow-up. *Epilepsia, 33*(1), 98–102.

Goldstein, L. H. (1990). Behavioural and cognitive-behavioural treatments for epilepsy: A progress review. *British Journal of Clinical Psychology, 29,* 257–269.

12 Assessment of Psychosocial and Emotional Factors in Epilepsy

Carl B. Dodrill
Lawrence W. Batzel
Regional Epilepsy Center, Department of Neurological Surgery, University of Washington School of Medicine

Although it is recognized universally that the brain is dysfunctional during an epileptic seizure, it is appreciated less frequently that brain dysfunction continues to exist between attacks in many people with epilepsy. This is demonstrated by the electroencephalogram (EEG), which often shows epileptiform abnormalities interictally in patients with epilepsy. Indeed, were this not the case, the EEG would be of little value except when seizures were recorded. Because the brain is the basis for a person's ability to adjust to the stresses and strains of everyday life, it is reasonable to expect that difficulties in adjustment may be found even between attacks in a number of people with epilepsy. This has been demonstrated, with 77% of people with epilepsy showing behavioral, intellectual, or neurological problems beyond their seizure disorders (Rodin, 1977). This study and many others cited within this chapter show that psychosocial and emotional factors represent a substantial proportion of the complicating concerns found in epilepsy.

In this chapter, the literature pertaining to *psychosocial* and *emotional* problems is summarized, the effective assessment of these problems is illustrated, and some of the most important treatment approaches are identified.

PSYCHOSOCIAL ADJUSTMENT IN EPILEPSY

Psychosocial functioning deals with the effectiveness of the individual in the social environment. The emphasis here is on how well the person functions in a myriad of people-related situations, including those pertaining to education, employment, finances, and a host of interpersonal relationships inside and outside the home. In the case of people with epilepsy, this area also includes adjustment to seizures, medication, and the need to relate to physicians. Emotional factors are related to these psychosocial areas, but are not central to it.

Procedures Used in Assessment

A review of the literature soon reveals that there is no classification system of psychosocial problems in epilepsy. The importance of this point is clear. If there were no formal classification system of epileptic seizures, it is unlikely that medical treatment for epilepsy would be systematically and efficiently directed. Drugs would tend to be given at random, and little progress would be made toward controlling seizures. In evaluating patients for psychosocial problems that will lead to an effective treatment plan, one also needs a psychosocial assessment method that will provide that guidance.

Two general procedures have been used commonly to evaluate psychosocial problems in epilepsy. The first of these is *ratings*. Ratings can be accomplished by the patient, by the patient's family or friends, and by treating professionals. Ratings have the advantages of being able to reflect the uniqueness of the patient's situation, of utilizing the accumulated experience of professionals, of flexibility in that their content can be adjusted easily to meet particular needs, and of adaptability for children and others who cannot complete tests and inventories.

Although ratings have important advantages, a review of the literature reveals their disadvantages when actually applied. Ratings often are used without any real effort to establish reliability either across raters or over time. Rarely is an effort made to establish validity by any type of external criterion. In addition, ratings often are accomplished for specific purposes in particular studies, and therefore lack generalizability. Should rating procedures seem similar in more than one study, it is likely that the ways in which the ratings were made probably varied significantly. Thus, comparability across studies is almost nonexistent. Finally, ratings by professionals are time consuming.

Given all of these factors, we have chosen not to review studies based on ratings. However, summaries of studies based in significant part on ratings have emerged, such as in connection with interictal behavioral changes (Devinsky, 1991), antiepileptic drugs effects (Dodrill, 1991), and overall psychosocial adjustment (Levin, Banks, & Berg, 1988).

The second general method of assessment of psychosocial problems in epilepsy is to utilize *tests* or *inventories*. Properly applied, this approach answers a number of the objections just mentioned with respect to ratings. Indices of reliability and validity commonly are reported. Also, if time is taken to develop a test or inventory, it is typically not for a highly specific purpose, and therefore tends to be broader in scope and have greater generalizability. This permits and actually encourages comparative studies. The consistency with which these procedures are applied is also likely to be greater than for ratings, both across sites and over time. Finally, less professional time is required routinely.

For all of these reasons, we favor the use of tests and inventories rather than ratings in assessing psychosocial problems in everyday practice. Ratings are still helpful with persons who cannot take tests, and in research contexts when used to appraise a limited number of psychosocial areas, or when they serve as the basis for the development of a test or inventory.

Psychosocial Tests and Inventories

Unfortunately, few tests and inventories to evaluate psychosocial problems in epilepsy have been available. In fact, no general inventory for this purpose was published prior to 1980. The most commonly used measure of general adjustment in epilepsy prior to that time was the Minnesota Multiphasic Personality Inventory (MMPI; Whitman, Hermann, & Gordon, 1984). Unfortunately, there is little in the MMPI that deals directly with the psychosocial implications of epilepsy. Furthermore, there are no MMPI norms for this group. Although other tests and inventories have been used (Rennick, 1975), none has been developed for people with epilepsy or standardized on that group.

For these reasons, the authors and their colleagues developed the Washington Psychosocial Seizure Inventory (WPSI) for adults with epilepsy (Dodrill, Batzel, Queisser, & Temkin, 1980), and the Adolescent Psychosocial Seizure Inventory (APSI) for teenagers with epilepsy (Batzel et al., 1991). Unfortunately, to date, these remain the only psychosocial inventories specifically directed toward people with epilepsy and standardized on this group. Therefore, they are the primary focus of the discussion here.

In the development of both the WPSI and the APSI, a premium was placed on objectivity and establishing a firm empirical basis for the placement of each item in every scale. In particular, subjective perceptions as to what an item is believed to measure were rejected as a basis for inclusion of an item in the inventory or for placement of it on a particular scale. Likewise, a factor analytic approach was rejected, because of the subjectivity involved in establishing the statistical criteria for factor determination and factor naming, and because of the lack of external validational criteria. Instead, items were placed on scales only when they significantly correlated with the adequacy of psychosocial functioning in that area in life, as judged by trained professionals. Although the WPSI is emphasized in the discussion that follows, the APSI was developed in a similar manner. To a considerable degree, both inventories replicate the judgments of professionals in identifying psychosocial problems in the patients to whom they are given.

Each of the following areas are evaluated with the WPSI:

- *Family Background.* Concerns are sought out in one's family of origin that can contribute to later psychosocial problems.

- *Emotional Adjustment.* General emotional difficulties (depression, anxiety, personal insecurity, etc.) are evaluated to provide an index of overall emotional adjustment.
- *Interpersonal Adjustment.* A person's ability to effectively relate to others in a variety of situations is assessed, as well as adequacy of number and quality of daily contacts with people.
- *Vocational Adjustment.* Ability to obtain and maintain employment and satisfaction with work are the focus.
- *Financial Status.* The extent to which the person has adequate money for basic needs is appraised by this scale.
- *Adjustment to Seizures.* Responses to seizures are sought out including feelings of embarrassment, resentment, and so on.
- *Medicine and Medical Management.* Reactions to the physician and acceptance of the need to take medication are examined.
- *Overall Psychosocial Functioning.* This overall adjustment indicator is not merely a summary of the other areas, but was developed to reflect the weighted importance of each area for each patient.

In addition to these eight scales, three validity scales (Number of Unanswered Items, Lie, Rare Items) permit an assessment of whether the inventory was completed adequately.

Presentation of the results is done by a profile that was developed with the same empirical emphasis as the inventory itself. Using multiple regression, scales were placed on the profile directly dependent on their relationship with professional ratings of adequacy of adjustment. Higher scores indicate poorer adjustment, with four areas of profile elevation indicated on the far right that have the following approximate meanings: Area 1—No problems; Area 2—Possible/slight difficulties; Area 3—Definite problems; Area 4—Severe/major problems. Using this profile, both the relative and absolute degrees of difficulties are conveyed for the various psychosocial areas.

To illustrate the uses of the profile, a large group of cases was drawn from the Neuropsychological Laboratory of the Regional Epilepsy Center in Seattle, Washington. The group consisted of 447 adults (238 women, 209 men) who averaged 29.22 years of age (*SD* = 9.92; range 16–66) and 11.53 years of education (*SD* = 2.68; range 3–20). Racial backgrounds were White in 425 cases, Black in 10, and other in 12. A total of 230 were unemployed, 110 were employed, 55 were students, 45 were housewives, 5 were retired, and 2 were unclassified. Average age at onset of epilepsy was 14.18 years (*SD* = 10.82; range 0–63). Primary seizure types were as follows: 44 simple partial, 231 complex partial, 75 generalized tonic–clonic, 53 generalized other than tonic–clonic, 43 combinations of these, and 1 unclassified. In addition, 231 persons also had secondarily generalized tonic–clonic seizures. Etiology was known in

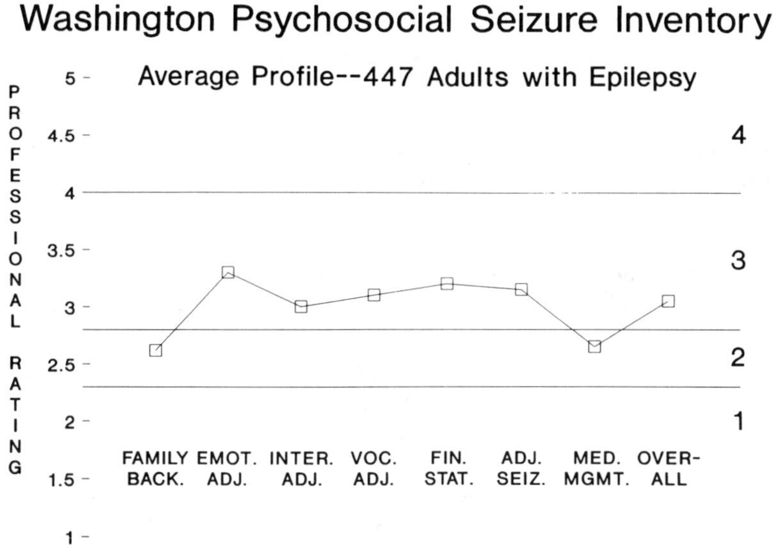

FIG. 12.1. Average WPSI profile for 477 adults with epilepsy seen at the Regional Epilepsy Center, University of Washington School of Medicine, Seattle.

199 cases. The average number of antiepileptic medications was 1.93 (SD = 0.82; range 0–4).

The average WPSI profile for this large group of patients is presented in Fig. 12.1. This figure shows that, for the typical patients whom we see, there are definite emotional, vocational, financial, and interpersonal problems, as well as difficulties in dealing with their seizure disorders.

Literature Review

Because the area of psychosocial adjustment in epilepsy is not well defined, a precise survey of it is difficult. Levin, Banks, and Berg (1988), in a fairly recent review of the literature on psychosocial problems in epilepsy, chose to resolve this matter by using the framework for psychosocial difficulties set up by the WPSI. Their review covered more than 150 papers, of which the results are organized according to the areas covered by the WPSI scales. This review provided a great deal of information about basic findings in each psychosocial area. Because this general review is available, the focus here is on highlighting important issues and providing recent findings.

First, the types of psychosocial concerns noted on an inventory such as the WPSI show a substantial degree of consistency across subject samples. The first multisite study compared WPSI results on 315 adults with epilepsy evaluated at five different places across the United States (Dodrill, Breyer, Diamond, Dubinsky, & Geary, 1984). Four of the five samples were obtained from epilepsy centers or epilepsy societies that tend to attract individuals with special needs. Despite wide geographical distribution, these four samples had almost identical WPSI profiles, with significant problems noted in the areas of Emotional Adjustment, Financial Status, Vocational Adjustment, Interpersonal Adjustment, and Adjustment to Seizures. The fifth sample consisted, in significant part, of private practice neurology patients who showed fewer problems in Vocational Adjustment, Financial Status, and Family Background than the other groups. Otherwise, their profiles were similar. Thus, there are important commonalties in psychosocial problems in epilepsy across groups, and this finding may lead to treatment interventions with significant generalizability.

Second, despite the conclusion just reached, the degree of psychosocial concerns is related to how the subject sampling is conducted. This point is illustrated by a study that began with an unbiased sample of 235 individuals who had active seizures in one community 5 years previously (Trostle, Hauser, & Sharbrough, 1989). The community was above average socioeconomically and intellectually, and retarded persons were excluded. Results showed that persons with the best WPSI profiles at follow-up were seizure-free and off medication, next best if they were seizure-free but on medication, and worst if they had both medication and seizures in the 12 months prior to follow-up. However, all groups had fewer problems than any of the groups in the five sample comparative study reported earlier (Dodrill et al., 1984). Differences in sampling are likely responsible for these findings, and it is clear that care is required in making generalizations from any particular subject group.

Third, intelligence and neuropsychological functioning are related to extent of psychosocial problems in epilepsy, with brighter and less neuropsychologically impaired persons showing fewer psychosocial concerns (Dodrill, 1981). This relationship has permitted the development of Intelligence and Neuropsychological Impairment scales for the WPSI, by which functioning in these areas can be estimated (Dodrill, 1983).

Fourth, the psychosocial response to treatment is highly variable depending on the type of treatment involved. Changes in medication typically are not associated with significant psychosocial changes at least as evaluated by the WPSI, apparently because the seizure frequency changes are routinely less than 50% (Loiseau, Strube, Tor, Levy, & Dodrill, 1988; Wilensky et al., 1983). However, surgery for epilepsy usually produces greater relief from seizures (> 75%), and it is more typically associated with a positive psychosocial change (Dodrill, 1987; Rausch, 1991). Cognitive behavioral therapy has been less effective in producing psychosocial change (Tan & Bruni, 1986) than family counseling (Earl, 1986) or intensive educational efforts (Helgeson, Mittan, Tan, & Chayasirisobhon, 1990). We conclude that to obtain a measurable improvement in psychosocial functioning, one must have an intervention that either produces substantial seizure relief *or* is intense and well directed toward psychosocial problems.

EMOTIONAL ADJUSTMENT IN EPILEPSY

The area of emotional factors in epilepsy has been of interest for decades. Whereas a number of issues has been raised, matters pertaining to (a) the temporal lobe syndrome, (b) types of emotional problems commonly encountered, and (c) treatment considerations are among the most important, and they are discussed here.

Temporal Lobe Syndrome

Investigators addressing emotional factors in epilepsy often refer to the so-called *temporal lobe syndrome*. This term is used to apply to a series of behavioral characteristics thought to be present in patients with complex partial seizures who often have involvement of the temporal lobes. These characteristics include altered sexuality, deepened emotionality, anger, sadness, circumstantiality, hypergraphia, hyperreligiosity, and humorless sobriety. Although postulated for decades, it was Bear and Fedio (1977) who initially popularized studies in this area. Later, Fedio and Martin (1983) raised the possibility that the characteristics shown might relate to the side of the epileptic focus. Although this syndrome is intrinsically interesting, measures of it fail to demonstrate uniqueness and instead appear to be indicators of general maladjustment (Master, Toone, & Scott, 1984; Mungas, 1982; Rodin & Schmaltz, 1984). Also, studies of groups of patients do not support consistently the existence of a general syndrome (Sorensen & Bolwig, 1987; Tucker, Novelly, & Walker, 1987). Although it likely exists in a few patients with epilepsy, it is more of a curiosity than a syndrome that requires therapeutic intervention. Indeed, no particular intervention program for it has been advanced, and it is viewed as an enduring set of characteristics of clinical and theoretical interest.

Types of Emotional Problems

Several types of emotional problems in epilepsy have been reported repeatedly and are of adjustmental significance. These difficulties constitute the primary areas of concern for professionals working with people with epilepsy. The most common of these problems are reviewed in summary form next.

Depression. This may be the most common emotional concern found in epilepsy (Altshuler, 1991). Recent substantial reviews of the problem are available (Altshuler, 1991; Hauser & Hesdorffer, 1990; Robertson, 1989). Biochemical imbalances found in depressed people also are found in persons with epilepsy and may be in part responsible for its high incidence (Hauser & Hesdorffer, 1990). Depression is more likely to be found with lesions related to the left hemisphere, at least among men (Strauss, Wada, & Moll, 1992). Stressful life events, poor adjustment to seizures, financial stress, and female gender are also predisposing factors (Hermann & Whitman, 1989), and there are others as well (Robertson, 1989). In addition, the stresses of the disorder, with its intermittent and often unforetold emotional and psychosocial crises, represent an obvious source of distress. Not only is the rate of depression higher than for normal persons, but the suicide rate is also from two to seven times higher (Hauser & Hesdorffer, 1990). Finally, the D Scale is usually one of the two highest scales (along with Sc) on the MMPI in many studies reviewed (Dodrill & Batzel, 1986). Thus, the importance of this problem is great.

Psychosis or Psychoticlike Conditions. Psychosis in epilepsy has been studied for many years, and important reviews of the phenomenon have appeared recently (Schmitz & Wolf, 1991; Trimble, 1992). Circumstances at times thought to be risk factors for psychosis include left-sided lesion, left handedness, onset of epilepsy in adolescence, and temporal lobe location of pathology (Trimble, 1992). However, attention is drawn to significant differences in definition of psychosis from one study to the next, and also to sampling differences. For example, beginning with a sample from a psychiatric setting and looking for people who also have epilepsy often results in higher rates of psychosis being reported than beginning in a neurological setting and looking for patients who are also psychotic (Schmitz & Wolf, 1991). Personality inventories also present increased evidence for unusual or psychoticlike thinking, but no more so than that found in other disorders associated with brain dysfunction (Dodrill & Batzel, 1986). This finding argues against epilepsy being identified with a unique set of emotional concerns. Indeed, it appears likely that the basis for many of these unusual thought patterns is in underlying brain dysfunction (Conlon, Trimble, & Rogers, 1990; Csernansky, Leiderman, Mandabach, & Moses, 1990), and this holds true whether it is epilepsy or some other brain-related problem that is under examination (Beckson & Cummings, 1992; Filley & Gross, 1992).

Aggression. The belief that aggression is a major manifestation of epilepsy commonly is accepted and dates back to antiquity (Fenwick, 1991). Epilepsy symptomized by aggressive or violent behavior is all too often used as a defense in court cases, but an extensive review of the literature reveals very little evidence to support a connection between aggression and epilepsy (Treiman, 1986). Studies cited to support such a relationship often have subject selection biases (Hauser & Hesdorffer, 1990). Patients who experience a seizure may subsequently appear aggressive during postictal confusion, but neither during the seizure nor afterward do their actions demonstrate planned or purposeful behavior (Treiman, 1986). The behavior is generally nonspecific and lacking in direction unless the patient's movements are restrained (Neppe & Tucker, 1988).

Nonepileptic Seizures. Nonepileptic seizures are events that mimic epilepsy, but that have an origin not epileptic in nature. There are several synonyms for this group of problems including *pseudoseizures, hysterical seizures,* and *psychogenic seizures.* These attacks are quite common, and 5%–36% of patients thought to have epilepsy actually may have nonepileptic seizures rather than or in addition to epilepsy (Wilkes, Dodrill, & Thompson, 1984). Unfortunately, and in contrast to epilepsy, the diagnosis is often one of exclusion (Porter, 1991), and one that is made after several typical attacks have been recorded by both EEG and videotape with no indication of epileptic EEG activity or seizures typical for epilepsy. The characteristics of these spells, in contrast to epileptic seizures, have been described, and a classification system has been set up (Gates, Luciano, & Devinsky, 1991). Somatoform disorders are common, but several other different types of spells are also present and *hysteria* should by no means be viewed as synonymous with nonepileptic seizures. Differential diagnosis is frequently challenging (Neppe & Tucker, 1988) and is made more difficult by the finding that some patients have both kinds of disorders. Patients with nonepileptic seizures represent a significant public health problem, because they frequently are treated as if they had epilepsy and are chronically consuming diminishing health-care dollars (Gumnit & Gates, 1986). It is common for them to be referred to epilepsy centers as possible surgical candidates due to the intractability of their seizures. Two reviews of this complex disorder with particular ramifications for treatment are available (Blumer, 1990; Lowman & Richards, 1987).

TREATMENT

As was indicated earlier, the lack of a classification system for adjustmental problems in epilepsy has represented a major obstacle to treatment planning. Rodin (1977) recognized this and attempted to outline a classification system "that addresses itself specifically to the type and degree of handicap a given patient has, which could be of help to social workers, vocational rehabilitation service counselors, teachers, parents, etc." (p. 74). By this system, each person with epilepsy can be classified as having (a) epilepsy only, (b) epilepsy with behavioral problems, (c) epilepsy with brain impairment and/or organic mental changes, and (d) epilepsy with other neurological handicaps. Unless placed within the first group, a person might fall into more than one category. The percentages of 369 individuals seen at the Epilepsy Center of Michigan falling in each classification were 23%, 54%, 48%, and 10%, respectively. Patients in the last three groups also may be classified on a 4-point severity scale, but details for this were not provided.

Rodin's (1977) approach has merit because it provides basic guidelines toward rehabilitation in the emotional and psychosocial areas. In another study (Rodin, Shapiro, & Lennox, 1977), for example, it was shown that the epilepsy-only group was substantially different from the remaining groups on a host of variables, many with relevance to rehabilitation (employment prognosis, behavior prognosis, personality problems, history of social withdrawal, anxiety, medication compliance, etc.). Furthermore, Rodin's (1977) idea of a 4-point severity rating is sound, because degree of difficulty varies remarkably from one case to the next. In fact, the idea is similar to the four levels of profile classification on the WPSI.

We now briefly present three cases that are illustrative of common psychosocial and emotional problems in epilepsy, along with treatment ramifications arising from the psychosocial and emotional assessment procedures.

Case 1: (#4893)

The first case was a 49-year-old man with seizures of unknown etiology since age 20. True absence seizures occurred at the rate of four to six per month, with occasional generalized tonic–clonic attacks. The patient was taking 1,000 mg of Tegretol (serum level 10.7 μg/ml), to which ethosuximide was later added. He completed high school in normal classes. He was cooperative and quick through a 6–7 hour neuropsychological evaluation, which resulted in a WAIS-R Full Scale IQ score of 98 and evidence for mild nonspecific impairment on neuropsychological tests. Although he seemed to be somewhat socially retiring, observations of him did not reveal any obvious psychosocial concerns. He had been unemployed for the last 2 years, however, a circumstance that he related to his frequent attacks.

This man's MMPI profile was normal except for mild depression apparently related to his fianceé's health problems. As Fig. 12.2, reveals, his WPSI showed problems only in the vocational and financial areas other than his tendency to be socially reserved (Interpersonal Adjustment Scale).

This man demonstrated "epilepsy only," because there were no significant behavioral, intellectual, or neurological problems beyond his epilepsy. Thus, extensive psychotherapeutic or psychosocial intervention is not indicated by the tests. His lack of employment represented his one outstanding area of concern. A vocational rehabilitation program directed toward people with epilepsy (Fraser, 1980; Fraser, Clemmons, Trejo, & Temkin, 1983) was needed. Therefore, referral to such a program was made, but no other intervention was initiated.

We now turn to a case that is much more typical of patients requiring psychological intervention, because it involves a broader range of difficulties.

Case 2: (#5162)

Case 2 was a 39-year-old man with seizures dating from 18 months of age during a high fever. He had simple partial, complex partial, and generalized tonic–

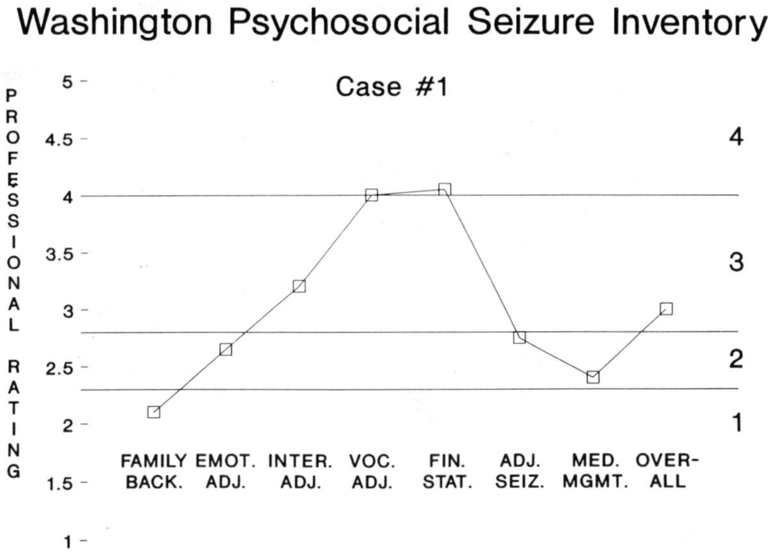

FIG. 12.2. WPSI profile for Case 1. Note the elevations on the Vocational Adjustment and Financial Status Scales.

clonic seizures, and was on Dilantin (serum level 7.0 μg/ml) and phenobarbital (serum level 13.2 μg/ml). He had not done well in school, but had not required special education. He had been unemployed for the last 5 years, and had only done odd jobs prior to that time on a part-time basis. He had seen a psychologist or psychiatrist weekly for a year while in high school for severe depression with suicidal ideation. He was cooperative, but slow during an 11-hour neuropsychological evaluation. He often had difficulty understanding instructions, chose inappropriate approaches toward problems, gave unusual responses, and could not effectively utilize feedback given to him to improve his responses. He obtained a WAIS-R Full Scale IQ score of 88, but there were many problems on the neuropsychological tests that pointed to moderate bilateral impairment in brain functions.

This man's MMPI profile showed a significant number of elevations (Fig. 12.3). He tended to amplify or otherwise exaggerate what are probably genuine concerns. The Sc scale of the MMPI must be interpreted carefully in people with epilepsy, because reports of genuine epileptic seizures often raise the scale score by several points. However, this man endorsed numerous items that raised questions about fundamental reality testing. A thought disorder with a paranoid flavor seemed likely. Also, he demonstrated a somatic focus in his thinking, and he clearly saw himself as unable to function due to physical problems. Anger, bitterness, anxiety, and hypersensitivity also were noted.

Figure 12.4 presents his WPSI. Psychosocial problems of significance were

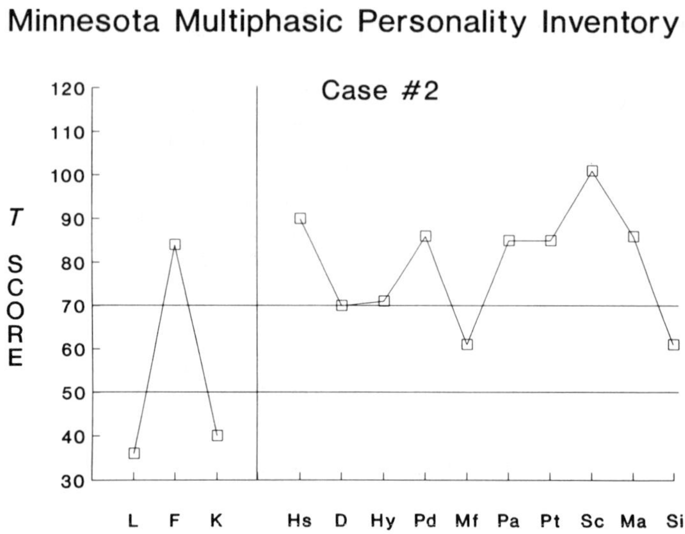

FIG. 12.3. MMPI profile for Case 2. Profile shows a variety of important emotional concerns.

observed in every area evaluated. This included his lack of employment (which he related to seizures) and consequent financial difficulties. His inability to come to grips with his attacks were very important in this case, and the WPSI revealed that he was resentful about them and that he felt that they had ruined his life. In addition, he reported much ambivalence about his previous medical care (Medicine and Medical Management Scale). In fact, he was reluctant to take advice from his current physician. Finally, there was evidence of interpersonal concerns that date back to his family of origin (Family Background Scale) and undoubtedly impact his current social functioning.

Using Rodin's system, this man would be identified as having both behavioral (emotional, psychosocial) problems as well as intellectual and cognitive limitations. Because his problems are both multifactorial and longstanding, the prognosis is guarded at best. With this many MMPI and WPSI scale elevations, our experience has been that only an intense program of intervention has any hope of resulting in a significant change. Dealing with his emotional problems appears to be the first line of action, and this might best begin with a psychiatric evaluation, because of the question of a thought disorder. Psychotherapy certainly is indicated and possibly medication, but attention must be paid to selecting a therapist who can build a trusting relationship with a distrusting patient. Also, his cognitive limitations are such that goals must be limited and practical by nature, and perhaps should include anger management, diminishing his focus on somatic concerns, providing guidelines for reality testing, and stress management. Presuming that some basic goals can be met in these areas, vocational guidance

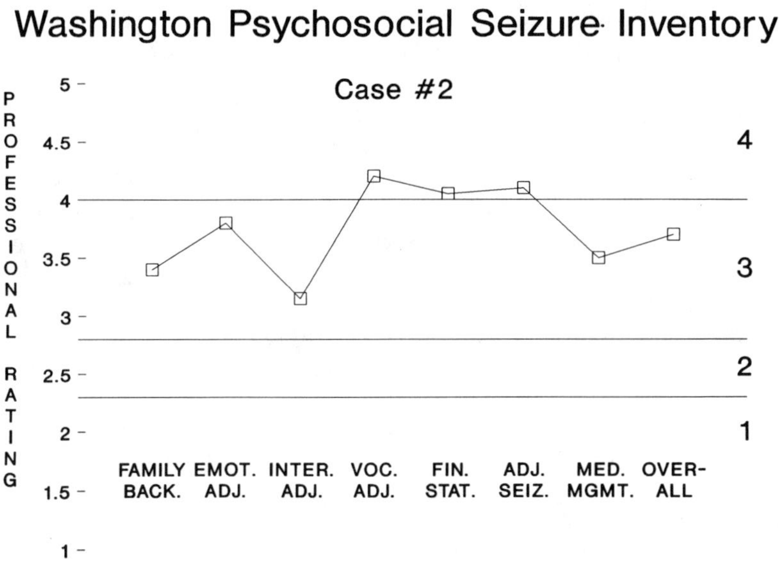

FIG. 12.4. WPSI profile for Case 2. Profile shows a variety of significant psychosocial concerns.

should be considered with his cognitive strengths and weaknesses in mind. It is likely that he will be capable of only unskilled work, and he may require a semisheltered setting. If seizure frequency can be reduced, this would certainly be favorable, but it should be understood that the problems that prevent better functioning in life are primarily emotional/psychosocial and cognitive/intellectual in nature.

The final case is one in which the emotional and psychosocial difficulties are not merely accompaniments of the spells, but they constitute the basis for the spells as well.

Case 3: (#5081)

The final case was a 39-year-old woman who, for the last 3 years, had episodes of disorientation and confusion that were precipitated among other things by flashing lights. They lasted for more than 15 minutes at a time. She was taking Dilantin (serum level 16.9 μg/ml). She did poorly in school, but managed to complete high school with some special assistance in math. She reported numerous medical problems over the years, including eight surgeries, fainting spells beyond her seizures, various blows to the head, decreased sensation on one side of the body with increased sensation on the other side, a possible stroke, and so on. She was sexually molested by an uncle from approximately age 8 to age 12, and allegedly was called "crazy" by her alcoholic mother, who beat her repeat edly with belts and shoes. She has received both inpatient and outpatient psychiatric care. Despite these factors, she had an employment record as a bookkeeper and bank loan officer, although she had been placed on disability leave for the last 2 years.

Results on a 7-hour neuropsychological evaluation appeared to be valid, except possibly for the hand dynamometer where her scores were low because she reported pain when squeezing the instrument. The evaluation revealed a WAIS-R Full Scale IQ score of 99 and mild nonlateralized impairment on the neuropsychological tests, with diminished scores on tests of motor speed, memory, and attention/concentration.

Her MMPI profile is presented in Fig. 12.5. The profile is characteristic of a somatoform or hysterical reaction. An excessive use of repression and denial was indicated, and there was a tendency for unresolved emotional conflicts to be expressed in physical symptoms. This type of profile is seen much more commonly in psychogenic or nonepileptic seizures than with genuine epilepsy (Wilkes et al., 1984), and, in the majority of such individuals, psychological factors ultimately are identified as likely causes of the spells.

Figure 12.6 presents her WPSI profile. The highest score is on the Family Background Scale. From clinical work, we have found that women who have scores this high on this scale have a likelihood of having been sexually molested. Such women routinely come from dysfunctional homes, and this may set the basis for the development of both nonepileptic spells and defective interpersonal relationships. This is true in this case, as is shown by the WPSI Interpersonal

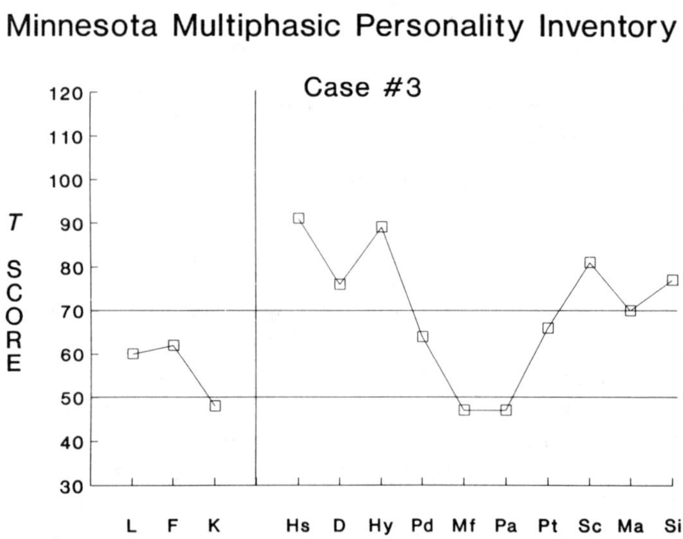

FIG. 12.5. MMPI profile for Case 3. Note the elevations on Hs and Hy relative to D. Elevations on Sc and Si are of secondary importance.

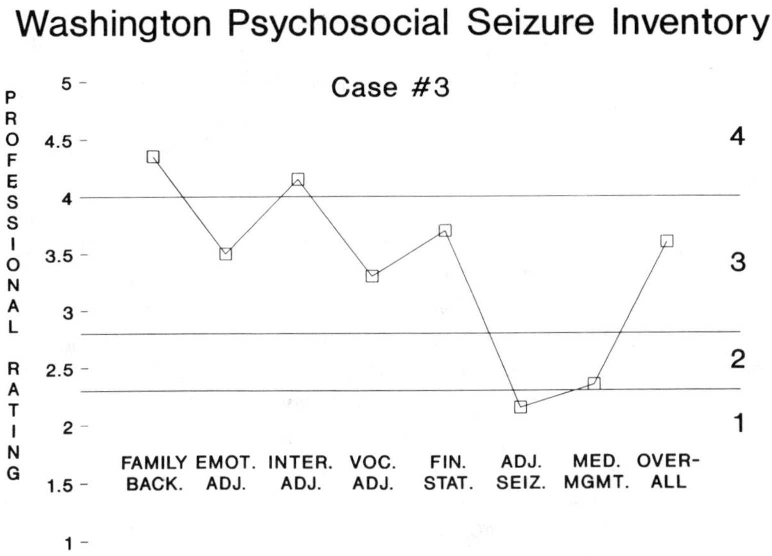

FIG. 12.6. WPSI profile for Case 3. Note the high elevation on the Family Background Scale with a secondary elevation on the Interpersonal Adjustment Scale.

Adjustment Scale and the MMPI Si Scale. Social withdrawal and diminished social skills are indicated.

To determine if her spells represented true epilepsy, she underwent long-term EEG/CCTV monitoring and a number of her typical episodes were recorded. These showed no EEG changes characteristic of epilepsy, and it was concluded that she had nonepileptic spells. Psychiatric intervention was recommended, and treatment in a sexual assault center was deemed to be particularly appropriate. Social skills training also was in order for this patient, because she seemed to have a substantial amount of difficulty in relating smoothly with others.

Comment

The three cases cited represent only a sample of the diversity of psychosocial and emotional problems seen in patients referred for seizure disorders, at least in specialized epilepsy centers. Our experience has been much like that of Rodin (1977), in that most of our patients have significant problems beyond epilepsy. Furthermore, the additional problems frequently constitute the greatest concerns.

In providing psychosocial and emotional assistance to people with epilepsy, we have found it best to begin with a solid assessment of intelligence, neuropsychological functioning, emotional problems, and psychosocial adjustment. This provides a basis on which to tailor an intervention plan. Treatment plans with demonstrated effectiveness include psychotherapy or counseling (Blumer, 1990;

Ramani & Gumnit, 1982), vocational guidance (Fraser, 1980; Fraser & Clemmons, 1989), social skills training (Davis, Armstrong, Donovan, & Temkin, 1984), family therapy (Earl, 1986; Pond, 1981), behavior modification (Goldstein, 1990; Henriksen, 1977), cognitive behavior therapy (Tan & Bruni, 1986), and methods with special relevance to children (Soboloff, 1978). Other valuable procedures may exist as well.

At the present time, empirical guidance is often lacking to direct professionals in terms of treatment methods of choice. This has been especially frustrating to the authors of this chapter, because specific treatment recommendations often cannot be made. Currently, such professionals often must make decisions more on the basis of judgment rather than data. The application of psychiatric and psychological treatment to patients, as if they had emotional problems that are unrelated to their epilepsy, may not result in favorable change (Blumer, 1990; Rodin, 1977). Clearly, there is a need for a classification of adjustmental problems in epilepsy that would help in assessment and treatment planning. It appears that the system devised by Rodin (1977), perhaps coupled with more refined methods in the psychosocial and emotional areas, could be developed into such a classification method. Research toward this end is to be encouraged strongly.

ACKNOWLEDGMENTS

Preparation of this chapter was supported by NIH grants NS 17111 and NS 24823 awarded by the National Institute of Neurological Disorders and Stroke, PHS/DDHS, USA. The WPSI was developed with the assistance of a grant from the Epilepsy Foundation of America.

REFERENCES

Altshuler, L. (1991). Depression and epilepsy. In O. Devinsky & W. Theodore (Eds.), *Epilepsy and behavior* (pp. 47–65). New York: Wiley-Liss.

Batzel, L. W., Dodrill, C. B., Dubinsky, B. L., Ziegler, R. G., Connolly, J. E., Freeman, R. D., Farwell, J. R., & Vining, E. P. G. (1991). An objective method for the assessment of psychosocial problems in adolescents with epilepsy. *Epilepsia, 32,* 202–211.

Bear, D. M., & Fedio, P. (1977). Quantitative analysis of interictal behavior in temporal lobe epilepsy. *Archives of Neurology, 34,* 454–467.

Beckson, M., & Cummings, J. L. (1992). Psychosis in basal ganglia disorders. *Neuropsychiatry, Neuropsychology, and Behavioral Neurology, 5,* 126–131.

Blumer, D. (1990). Diagnosis and treatment of psychiatric problems associated with epilepsy. In D. B. Smith (Ed.), *Epilepsy: Current approaches to diagnosis and treatment* (pp. 193–209). New York: Raven.

Conlon, P., Trimble, M. R., & Rogers, D. (1990). A study of epileptic psychosis using magnetic resonance imaging. *British Journal of Psychiatry, 156,* 231–235.

Csernansky, J. G., Leiderman, D. B., Mandabach, M., & Moses, J. A., Jr. (1990). Psychopathology and limbic epilepsy: Relationship to seizure variables and neuropsychological function. *Epilepsia, 31,* 275–280.

Davis, G. R., Armstrong, H., Donovan, D., & Temkin, N. R. (1984). Cognitive-behavioral skills training with clinically depressed epileptics. *Journal of Clinical Psychology, 40,* 930–935.

Devinsky, O. (1991). Interictal behavioral changes in epilepsy. In O. Devinsky & W. Theodore (Eds.), *Epilepsy and behavior* (pp. 1–21). New York: Wiley-Liss.

Dodrill, C. B. (1981). Neuropsychology of epilepsy. In S. B. Filskov & T. J. Boll (Eds.), *Handbook of clinical neuropsychology* (pp. 366–395). New York: Wiley.

Dodrill, C. B. (1983). Development of intelligence and neuropsychological impairment scales for the Washington Psychosocial Seizure Inventory. *Epilepsia, 24,* 1–10.

Dodrill, C. B. (1987). Commentary: Psychological evaluation (psychosocial changes following surgery). In J. Engel, Jr. (Ed.), *Surgical treatment of the epilepsies* (pp. 197–201). New York: Raven.

Dodrill, C. B. (1991). Effects of antiepileptic drugs on behavior. In O. Devinsky & W. Theodore (Eds.), *Epilepsy and behavior* (pp. 37–46). New York: Wiley-Liss.

Dodrill, C. B., & Batzel, L. W. (1986). Interictal behavioral features of patients with epilepsy. *Epilepsia, 27,* S64–S76.

Dodrill, C. B., Batzel, L. W., Queisser, H. R., & Temkin, N. (1980). An objective method for the assessment of psychological and social problems among epileptics. *Epilepsia, 21,* 123–135.

Dodrill, C. B., Breyer, D. N., Diamond, M. B., Dubinsky, B. L., & Geary, B. B. (1984). Psychosocial problems among adults with epilepsy. *Epilepsia, 25,* 168–175.

Earl, W. L. (1986). Job stability and family counseling. *Epilepsia, 27,* 215–219.

Fedio, P., & Martin, A. (1983). Ideative–emotive behavioral characteristics of patients following left or right temporal lobectomy. *Epilepsia, 24,* S117–S130.

Fenwick, P. (1991). Aggression and epilepsy. In O. Devinsky & W. Theodore (Eds.), *Epilepsy and behavior* (pp. 85–96). New York: Wiley-Liss.

Filley, C. M., & Gross, K. F. (1992). Psychosis with cerebral white matter disease. *Neuropsychiatry, Neuropsychology, and Behavioral Neurology, 5,* 119–125.

Fraser, R. T. (1980). Vocational aspects of epilepsy. In B. P. Hermann (Ed.), *A multidisciplinary handbook of epilepsy* (pp. 74–105). Springfield, IL: Charles C. Thomas.

Fraser, R. T., & Clemmons, D. (1989). Vocational and psychosocial interventions for youths with seizure disorders. In B. Hermann & M. Seidenberg (Eds.), *Childhood epilepsies: Neuropsychological, psychosocial and intervention aspects* (pp. 201–219). New York: Wiley.

Fraser, R. T., Clemmons, D., Trejo, W., & Temkin, N. R. (1983). Program evaluation in epilepsy rehabilitation. *Epilepsia, 24,* 734–746.

Gates, J. R., Luciano, D., & Devinsky, O. (1991). The classification and treatment of nonepileptic events. In O. Devinsky & W. Theodore (Eds.), *Epilepsy and behavior* (pp. 251–263). New York: Wiley-Liss.

Goldstein, L. H. (1990). Behavioural and cognitive-behavioural treatment for epilepsy: A progress review. *British Journal of Clinical Psychology, 29,* 257–269.

Gumnit, R. J., & Gates, J. R. (1986). Psychogenic seizures. *Epilepsia, 27,* S124–S128.

Hauser, W. A., & Hesdorffer, D. C. (1990). *Epilepsy: Frequency, causes and consequences.* New York: Demos.

Helgeson, D. C., Mittan, R., Tan, S.-Y., & Chayasirisobhon, S. (1990). Sepulveda epilepsy education: The efficacy of a psychoeducational treatment program in treating medical and psychosocial aspects of epilepsy. *Epilepsia, 31,* 75–82.

Henriksen, O. (1977). Behavior modification and rehabilitation of patients with epilepsy. In J. K. Penry (Ed.), *Epilepsy, the Eighth International Symposium* (pp. 225–233). New York: Raven.

Hermann, B. P., & Whitman, S. (1989). Psychosocial predictors of interictal depression. *Journal of Epilepsy, 2,* 231–237.

Levin, R., Banks, S., & Berg, B. (1988). Psychosocial dimensions of epilepsy: A review of the literature. *Epilepsia, 29,* 805–816.

Loiseau, P., Strube, E., Tor, J., Levy, R. H., & Dodrill, C. B. (1988). Evaluation neuropsychologique et therapeutique du stiripentol dans l'epilepsie (Neuropsychological and efficacy evaluation of stiripentol in epileptic patients). *Revue Neurologique, 144,* 165–172.

Lowman, R. L., & Richardson, L. M. (1987). Pseudoepileptic seizures of psychogenic origin: A review of the literature. *Clinical Psychology Review, 7,* 363–389.

Master, D. R., Toone, B. K., & Scott, D. F. (1984). In R. J. Porter, A. A. Ward, Jr., R. H. Mattson, & M. Dam (Eds.), *Advances in epileptology: XVth Epilepsy International Symposium* (pp. 557–565). New York: Raven.

Mungas, D. (1982). Interictal behavior abnormality in temporal lobe epilepsy. *Archives of General Psychiatry, 39,* 108–111.

Neppe, B. M., & Tucker, G. J. (1988). Modern perspectives on epilepsy in relation to psychiatry: Classification and education. *Hospital and Community Psychiatry, 39,* 263–271.

Pond, D. (1981). Psycho-social aspects of epilepsy—the family. In E. H. Reynolds & M. R. Trimble (Eds.), *Epilepsy and psychiatry* (pp. 291–295). Edinburgh: Churchill Livingstone.

Porter, R. J. (1991). Diagnosis of psychogenic and other nonepileptic seizures in adults. In O. Devinsky & W. Theodore (Eds.), *Epilepsy and behavior* (pp. 237–249). New York: Wiley-Liss.

Rami, V., & Gumnit, R. J. (1982). Management of hysterical seizures in epileptic patients. *Archives of Neurology, 39,* 78–81.

Rausch R. (1991). Factors affecting neuropsychological and psychosocial outcome of epilepsy surgery. In H. Lüders (Ed.), *Epilepsy surgery* (pp. 487–493). New York: Raven.

Rennick, P. M. (1975). Psychosocial evaluation of individuals with epilepsy. In G. N. Wright (Ed.), *Epilepsy rehabilitation* (pp. 81–103). Boston: Little, Brown.

Robertson, M. M. (1989). The organic contribution to depressive illness in patients with epilepsy. *Journal of Epilepsy, 2,* 189–230.

Rodin, E. A. (1977). Psychosocial management of patients with seizure disorders. *McLean Hospital Journal,* 74–84.

Rodin, E. A., & Schmaltz, S. (1984). The Bear-Fedio personality inventory and temporal lobe epilepsy. *Neurology, 34,* 591–596.

Rodin, E. A., Shapiro, H. L., & Lennox, K. (1977). Epilepsy and life performance. *Rehabilitation Literature, 38,* 34–39.

Schmitz, B., & Wolf, P. (1991). Psychoses in epilepsy. In O. Devinsky & W. Theodore (Eds.), *Epilepsy and behavior* (pp. 97–128). New York: Wiley-Liss.

Soboloff, M. (1978). Treatment of psychosocial problems. In G. S. Ferris (Ed.), *Treatment of epilepsy today* (pp. 115–125). Oradell, NJ: Medical Economics Company, Book Division.

Sorensen, A. S., & Bolwig, T. G. (1987). Personality and epilepsy: New evidence for a relationship? A review. *Comprehensive Psychiatry, 28,* 369–383.

Strauss, E., Wada, J., & Moll, A. (1992). Depression in male and female subjects with complex partial seizures. *Archives of Neurology, 49,* 391–392.

Tan, S.-Y., & Bruni, J. (1986). Cognitive behavioral therapy with adult patients with epilepsy: A controlled outcome study. *Epilepsia, 27,* 225–233.

Treiman, D. M. (1986). Epilepsy and violence: Medical and legal issues. *Epilepsia, 27* (Suppl. 2), S77–S104.

Trimble, M. R. (1992). The schizophrenia-like psychosis of epilepsy. *Neuropsychiatry, Neuropsychology, and Behavioral Neurology, 5,* 103–107.

Trostle, J. A., Hauser, A., & Sharbrough, F. W. (1989). Psychologic and social adjustment to epilepsy in Rochester, Minnesota. *Neurology, 39,* 633–637.

Tucker, D. M., Novelly, R. A., & Walker, P. J. (1987). Hyperreligiosity in temporal lobe epilepsy: Redifining the relationship. *Journal of Nervous and Mental Disease, 175,* 181–184.

Whitman, S., Hermann, B. P., & Gordon, A. C. (1984). Psychopathology in epilepsy: How great is the risk? *Biological Psychiatry, 19,* 213–236.

Wilensky, A. J., Ojemann, L. J., Friel, P. N., Almes, M. J., Levy, R. H., & Dodrill, C. B. (1983). Cinromide in epilepsy: A pilot study. *Epilepsia, 24,* 401–409.

Wilkus, R. J., Dodrill, C., & Thompson, P. M. (1984). Intensive EEG monitoring and psychological studies of patients with pseudoepileptic seizures. *Epilepsia, 25,* 100–107.

13 Methodology

Lee Sechrest
Susan Maller
University of Arizona

In the treatment of epilepsy, the primary goal is the reduction of seizure activity. In a few cases, it seems possible to ameliorate seizure activity completely. The two major treatments in the management of epilepsy are drug therapy and surgery. Numerous studies annually provide persuasive evidence that these two interventions may elicit both therapeutic and detrimental outcomes or, often, both. The primary focus of quantitative research on epilepsy is the efficacy of treatment methods. It is imperative to quantify the effects of treatments to ensure that the most effective treatments are employed in clinical practice and to safeguard against the risk of the use of potentially harmful treatments. The importance of the quantification of outcomes in health-care research has been highlighted by Sechrest and Cohen (1979): (a) potential harm of interventions, (b) failure to develop more effective measures, (c) reduction of costs, (d) accountability, and (e) verification of improvement. Unfortunately, several factors frequently confound or weaken the findings of these evaluation studies. The standardization of a treatment program often is open to question, because treatments tend to be complex, delivered by poorly trained or unmotivated people, and can be disrupted totally by events in the real world (Sechrest, West, Phillips, Redner, & Yeaton, 1979).

METHODOLOGY IN EPILEPSY TREATMENT STUDIES

No special justification exists for writing a paper on methodological problems in research on treatment of epilepsy. Methodological problems at more than a superficial level differ only marginally from one field or problem area to another.

Some of the problems are more salient in one area than another, and some are more difficult to deal with, but at bottom they are the same. One does not need to be a subject matter specialist to set forth principles of research methodology and deal with the problems they raise. However, only a subject matter specialist may know which problems are especially salient and which ones threaten to be intractable.

Our aim in this chapter is to summarize a set of methodological issues that have proven widely troublesome, and to give our impressions, admittedly as outsiders, of their applicability to research on management and treatment of epilepsy. At the same time, we want to sketch out an overall research strategy that we believe could be helpful in the field of epilepsy as it is proving to be in other fields. We do not think that the difficult problems in devising and testing interventions for complex problems can be dealt with effectively by a "bag of tricks" methodological approach that considers first this design and then that one. Rather, we need a strategic approach that is based firmly in a coherent "logic of inquiry," an approach that is strategic in nature.

GENERALIZABLE KNOWLEDGE

We begin with the assumption that our aim, as scientists, is to produce knowledge that is generalizable beyond the specific context and circumstances of its production. As wonderful as it might be to know that one apparently had cured a patient of seizures by a novel surgical procedure, our satisfaction as scientists would be minimal unless we had some confidence that we could do the same thing over and over again, with other patients, in other locations, at other times, and, most likely, replicate that success by teaching others to do the same thing.

Many dimensions of generalizability can be, and should be, imagined. To return to our example of a surgical cure for seizure disorder, we may think not only of patients, but of an array of patient characteristics, such as age, gender, general health status, educational level, and so on. We also would think of specific characteristics of the brain lesion, such as its exact type, size, location, and time of onset. We might think of the measure used to assess outcome. The specific measure chosen might be frequency of seizures, but surely we would be interested in generalizing the idea of "successful treatment" to such other functions as cognitive functioning, affective stability, and overall quality of life. Finally, but without having exhausted the possibilities, we would, if we thought about it, want to be able to generalize across specifics of the surgery (e.g., to expect that the results would be largely the same even if the surgery were performed by another team, in another place, with somewhat different equipment, and with reasonable modifications of technique).

A powerful conceptual and analytic framework for thinking about generalizing research findings is provided by generalizability theory (Cronbach, Gleser,

Nanda, & Rajaratnam 1972), although it has not been applied widely. In generalizability theory, each potentially relevant aspect of a total research problem and setting that could vary is termed a *facet* of the research. Many facets of a research setting are fixed within the context of any one study. For example, a surgical procedure might be tested across a number of different patients, but with the surgery always being performed by the same surgical team. In such a series of cases, surgical team would be a fixed facet, and the research would not provide any basis for generalizing to other surgical teams. Other aspects of the overall problem might be variable and a foci of interest. For example, the surgical series might include both younger and older patients, and the results might indicate that generalization across age would be justified (i.e., results did not differ by age). If facets are varied and systematically studied, estimates may be made of the extent of any limits on generalizability. Still other aspects of the research problem might be allowed to vary, perhaps even without any deliberate plan to do so (e.g., different surgical suites might be used, surgeries might be done at different times of the day, and the like). Such variability within, or even across, studies has been termed *heterogeneity of irrelevancies* (Cook & Campbell, 1979), because no reason exists to suppose, a priori, that the variables involved are in any way critical to the outcomes. If variables are allowed to be heterogeneous, then, to that extent, their specific values do not represent limitations on the generalizability of research findings. On the other hand, variance associated with irrelevant variables does constitute noise and can reduce the likelihood that true effects will be detected. If supposedly irrelevant variables are not measured, then their effects, if any, cannot be estimated and partialed out of any differences between groups.

Still, one cannot deal with every possible variable in the context of any one study. From the standpoint of generalizability, it is preferable that variables not specifically to be measured and analyzed should be allowed to vary in a reasonably normal way. Every potential variable that is fixed at some one value in an experiment or other study is a potential limitation on the generalizability of the findings. To some extent, that idea goes against the grain of what often is taught as proper scientific methodology. The latter is frequently taken to require that all variables, save the critical experimental variable, be as carefully and completely controlled as possible. But if, in the real world, surgery is sometimes done very early in the morning, sometimes later, and occasionally in the afternoon period, then no persuasive argument exists for setting the time for surgery at 8:00 a.m. for all study patients. If assessments are sometimes done by male and sometimes by female examiners, then to require that all assessments in an experiment be done by male examiners would not be a good idea. Every variable—facet—of a study that is constrained in any way that would not be a constraint in a wider set of potential observations to which one would like to generalize is a constraint on that generalization.

In fact, every constraint imposed on variables is an implicit acceptance by the investigator that generalization may be limited. For example, why would a researcher specify that "patients were given 2ml of XYZ brand analgesic upon return to their postoperative care beds"? The aim of such description in science is to enable other researchers to replicate the work of the first investigator (i.e., to maximize the probability that the results will *generalize* to other occasions). The very act of specification implies that results *might* not be the same if, say, the dose were 1ml or 3ml, if another brand of analgesic were used, or if the dose were given at a different time. To see that the argument presented here makes sense, think about what is *not* specified: whether the dose was given by spoon or by another container, whether the person administering the dose was male or female, what that person said to the patient while giving the medication, and so on.

Aside from carelessness, three reasons exist for omitting some details from descriptions of scientific methodology. First, some details, particularly those pertaining to individual persons, are omitted because their presentation would be offensive in some way. For example, one would never find in the description of research methodology a statement such as "the phlebotomist employed on the project was physically quite unattractive," although that fact might have some bearing on reactions of research subjects to having blood drawn. Second, some details may be omitted because it may be assumed that they refer to phenomena that are sufficiently standardized in the field that they can be assumed to be invariant. Thus, one would not need to describe in detail just how the phlebotomist goes about drawing blood, or one might not need to describe the origin of doses of aspirin. The third reason for not omitting descriptions of details of research procedures and settings is that it is not readily imaginable that they should have any effect on results. Physical characteristics of research facilities (e.g., color of walls, type of floor covering) are never described unless the investigator wants specifically to call attention to them. To note that "the waiting room was not brightly lit and was decorated and furnished in such a way as to be soothing and restful" would only be relevant if the researcher meant to imply that some other sort of waiting room might have resulted in different research outcomes.

Generalizability theory as set forth by Cronbach et al. (1972) provides a way of estimating parameters reflecting generalizability (e.g., generalizability coefficients). Although estimating such coefficients might be beyond the interests of many investigators, and beyond the possibilities of data actually available for analysis, the conceptual framework provided by generalizability theory is extraordinarily useful. In the planning of any research enterprise, investigators would do well to consider carefully across just what facets they will want to generalize, and then to consider how they would make such generalizations plausible when the research is completed.

CRITICAL MULTIPLISM

A constructive framework from which to plan research that will enhance generalizability of research findings, particularly across sets of studies, is *critical multiplism* (Cook, 1985; Shadish, 1989). That framework constitutes the combination of two prescriptions for research planning: critical thinking and multiple representation.

The critical part refers to the fact that in planning a research effort, decisions about how to carry out the research should be made critically; the opposite would presumably be mindlessly (Shadish, 1991). For instance, one must decide what the outcome measure will be for an intervention study. One might simply elect to use whatever outcome measure is common in the field and let it go at that. That could be fairly mindless decision making if one knew that the common outcome measure had deficiencies or if it were unlikely to capture exactly the outcomes intended from the intervention. If one were interested in the effects of treatment of seizure disorders on reading ability of children, one would use as research subjects children of one gender or the other, or else children of both genders. Critical thinking would lead to an active, rather than a passive, decision about what to do, along with the articulated reasons for doing it that way. Less critical approaches would be of the "convenient," or "seemed like a good idea at the time" variety.

The multiplism component has to do with the fact that only if facets of research are allowed to vary or are planned to vary will we have good grounds for generalizing findings. Multiplism is precisely the thinking behind recent federal legislation that mandates that research supported by National Institute of Health (NIH) will be expected, unless otherwise justified, to include both male and female subjects and subjects from minority groups as well as from Whites. Too much important biomedical research was being done on White males and was regarded as dubiously applicable to females and minorities. That thinking, multiplism, is also behind frequent complaints that so much of psychological research is done on college sophomores.

Any facet of research across which generalizations are desired is subject to the same concerns for narrow representation. For example, drugs used to treat cancer too often are evaluated exclusively in terms of their fairly short-term effects on characteristics of tumors, such as size of the tumor, without regard to effects of other kinds, quality of life being a notable alternative concern. Sometimes it turns out that research findings obtained in one laboratory or treatment center are seemingly not replicable elsewhere. Occasionally it is even the case that a result evident in one statistical analysis is not so in another. Devine and Cook (1983) found that the effect of psychological preparation for surgery had an effect on length of hospital stay, but that effect was considerably reduced in studies done toward the latter part of the period covered by their meta-analysis. They speculated the reason was that changes in policies about reimbursement for hospital care had, by that time, squeezed most of any discretionary variance out of length of stay. Thus, the results of studies were only modestly generalizable over time.

The opposite of multiplism is singularity (Shadish, 1989), fixing facets at single values. Many facets of studies could be vulnerable to the limitations of singular approaches: population, time, place, laboratory, outcome, statistical analysis, interpreters of findings, and so on. That is, results might not be generalizable to other populations, other times, places, laboratories, outcome measures, statistical analyses, and interpreters. A facet that is of great importance in many areas of investigation, but one often neglected almost completely, is representation of treatment. For example, the inclination to employ standard doses of drugs in clinical trials of their efficacy may limit generalization of findings to extra-trial situations, in which drug doses are varied to fit circumstances and characteristics of patients. For instance, some years back, a substantial controversy about the effectiveness of oral hypoglycemics hinged in part on the fact that the clinical trial employed standard doses and found little evidence of efficacy, but proponents of the drugs insisted that they should have been given in flexible doses (e.g., taking into account body weight of patients; Canivet et al., 1971). Various problem areas in social and behavioral sciences, but probably other fields as well, have been limited over periods of time by the dominance of one research paradigm (not in the Kuhnian sense), often with subsequent discovery that findings did not generalize well when aspects of the paradigm were changed.

A patient education program that is defined too precisely and controlled may not yield results that are very generalizable (e.g., if the program is tried with other personnel, in other settings, with a different time schedule, and the like). Somewhat paradoxically, a sloppier version of an intervention may produce results that are actually more generalizable. Thus, if, in a particular experimental study of patient education, the researchers admit that on occasion they had to produce a substitute for the person actually scheduled to run sessions, if they had to change the order of topics for some groups, if some groups had one 2-hour session per week, whereas others had two 1-hour sessions, and if the results of the intervention were still impressive, they should be regarded as even more impressive for their robustness.

If it is possible to assess strength of treatment (e.g., amount, intensity, quality; Sechrest et al., 1979), then variations in strength of treatment become a highly useful and potentially informative variable in the analyses of data. In particular, one may be able to make use of the concept of the *dose-response relationship* to strengthen interpretation of findings. The finding of a reasonably regular relationship between the strength (dose) of a treatment delivered and the outcome achieved is a powerful argument for the causal effect of the treatment.

An obvious objection to the idea of multiplism is that a researcher cannot possibly be expected to do studies with multiple populations, in multiple places, at multiple times, with multiple treatment representations, and so on. That is true, but it is also true that scarcely anything of genuine interest is ever settled by a single study. We look instead to a series of studies to find useful multiplism. However, that multiplism will not be found if a field has settled too narrowly on a set of fixed facets defining the correct properties of studies. We want, over a series of studies, preferably done by multiple investigators, to find variations in samples that result in a range of populations being represented, to find variations in specific circumstances of the studies, in definitions of treatments, in choice of outcome variables, in approaches to analysis, in theoretical orientation taken in interpreting findings, and in many other facets of the overall research enterprise.

What the critical multiplist investigator needs to do is think analytically and critically about the problem being attacked and the field in which it resides and then, to the extent possible, shape his or her own study in such a way as to contribute maximally to generalizability of findings. For example, that means that the critical multiplist should try to discover lurking invariances in the way previous studies have been done, such as restrictions on populations sampled, constraints on definitions of treatments, and narrow conceptions of outcomes. Then the critical multiplist investigator should plan his or her own research to enhance multiplism. The critical multiplist will not want to change everything at once, for then the results, if different from those previously obtained in the field, might not be readily interpretable. The critical part of the critical multiplist prescription comes in trying to determine just how the greatest gain in understanding might be achieved by introduction of careful, systematic, and limited variations into the prevailing research paradigm. Try to determine the potentially important facets that have not been varied in the work of other researchers, and then introduce that variation into studies to be undertaken.

MEASUREMENT MODELS

Good science begins with good measurement. That statement represents such an obvious fact that it is often taken to be either platitudinous or a truism. If either view is correct, then we have to ask why our measurement efforts are not much better than they are and why measurement tasks are not taken more seriously. Meehl (1967) pointed out that, in the physical sciences, when the measurement of some construct is found to be inadequate, every effort is bent toward improving instrumentation, whether by improving an existing instrument or building a new one.

It is customary in discussions of measurement to distinguish between validity and reliability of measures. That distinction is unnecessary, because, as generalizability theory (Cronbach et al., 1972) makes clear, the one central question to be asked of any measure is to what other performances it can be generalized. To the extent that other performances involved the same or highly similar instruments (or other observations), the usual view is that reliability is at stake. To the extent that the other performances are quite different from the one at hand, the issue is more likely to be construed as validity. Thus, if we give a person a self-esteem measure one day and give him or her the same one, or a very similar one, the next day, we usually have in mind test–retest reliability. However, if the next day we give the person the opportunity to name him or herself as leader of a small group, thinking that such behavior reflects self-esteem, we are inclined to think of validity. In fact, both tasks simply tell us something about the generalizability of the self-esteem measure: will it generalize to another administration on another day? will it generalize to a somewhat different task on another day?

Ordinarily, of course, we prefer a high level of generalizability for our measures, but we should not always have that preference. One such limitation is that we want measure that are sensitive to change, particularly to deliberately induced change (i.e., treatment; Sechrest & Cohen, 1979). Hence, we do not want measures that generalize over time if events have occurred during the intervening time that should attenuate generalizability. For example, if clinicians become accustomed to recording blood pressure routinely and are biased by previously recorded values, we may achieve high, but unwanted, consistency over time. When blood pressure changes, we want clinicians to notice. Similarly, a measure of mood states should not be too consistent over time, because moods are supposed to change. However, a measure that is slow to change, or that changes only in very minute ways, is unsatisfactory for evaluating effects of interventions. Thus, to evaluate the effects of interventions, one must select outcome measures for which there is some chance of detecting change.

A second limitation on our preference for generalizability is that we want measures to have *discriminant* generalizability (or discriminant validity). For example, a measure of depression that correlates too well with (generalizes to) trait anxiety would not be optimal. Similarly, we do not want measures that generalize too well to a measure of social desirability. Unfortunately, the discriminant generalizability of measures rarely is assessed. We are faced every year with reports in the literature of numerous new scales, instruments, measure, and so on, with almost no evidence at all about how any of them differs from any previous measures nor from any currently popular measures. Craik (1986) suggested that every study making use of any given measure should include a previously developed measure against which the new one can be calibrated. Absent such a concerted attempt to determine generalizability across diverse measures, we only can assume that we have a lot of differently, often exotically, labeled measures that represent substantial redundancy.

A third limit on the desired generalizability of measures is that we want minimal generalizability on account of shared method(s) of measurement. Whenever any two or more measures are similar in the methods and circumstances of their measurement, they are likely to correlate for that reason, whether they share any conceptual similarity at all. Meehl (1990) wrote about the "crud factor," the tendency for all of our measures to correlate around .3 to .4. Those correlations mean that measures are to some extent generalizable to other measures, but not for reasons that are desirable.

Campbell and Fiske (1959) proposed the multitrait–multimethod matrix (MTMM) as a way of assessing overlap of measures attributable to trait (i.e., substantive variance as opposed to method variance). For example, if the correlations between measures of two different traits by a common method are about as high as the correlations between measures of the same trait by different methods, then one must question the usefulness of the trait measures. The MTMM has not been implemented very often, in part because the data requirements—multiple traits measured by multiple methods—are demanding. Another reason, however, is that no very satisfactory method for analysis of MTMMs was available. Recent approaches by confirmatory factor analysis have proved conceptually and analytically straightforward, with easily interpretable variance estimates resulting (Ferketich, Figueredo, & Knapp, 1991; Figueredo, Ferketich, & Knapp, 1991).

Implementing MTMM methodology will be difficult in a field such as epilepsy. It will not be easy to acquire so much data from sufficiently large samples of subjects to provide stable parameter estimates for variance components. It is likely that the only solution will be for individual investigators to develop plans for cooperative studies. No field should permit itself to be handicapped by inadequate measures, simply because it is difficult to get organized to improve them.

One of the most common sources of method variance is *reactivity,* which is the tendency for values on measures to be affected by the fact of measurement. For example, if someone asks, "How do you like my new haircut?", a strong social pressure exists to respond favorably, "Oh, it's very nice." Similarly, if a person is asked to respond to questions about a treatment that he or she has just undergone, a strong pressure usually exists to respond positively. Usually reactive effects are specific to the circumstances of measurement (e.g., the person might not describe treatment so favorably to an inquiring friend,) and short-lived (e.g., if asked 6 weeks after termination of treatment, the person might not rate it so favorably). Under some circumstances, however, measurement of some phenomenon may change it in an enduring way. Schwartz and Orleans (1967) found that interviewing people about their attitudes toward income taxes could bias their tax returns at a later time. If people were asked questions about penalties for failing to pay the correct amount of taxes, they tended to report more income, although also more deductions, than if they were asked questions about the duty of a citizen to pay taxes and the social use made of taxes.

Researchers employ a variety of strategies to reduce reactivity, often without any explicit recognition that they are doing so. Respondents to questionnaires often are told that the "results are for science," that responses will be kept confidential, that there are no right or wrong answers, or that names need not be put on the answer sheets. It seems reasonable that such strategies should reduce reactivity to at least some extent.

Another approach is to try to use measures that do not require the awareness of people that they are being measured, what are called *unobtrusive measures,* or to use measures that are inherently not reactive. Space does not permit any further explication of nonreactive measures, but a standard reference can be consulted (Webb, Campbell, Schwartz, & Sechrest, 1966; Webb, Campbell, Schwartz, Sechrest, & Grove, 1981). Suffice it to say that reliance on measures that are even moderately reactive can be highly misleading, so much that little credence should be given to such measures, at least when they are used alone. Findings that studies employing reactive measures regularly report better outcomes for a wide range of treatments (e.g., Shadish, 1991; Smith, Glass, & Miller, 1980) are cause for concern. What that means is that conclusions about the favorableness of outcomes of therapies do not generalize well across outcome measures.

If not a solution, at least a major help with many measurement problems is provision for obtaining multiple measures of constructs. Multiple measures, to the extent that they do not share the same sources of error, make possible a triangulation process that should provide better estimates of variables than would be likely from any one, flawed measure. That measures will be flawed must be taken for granted, but only with multiple measures can some estimate be made of the magnitude and direction of error. Of course, if all measures are flawed in the same way and to the same degree, no great advantage is obtained, which is why we ought to strive to use measures that differ as much as possible in all ways except the focal construct of interest. Selection or development of such measures requires a keen awareness of sources of variance in measures so that measures can be identified that do not share, or at least overlap minimally, in extraneous sources.

The term *error* in relation to measurement has a venerable status, but preferable terms might be *unexplained variance* or *residual.* The term *error* implies an indeterministic process that is not entirely appropriate for our problems, because most of the variance in our measures that is residual is probably determined, albeit in ways we may not know, but also albeit in ways that are often discoverable.

Two types of residual effects in measures can be distinguished: bias and random. Bias refers to consistent effects that are, by definition, deterministic in nature. Reactivity of measurements results in bias, that is, consistent tendencies for measures to be higher or lower than they should be (not necessarily better, because malingering would produce bias in a worse direction). Bias would not be a problem if we knew how to detect it, because we could adjust for it. We constantly make such adjustments in our everyday lives (e.g., discounting somewhat the adjectives employed by a commentator who cannot be considered disinterested). However, in research, bias is often a serious problem, because accurate measurement requires that bias be estimated with some precision. Although we may suppose, or even know, that bias exists in some set of measures, estimating the degree of bias with any precision is extremely difficult. For example, suppose in a sample of epilepsy patients, they rate their satisfaction with their physicians at a mean of 4.45 on a 5-point scale, indicating high satisfaction. Suppose also, however, that we discover that 25% of those patients unaccountably change physicians during the subsequent year. We may suspect that the rating of 4.45 was an overestimate of satisfaction, but it would be difficult to know where to set a value that would not be biased. Often the best that additional measures can do, with respect to dealing with bias, is to warn that bias probably exists and suggest that interpretations of finding should be guarded.

What usually is called *random error* is called that exactly because it is, within the context of the study involved, unpredictable; *stochastic* is the term often used. Random error may be deterministic in the long run, but that does not matter for a given study. For example, if persons in two groups are asked to keep a food diary, those who conscientiously fill it out after each meal may produce results somewhat different from those reflecting responses of persons who fill the diary out sporadically or at the end of each day. That variance, although potentially discoverable and subject to estimation, would be random with respect to the intervention differences between groups (*if* subjects had been assigned randomly to the two groups; if assignment had not been random, e.g., people volunteered for the two groups, then that nonrandomness easily could be correlated with variations in diary completion habits such as conscientiousness).

The idea of randomness means that observed scores for some persons are variably higher than they should be, whereas others are variably lower. Randomness also means that scores for a particular individual are likely to be higher than they should be on some measures and lower on others. Measurement precision can, then, be improved by obtaining additional measures whose error component is uncorrelated with the initial measure (i.e., because the second measure, or any additional measures, will have errors unrelated to the original ones, when added, they will tend to cancel out, providing an improved estimate of the true value). The larger the error component, the greater the advantage in having multiple estimates. Consider that one has judgments, let us say of functional capacity, for patients rated by two raters who, in a previous test, have been shown to produce ratings that correlate .80. That means that 80% of the variance in the ratings can be considered dependable. If one decided to have each rater rate each patient, by the Spearman-Brown prophecy formula (Lord & Novick, 1968), their combined ratings would have a reliability of .89, a gain of 9% in dependable variance. But suppose for another task, one had two raters whose ratings correlated only .40; if their ratings were combined, the resulting reliability would be .57—a very substantial gain of 17% in dependable variance. In fact, if one could afford to have six raters, their combined ratings would have a reliability of .80, even though their individual ratings were only .40.

Effects of Unreliable Measures

It should be obvious, but it seems often forgotten, that measures are useful only to the extent that they are dependable (reliable). That truth is, importantly, symmetrical around the equal sign in our equations. Nearly everyone comprehends that one cannot use throws of dice to predict anything, because the results of tosses of the dice are unreliable. Concern is expressed for the reliability of measures of personality, cognitive functioning, and so on that are used to predict behavior of some sort.

Equally important, however, is that unreliable measures cannot be predicted; dice throws are as unpredictable as they are unpredictive. Sutcliffe (1980) presented a particularly cogent discussion of the relationship between reliability of measures and the likelihood that one will find significant effects involving them. For example, if reports of seizure activity are not very reliable, then interventions meant to affect seizures will not produce notable outcomes. The data presented in Table 13.1 illustrate the effects of measurement error on outcomes of interventions.

Column 1 indicates whether cases are experimentals or controls, and Column 2 shows true experimental outcomes measured without error. The correlation between experimental condition and outcome is 1.00. But, when 50% error variance is introduced, as in Column 3, with the resultant observed outcome

TABLE 13.1
Illustration of Consequences of Measurement Error in Dependent Variables

Exper. cond.	*Expect. outcome*	*Error*	*Observ. outcome*
E = 1	5	5	10
1	5	1	6
1	5	1	6
1	5	5	10
1	5	5	10
1	5	1	6
C = 0	1	1	2
0	1	1	2
0	1	5	6
0	1	1	2
0	1	5	6
0	1	5	6
X = 6	Y = 36	E = 36	Y′ = 72
$X^2 = 6$	$Y^2 = 156$	$E^2 = 156$	$Y'^2 = 528$
	XY = 30	XE = 0	XY′ = 264
	var = 4.0	var = 4.0	var = 8.0

$r_{xy} = 1.00$ $r_{xo} = .00$ $r_{xy} = .71$
$R_2 = 1.00$ $R^2 = .50$

given in Column 4, the correlation between experimental condition and outcome is reduced to .71. Instead of 100% of the variance in the dependent variable being attributable to the treatment condition, that variance is reduced to 50%. If only a part of the variance in an outcome measure is dependable, then the possible effect of any intervention will be attenuated correspondingly.

If the reliability of measures (i.e., outcome measures) differs substantially from one sample to another, or from one research paradigm to another, then estimates of treatment effects will vary, even if no true differences exist (Sutcliffe, 1980). For example, if estimates of seizure frequency for children are obtained from parents, whereas those for adolescents are obtained by self-report, and if the latter are more reliable than the former, then a drug used to treat seizures will appear more effective with adolescents than with children. Or, if outcome measures used with surgery are different from those used with drug treatments and are, in particular, more reliable, then surgery will appear to be a more effective treatment than drugs, even if both are equally effective. Most comparisons of interventions of any kind, whether considered across samples, across time, across conditions, and so on, ignore the potential influence of differential reliability altogether.

Measurement Models

The most satisfactory way to deal with measurement problems is to incorporate measurement models into plans for data collection and analysis. A measurement model is a specific conception of variance in measures that is attributable to the way in which they are measured. The assumption of a measurement model can scarcely be avoided; the issue is whether the model is to be explicit and its effects allowed for in analysis and interpretation of findings. For example, multiple regression analyses assume that variables are measured without error; that is a measurement model. The result of applying such a model is that the effects of variables on each other are underestimated. One example is the estimate in one sample that more than 60% of the variance in social skills was accounted for by depression when one took error of measurement of both variables into account, whereas the straight regression (no error) model estimated only about 16% variance overlap between the two attributes.

To the extent that any variable is measured with error, any estimates of its relationships with other variables will be too low. Of course, that statement is true only at the level of theoretical relationships. At an observed level, two variables are related only as well as they are related. They can be made to be better related only by reducing the error. However, at a theoretical level, one wants to know a different sort of thing. If one knows that the relationship between stress and probability of seizures is .3, then, for purposes of predicting seizures, that correlation is all one has. On the other hand, for purposes of planning an intervention to reduce seizures, such as stress management, if one knows that both stress and seizure probability are measured with only 60% reliable variance, then the two variables can have only 36% reliable variance in common. Therefore, a correlation between stress and seizure frequency of .50 would be fairly remarkable, because it would indicate that about 70% of the reliable variance (.25/.36) had been accounted for—nearly three times as much as the .25 implied by the raw correlation of .50.

Observed and Latent Variables

If a person is going out to lunch and decides to check his or her monetary resources before doing so, the actual count of money totaling $15.45 is of interest in its own right. That is how much money he or she has with which to pay for his or her lunch. On the other hand, if that same person, a researcher, includes a question in an interview about the income of a family, he or she may not be interested exactly in the number of dollars the family has coming in each year. Rather, he or she may want to use reported income to infer something about the security of the family or about its social status. Similarly, an inventory item like "I have nightmares frequently" might be of direct interest to a researcher wanting to identify persons to interview about nightmares, but it might instead be regarded as an indicator of anxiety or other distress. These examples illustrate the differences between *observed* and *latent* variables.

Observed variables are measured directly and are interpreted at a manifest level. They do not require inferences about what is being measured. Another important, in fact critical, feature of observed variables is that they are, by definition, *measured without error*. What is observed is observed. That does not mean that observed variables should not be a cause of concern. An important concern is implicit in their use. That concern, paradoxically, is whether the observed value is, in fact, accurate (i.e., without error). For example, if the person counting his or her money before going out to lunch misses a $5 bill and, therefore, actually has $20.45 instead of only $15.45, the observed value is in error. If observed values are so often or so seriously in error that they cannot be taken for what they seem, then they must become interpreted as *indicators* of some latent variable; they lose their status as observed variables. So a first consideration in making use of an observed variable in a model is whether it is plausible that the variable is substantially accurate with respect to what it is supposed to represent. If people cannot be depended on to count their money accurately, then their reported amounts have to be considered as an indicator of some underlying idea of monetary resources, rather than as a veridical statement of resources.

Latent variables are constructs that, in theory, account for variance in what actually is observed. "Money being carried" may be a latent variable that accounts for some, but not all, of the variance in "money reported." The latter value may vary not only because of money actually possessed, but also because of inaccuracies in counting, willingness to report truthfully, and so on. Put simply, latent variables are assumed to be measured with error, and it is the task of the data analyst to estimate and allow for that error. One obvious way of estimating the error is to use multiple measures of the latent variable, which is what is done when one uses multiple items in a questionnaire to measure the same thing or when one makes several observations converging on the same construct. The variability in those several estimates can be used to estimate error and, by inference, dependable variance. However, another possible approach is to use estimates of error obtained from other studies, from the extant literature. It is common for investigators to look into and report published information on the reliabilities of measures they use or consider using. Finally, one may use upper- and lower-bound estimates of reliabilities of measures, bracketing (Reichardt & Gollub, 1986), to do sensitivity analyses to determine the robustness of findings against inadequacies of poor measures.

A form of modeling and statistical analysis called *structural equations models with latent variables* (Bentler, 1989) has the advantage of explicitly incorporating measurement models into estimates of effects of variables on each other. Usually, previously published reliability coefficients for measures simply are reported, with the assurance that the measures are sufficiently reliable to be used in the proposed study. Formal measurement models make actual use of reliability estimates to correct (disattenuate) estimated relationships, most often expressed as path coefficients. However, no reason exists that either previously published estimates or bracketing estimates could not be entered into structural equations models to permit assessment of measurement effects. If one is using self-esteem as a latent variable in a study, one might estimate the error associated with its measurement either by the variability across two or more measures or by a value obtained from some previous study.

Many variables are allowed to enter into studies as if they were observed (i.e., error-free), whereas a little reflection shows that they are implicitly latent variables. Gender, race, age, income, and education are typical examples. Gender may seem like an observed variable because it is measured with virtually no error. But it is measured only as a biological variable; we are only occasionally interested literally in biological gender. More often, we are interested in gender as a proxy variable for a complex residue of cultural experience (i.e., a latent variable). Gender is a far from perfect measure of that residue; males and females differ considerably in the details of their experience and how that experience will have rubbed off on them. Similarly, race is usually of interest as a proxy for a similar kind of cultural residue, as is education. Age may be a proxy for some aspects of physical condition, experience, outlook, and so on.

When variables that are actually indicators—proxies—are entered into analyses as if they were in fact observed, they are assumed to have been measured without error. For example, gender as a proxy for experience is assumed to be a perfect proxy. When the analysis is done without allowing for that imperfection, the invariable result is that the coefficient for the latent variable, the estimate of the effect of the latent variable, will be underestimated. If age is used as a variable in a structural equations (or other) model with the unexplicated assumption that age is a proxy for physical decline, so that age is assumed to be a perfect indicator of that decline, the net result will be that the effect of physical decline, the actual latent variable, will be underestimated. The solution is to estimate, probably best by bracketing, the error inherent in age, or other such variables, as measures of latent variables of real interest.

Improving Measures Is Cost-Effective

In many instances, improvement in measurement is the most cost-effective way to improve a research undertaking. For example, improving measurement can increase statistical power by decreasing error terms, often at a considerably lower cost than obtaining additional subjects. Adding measures of different constructs may enable the testing of competing hypotheses, as recommended nearly 100 years ago by Chamberlain (1965), without necessitating any additional experimental arrangements. In fact, improvement of measurement should be a part of every overall research strategy for dealing with complex problems.

Effect Size Estimates

One further issue related to measurement, which is rarely addressed directly even in applied research, is the size of the effect achieved by intervention efforts (Sechrest & Yeaton, 1981). By *size of effect* we refer to the clinical or social, as opposed to the statistical significance of the effect. One might reduce seizures in an experimental group by an average of .25 seizures per week, and that might be statistically significant. Whether it would be important clinically or socially would be another matter.

How does the researcher measure an effect and determine whether it is a big effect or only a small one? A treatment effect is considered to be present when there is a difference between experimental groups and it is statistically significant. Unfortunately, the magnitude of a treatment effect usually is inferred from the p value; that is wrong, for reasons made clear elsewhere (Sechrest & Yeaton, 1981). In the case of an experimental design, the treatment effect is merely the difference between two means. However, when designs are not purely experimental, such as those often used in the study of epilepsy in humans, the assessment of treatment effects is less straightforward.

Several approaches to the evaluation of effect size may be considered when one is required to interpret the outcome of an intervention study. These may include the following: expert judges, norms, standards, and empirically derived statements of behavioral implications.

Expert Judges. Usually for clinical interventions, the statistical significance of an effect does not adequately reflect the importance of an effect in relation to a patient's welfare. In such situations, expert judges, such as physicians, may be asked to evaluate the clinical importance of an outcome based on their knowledge and experience. For example, clinicians might be asked to assess the importance to patients of having seizures reduced from four to three per week. Although experimental trials may have shown a drug to produce a significant effect, medical practitioners may agree that they do or do not see any clinical advantage in that amount of change.

Norms. It is often useful to judge the effectiveness of a treatment by comparing it to previous or alternative treatments in terms of the costs, risks, and benefits involved. For example, a new drug treatment may be introduced that reduces seizures due to vascular diseases in elderly patients. The magnitude of the reduction may be more meaningful if it is compared with effects obtained with other drugs, with other forms of treatment, or with the effects of treatments in general. A treatment effect may be larger than what might be obtained by other drugs used in the same condition, but if the effect is small in relation to effects achieved for other conditions, enthusiasm for the drug may be tempered.

Standards. For some kinds of conditions or interventions, standards may have been established for what are considered acceptable effect sizes. To illustrate, the common standard for extensively invasive surgeries is a complete ablation of seizure activity. This standard is appropriate, because otherwise the risks of the treatment would outweigh the benefits. Standards could be established for other categories of treatments (e.g., that epileptics of certain types should be managed with no more than X seizures per year). An intervention plan that did not achieve that result would be considered unacceptable no matter how significant the findings from a test of its effectiveness.

Behavioral Implications. An approach to evaluating the magnitudes of treatment effects that needs to be explored and developed is assessment of treatment effects in terms of their behavioral implications. For example, what (more or less) is the consequence of improving the quality of life of a patient by 6 points on a 100-point scale? This example illustrates that many of our outcome measures are not expressed in a metric that has any direct meaning. If we increased the assertiveness of a patient by some amount in a training program, what would that person be able to do that he or she would not have been able to do before? Until we have a better and more behaviorally oriented understanding of the meaning of the effects we produce in our studies, we will not be able to make fair judgments of the worth of efforts to produce them.

GENERALIZABILITY OF CAUSE

The aim of assessing the effects of interventions, or treatments, must be to arrive at causal generalizations, that address five issues (Cook, 1990): treatments, observations, cases, settings, and time.

First, we want to generalize about treatments (i.e., beyond the specific characteristics of the treatment actually implemented and observed). We do not want generalizations about surgery to be limited by the identity of a specific surgeon, the manufacturer of the equipment, the brand of anesthesia used, or the microdetails of how procedures were done.

Second, we want to generalize about observations beyond those specific to the study in question. Of necessity, we must limit our observations to particular measures, specific times, available interviewers, and so on. But we would be dissatisfied if we had to admit that our conclusions about the effectiveness of some intervention applied only to the XYZ Scale of Satisfaction or were limited to judgments made by Joe, Ellen, or George.

Third, any intervention study involves particular persons (or other units of observation and analysis, such as hospitals or groups). We would think our work nearly pointless if the results obtained could not be generalized to new cases. What would be the point of showing that Mr. Jones was helped by an intervention if that were no indication at all that anyone else could be helped?

Fourth, every intervention is carried out in a particular setting, in a complex context of variables thought to be (hoped to be) irrelevant. We want to generalize to other settings, institutions, surgical suites, cities, teams, times of day, and so on.

Fifth, we want to generalize over time. We want to believe that our findings from today will still be true tomorrow and next year. This latter potential restriction on generalization of causal connections is, at a logical level, the most troublesome. The first four issues can be dealt with, at least to some extent, by deliberate research design strategies. Generalization across time requires an act of faith, because we never can sample across time and only can respond inductively from our past experience. Still, for most treatment studies, generalization across time seems to pose no great problems, because we do not expect mechanisms of either problems or change to vary much over time. Comparisons of treatments may differ over time as more effective treatments are developed, but we do not expect the absolute effectiveness of old ones to change. Aspirin is effective as ever, we believe, although many new analgesic and antifebrile substances, some of which may be better than aspirin, have been discovered.

Local Molar Causal (Internal) Validity

The most basic, and obvious, limitation on the generalization of a causal connection has to do with the legitimacy of the claim that any causal connection between two events exists. A whole set of issues surrounding this problem was referred to initially as the problem of internal validity of experiments (Campbell & Stanley, 1966; Cook & Campbell, 1979). Later, Campbell (1986) relabeled the problem as local molar causal validity: did this complex treatment make a difference in this unique application in this particular time and place? A correct answer to that question is at the heart of the difficulties of designing and carrying out worthwhile research.

For a variety of reasons, answering the local molar causal validity question is not straightforward. The reasons have to do with what have become known as threats to validity, to alternative explanations for observed findings that might lead to mistaken conclusions about their actual causes. Good research design—and execution, because carelessness can result in good research going bad—minimizes the persuasiveness of alternative explanations. Space does not permit more than a cursory review of the threats to local molar causal validity, and excellent discussions of them easily are found elsewhere in any case (e.g., Campbell & Stanley, 1966; Cook & Campbell, 1979), but it may be useful to review them briefly here.

Local molar causal validity refers to the confidence that, given that a causal relationship between two variables appears reasonable to suppose, it is not mediated by some other extraneous variable(s). For example, consider a study from which it appears likely that a surgical procedure reduces partial seizures occurring in patients with a focal epilepsy. If cases had been assigned randomly to receive or not receive a surgical intervention, and if all patients were followed for later unbiased measurement, acceptance of the causal connection might readily be accepted. On the other hand, if randomization were not possible or various factors entered in to cause patients to be lost from the study, internal validity might have been compromised.

Selection is a threat to the causal interpretation if cases exposed to the treatment, or those available for later study, are different from those in the comparison group. For example, if subjects were selected for surgery because their lesions were more accessible, outcomes might differ because of that very selection difference. Children whose parents volunteer them for experimental treatments may be different from those whose parents are more cautious.

Differential attrition (sometimes called mortality) from groups also may represent a threat to causal inferences. If patients in one group are more difficult to find at follow-up, that may be because they are less satisfied with treatment or have left the community to seek treatment elsewhere.

History as a threat refers to events outside the experimental context that might explain research findings. If one were comparing two methods of training epileptic children implemented in separate communities, any unusual event in one community and not in the other (e.g., a community epilepsy awareness campaign, a widely publicized story about an epileptic criminal) could result in differences between groups that might, if the investigator were not fully informed, be mistaken for an experimental effect.

Testing is a threat to local molar causal validity if testing is reactive in any way, especially if testing differs between experimental conditions. In a study involving only one group with a simple before–after testing schedule, practice effects may result in improvement over the two testing times. Testing may sensitize patients in one condition to the intervention without affecting the other group in the same way, resulting in a later difference in responses that might appear to be a treatment effect.

Under some conditions, instrumentation differences may exist between groups or over time. A common instance is a research arrangement in which interviewers know which patients are in which research groups (i.e., the interviewers are not blinded). If surgical and nonsurgical patients must be interviewed, it may be difficult to keep interviewers from knowing which patients are which, and any biases of interviewers could be blatant. Or, interviewers may be calibrated differently from beginning to end of a study as they become wiser or more bored. For example, they may change their standards for what they are satisfied with as reports of seizure activity.

Maturation also may be mistaken for treatment effects by unwary researchers. Most fevers are self-limiting and will mature toward normal whether treated or not. Depression tends to be similarly self-limiting, but over a longer period of time. Any types of problems related to seizures that change over time put research at risk of drawing wrong inferences about treatments if protection, by some design feature, is not exercised against those normal change processes.

Statistical regression also may be a problem, especially with measures of limited reliability. The reason is that subjects often are selected for intervention specifically because they are exceptional (extreme) at some moment in time. That very exceptionality may be partly attributable to measurement error—the fact that the persons were "caught at a bad time" or that scores on some measure were deflected away from normal by a chance convergence of random sources of variance. On any subsequent measurement, including those taken after some intervention, such persons might appear to have improved.

Interactions between any of the threats to validity also may occur (e.g., between selection and maturation or selection and statistical regression). The only way to deal with threats to validity is to design and carry out studies so that the threats, often called plausible rival hypotheses, are less plausible than the preferred hypothesis.

Ruling in Causes

The philosophy of science underlying the weakening or ruling out of plausible rival hypotheses is the doctrine of *falsification,* the idea that hypotheses are strengthened by surviving attempts at falsification. However, Einhorn and Hogarth (1986) argued that we infer cause more positively also by insisting that causes must have certain features, such as temporal precedence and contiguity in time and space if they are to be plausible. Cordray (1986), in turn, argued for research strategies best described as "ruling in" causes. That is, we should design and carry out research so that the case for our preferred causal hypothesis is made as plausible as possible.

The aim of much research is to produce a persuasive conclusion about the effectiveness and utility of some diagnostic procedure or treatment. No single outcome study can deal effectively with the entire array of issues surrounding effectiveness and utility. That degree of comprehensiveness is unlikely in the extreme. Still, outcomes research must contribute to the resolution of uncertainty pertaining either to the effectiveness or utility of a medical procedure, or to both; otherwise, the research is pointless.

One critical link in the argument concerning the effectiveness of an intervention is the demonstration that the intervention was sufficient, a priori, to have produced an effect, and that it was implemented well enough to be an acceptable representation of the intended treatment (Sechrest et al., 1979). That is to say, one must demonstrate (rule in) that the treatment was a plausible cause in the first place. Unfortunately, the methodology for assessing strengths of interventions is not well developed, although that does not excuse failures to try. Although, if a treatment protocol can be specified, one can determine where and to what extent departures occurred and what the implications of those departures might be for conclusions about the wider effectiveness of the intervention. Before one concludes that something does not work, one should at least be sure that it has been tried (Sechrest, White, & Brown, 1979).

Strength of treatment refers to the intensity with which the treatment actually is delivered (Sechrest et al., 1979). In the study of the treatment effects of drug therapies, dosage is the most common measure of treatment strength. Making a useful assessment of the strength of a surgical treatment is more difficult, but presumably a conservative strategy that risked not removing all of a lesion would be weaker than a more extensive procedure. More extensive surgeries may be considered optimal, because they result in a complete ablation seizure producing tissue. Obviously, however, strong treatments may not be optimal for all epilepsies.

Integrity of treatment refers to the intensity with which the treatment actually is delivered. Any conclusions about whether a treatment is effective or not can be reached only in full knowledge of how strong the treatment actually was. The integrity of treatment can be assessed fully only after the treatment has been completed. For example, patients may have complied with prescribed drug regimens, but if an individual physician participating in the study altered the planned dosage, the integrity of treatment would have been compromised. For the integrity of a treatment to be maintained, a commitment from all parties involved in the execution of the planned treatment program should be obtained.

Mediating mechanisms are events thought to occur as a direct consequence of interventions and that form the basis for occurrence of longer range outcomes. For example, assertiveness training may be intended to help people attain more control over their lives, which in turn is expected to result in greater life satisfaction. If assertiveness training actually does not produce greater control, then failure to show greater longer range life satisfaction may be understandable. Mediating mechanisms may be particularly important in ruling in a cause when close contiguity in time or space is not evident. For example, if some seemingly modest event in a child's life is expected to result in better adult functioning, then the case for that event is likely to be stronger if it is possible to specify mediating mechanisms that can carry the effect from child to adult years. Even contiguity over space or occasions may be an issue to be resolved by mediating mechanisms if a strong case for causality is to be plausible. Thus, if a change in parental treatment of a child at home is to have an effect on the child's behavior at school, ordinarily one will need to rule in the causal inference by indicating the mediating construct that is meant to bridge the home–school gap.

Although a complete set of recommendations for ruling in causes cannot be specified here—indeed, a complete set has not been developed—researchers should pay more attention to that dimension of their research in early planning stages. Buttressing the positive argument for a preferred causal attribution is an important element of an overall research strategy.

OTHER VALIDITY ISSUES RELATED TO CAUSAL CONCLUSIONS

We do not have space here to give full consideration to two other important sets of issues related to the validity of causal inferences one would want to make from research findings. One set of issues concerns statistical conclusion validity; the other has to do with construct validity.

Statistical conclusion validity refers to the legitimacy of the data analyses as a basis for conclusions to be drawn. This type of validity often is threatened when, owing to small sample sizes, statistical power is compromised. With small samples, a study is biased in favor of acceptance of the null hypothesis, and potentially useful treatments may be abandoned. Unfortunately, when research is conducted on a low-incidence population, which is the case in epilepsy research, low statistical power is a distinct threat to statistical conclusion validity. A related problem is that small samples often result in an excessive number of statistical tests, because variables outnumber cases, and the result may be a serious slippage in alpha. Results may be accepted as significant, because, individually, they are associated with apparently significant test values, but the true value of alpha may be much larger than .05. Inappropriate statistical tests, inefficient tests (e.g., dichotomizing continuous variables), and outright statistical errors are among other common statistical conclusion validity problems.

Construct validity refers to the degree to which the constructs assumed to underlie the processes being studied actually are represented by the measures and procedures employed in the research. Construct validity is thought of most often in relation to measures of variables (e.g., whether a purported measure of self-esteem really measures self-esteem). Thus, construct validity may refer either to independent or dependent variables and their representation in the research. If seizure activity is used as an index of quality of life, and in reality seizure activity is related only weakly to quality of life, then that outcome measure would have poor construct validity. Construct validity also applies to treatments. A classical example is a drug that works because it is a placebo. That is, the researchers are mistaken in thinking that the chemical properties of the drug are the critical factor in treatment effectiveness. According to Sechrest et. al (1979), "problems with construct validity lead to misinterpretation of the results by the original experimenter or subsequent investigators because the experimental treatment is assumed to be something it is not" (p. 18). Consider the example given earlier of patients undergoing surgery for relief of partial seizures. Suppose some of the patients' physicians include add-on medications in the patient's treatment regimen. The resulting problem would be uncertainty about whether any improvement in patients' health status was the result of medication or, perhaps, both.

EXTERNAL VALIDITY

What usually is called *external validity* actually has been of central concern in this chapter, because external validity refers to the generalizability of causal inferences. Hence, we return only briefly to the problems of generalizability. However, they are worth some repetition in an area of applied research such as treatment of epilepsy. Findings that are limited distinctly with respect to specific conditions of their discovery are not of great value to the broader field.

One general recommendation that follows from concern for external validity is the superficially paradoxical notion that research should not be designed and controlled too tightly. What is wanted is heterogeneity of irrelevancies (Cook & Campbell, 1979). That is, all those features of research samples, arrangements, and setting that are regarded as irrelevant should be allowed to vary in a rather natural way. Or, if it is feared that they might be relevant, they should be varied in a perhaps unnatural way. For example, laboratory researchers often make use of white rats purchased from a supplier guaranteeing a high degree of uniformity. That uniformity reduces "noise" or error in experimentation, which jeopardizes detection of subtle experimental effects, but also reduces generalizability of findings to laboratory-reared white rats. No one imagines that findings on white rats would be generalizable to wild populations. A misguided researcher in epilepsy might think, by analogy, that it would be desirable to limit the samples exposed to treatments in a study to 19-year-old males living in St. Louis. That would be misguided, because the results, for reasons we may not understand readily, might be ungeneralizable to epileptics of other ages, to females, or to those in other geographic locales. Similarly, having all surgeries performed by the same surgical team, in the same suite, at the same time of day, and so on, might seem like wonderful experimental precision, but it also would run the risk of limiting generalizability to highly similar conditions, if not to the exact same ones.

Just as in the case of test items, if one wants to generalize across test items, one must provide for variability in those items; and if one wants to generalize across occasions, one must provide for variability in those occasions. If an epilepsy treatment researcher wants to generalize across any dimension, then variability in that dimension must be built into the study. Obviously, if variability can be controlled deliberately and introduced in known ways, then the influence of such variables can be estimated. Practically, however, one cannot control everything, and those variables that cannot be controlled and studied are best left to vary in natural ways and to natural degrees.

AN OVERALL STRATEGY

We have made scant mention of specific research designs to this point, although some examples are discussed briefly at a later point. Part of the reason for that omission is our view that research designs, as such, generally are accorded too much importance in writings on methodology. Some writers treat research design issues as if they could be encapsulated in something like a catalog of dress patterns, through which the consumer might browse until finding one that seems attractive and, perhaps, practical. We do not think that useful research can be produced simply by shopping for a suitable research design that can then be used like a template to cut out a research plan. Rather, what is needed first is a recognition of what the essential problem is, which we think of, in terms of information theory, as *the uncertainty,* and then how that problem may be addressed. We need overall research strategies, of which any particular design is only a part. Central roles must be accorded to the nature of the argument to be made and the type of evidence to which the audience is sensitive, the logic of the general inquiry, measurement, which we have discussed already, and theory. Only then does one get to the question of what tactics are to be followed in assembling a data set.

Theory needs to be mentioned explicitly, because its role, especially in applied research, often is overlooked. Under many circumstances, sound theory can, to some degree, substitute for method. The arguments presented by Lipsey (1990) are recommended, and we only briefly summarize the case for theory here. We do not have reference to high-flown, formal theory. We have in mind modest theory about what a problem is and how the intervention that is planned is supposed to deal with it—what Lipsey (1990) called "small theories of treatment." The better and stronger one's theories are about what is supposed to happen and how it is supposed to happen, the greater the flexibility one has in assembling the data meant to demonstrate those happenings. To take one admittedly extreme example, suppose one investigator proposed that doses of Vitamin C would be helpful to victims of panic disorder, and another investigator proposed that a new tricyclic drug would be helpful. Surely we would exact more stringent standards of evidence for the former than the latter. Supposedly Kurt Lewin, the eminent social psychologist, once opined that "Nothing is quite so practical as a good theory." Lewin had in mind the development of interventions for social problems, but his maxim applies as well to the development of sound research plans.

A satisfactory overall strategy for dealing with a research problem, such as the effectiveness of an intervention, must begin with a clear statement of the focal research issues, a seemingly obvious notion, but one that too often is sloughed over with fairly causal propositions about finding out whether some treatment works. The research issues have to be couched in specific expected outcomes, treatment parameters, populations, research settings, and so on. The strategy should be specific with respect to data to be collected, and every theoretical or other research construct must be represented by one or more variables, preferably more. Ideally, no data should be left over, either (i.e., no data collection should be envisioned for which there is not a place within the definition of some essential research construct). The temptation to throw in variables should be thrown out, as well. The research design and its subsequent analysis then should be formulated in terms of the data to be collected and the issues to be addressed. If the research issues have been specified clearly, the design and analyses that will be required will be almost inescapably evident. For example, if a critical issue has to do with change over time, then a longitudinal data collection effort is necessary, and measures must be chosen that are sensitive to change and not reactive to effects of testing. Then, the statistical analysis will similarly have to allow for analysis of change, whether by repeated measures, a structural equations model with time as a variable, or individual growth curve analysis. If change over time is not an issue, then a longitudinal design is not only not necessary, but may even be inappropriate. For a more complete discussion of these and other issues, see Sechrest and Figueredo (in press).

Sources of Data

We must distinguish between sources of data and types of research designs. Sources of data have to do with from where our observations or numbers come. Research designs are the strategies of obtaining or analyzing data in such a way as to make legitimate the causal interpretations that are wanted as the end result of the research. For example, data may come from existing medical or other records, from data sets collected for other purposes, from previously completed studies, or they may be collected *de novo*. In some cases, new variables may be created from recorded information not remotely related to the aims of the research at hand (e.g., analyses of personal diaries or family photographs to plot the progression of disability). Research designs are the basis for algorithms by which observations (numerical data) are allocated to particular statistical procedures aimed at determining the likelihood that variations in observations are attributable to some intervention. For example, in the case of a randomized experiment, the algorithm is simple: determine what experimental arrangement gave rise to the number and then assign that number directly to that arrangement. In the case of a quasiexperiment, the algorithm may be more complicated: determine the value for the observational unit before the intervention and subtract that number from the number observed after intervention and then assign that difference (gain) score to the arrangement giving rise to the observation. Different strategies may result in algorithms that "correct" observed numbers in diverse ways, or that assign them to subunits for analysis on the basis of diverse characteristics (e.g., gender, age, comorbidity, etc.).

We are more concerned here with research designs and strategies for analysis than with sources of data per se. It is true, however, that sources of data and research designs are confounded substantially along the major fissure of randomized versus nonrandomized designs. For example, in general, reliance on existing records results in data that require correction or allowance for differences that might have arisen for reasons other than the intervention of interest. Conversely, randomized experiments always require collection of data de novo. However, one may occasionally encounter an "as if random" (Lord, 1963) arrangement, which was made for administrative reasons or resulted from some more or less naturally occurring event, that may be explored by use of existing records or new data collection (Wood & Sechrest, 1992). For example, a clinic might have closed with its caseload being split between two other facilities in such a way that no bias would seem likely. If the two receiving facilities handled cases in interestingly different ways, one might interpret differences in outcomes fairly directly and confidently.

Data from almost any source could, however correctly or incorrectly, be subjected to the algorithms and analyses of almost any design. For instance, one could obtain data on temporal lobe surgery done in different ways by two surgeons and simply compare outcomes. To do so would be to treat the data as if they had resulted from a randomized experiment. Similarly, one could take the data from a randomized trial, break them out by patient characteristics such as seizure severity, and analyze them by correcting for any differences; that would represent the strategy of a quasiexperiment. Or one might obtain from medical records the daily incidence of seizures per patient over the previous 6 weeks (retrospective) and then initiate an intervention with a random half of patients followed by another 6 weeks of data collection (de novo and prospective). The resulting data might be treated as a simple randomized experiment using postintervention data only as a pre–posttreatment analysis of change scores, or as two-time series: one interrupted and one not.

Strategies for Generating Data

Four basic strategies exist for generating data relevant to arguments about treatment effectiveness, or any other causal argument. That is, one wishes to make the argument that a given treatment applied in the presence of a particular condition will result in a dependable change in that condition. (For the most part, in medical/health research, one wishes to demonstrate improvement, but the task of arguing cause and effect is the same whether one is arguing for salubrious or deleterious effects.) First, one may, at the simplest level, note the results of application of a treatment and argue that they are so obviously contrary to theoretical or intuitive expectations that they compel acceptance of the cause–effect relationship. Second, one may observe a systematic relationship between the amount or level of the treatment applied and the outcome—the dose response curve—and therefore argue that the treatment must have produced the outcome. Third, one may observe a case (patient, subject, etc.) in one condition, apply the treatment, and then observe that the condition has changed (i.e., precondition minus postcondition equals treatment effect). Finally, one may observe a case to which a treatment has been applied and observe another case to which no treatment has been applied and argue that any difference must have been due to the treatment.

But what of randomized experiments, case-control studies, nonequivalent comparison groups, regression–discontinuity analyses, and so on? Those and other design features of studies are all specific research tactics aimed at enhancing the interpretation (i.e., persuasiveness) of one or the other of the preceding strategies for developing data. For example, a randomized experiment is an attempt to buttress the comparison group strategy to make stronger the argument that the difference between groups is really attributable to the treatment. The addition of a pretest so that the design becomes a randomized trial with a pre–post comparison is aimed at even further strengthening the argument. Similarly, designs in which treatment dosages are varied deliberately, even with reversals, are attempts to strengthen raw, naturalistic observation.

From a more systematic perspective, elaborations on the four basic strategies described here are attempts to deal, in one way or another, with threats to validity of conclusions we draw from our studies (Cook & Campbell, 1979). Each of the four strategies can be implemented in diverse ways, nearly all of which will leave the conclusions from research vulnerable to one or more challenges to the causal interpretation of the relationship of the treatment to the outcome (threats to internal validity). Specific research tactics (e.g., blinding of observers to conditions, random assignment to groups) are directed at reducing vulnerability to one or more of the critical challenges (threats). Specific tactics may weaken one or more challenges in varying degrees and, hence, leave the causal interpretation relatively stronger.

The strategy of arguing from the obviousness of observed outcomes is not likely to be persuasive very often, in part because neither theory nor intuition provide sufficiently firm grounding for judging outcomes. Most often, arguing from the obviousness of observed outcomes is likely to be in the context of case studies or very small samples, adventitiously noted, and in exploratory stages of work. Many of the case studies in the *New England Journal of Medicine* (*NEJM*) depend, for their interpretations, on the argument that it is obvious that they should not have turned out as they did. Fleming's discovery of the antimicrobial effects of penicillin may be another example: In theory, the cultures in the dish should have been thriving. Surgeons may be led to look carefully at certain cases, because no reason exists for why they should have died, perhaps as in early observations of halothane anesthetic. Ordinarily, however, this strategy of arguing from expectations is not productive.

Correlations between administration of treatments and outcomes can be determined either when one or a small number of cases get several treatments whose outcomes can be observed, or when a larger number of cases get treatments that vary in some way that can be associated with outcomes. The multiple treatments (doses) per case instance requires fairly quick response to treatment and equally quick decay of treatment effects or else successive doses may build up or interfere with each other. Some treatments (e.g., surgeries, electroconvulsive shock) are irreversible (i.e., one cannot observe a return to baseline), and others (e.g., surgery) are not only usually irreversible, but they only can be given once and in one standard dosage. Many treatments would be very difficult to quantify in our present state of knowledge, and, therefore, dose–response relationships cannot be estimated readily. The interpretation of observed correlation between treatment and outcome is enhanced by such research tactics as blinding and double-blinding, use of nonreactive outcome measures, alternating treatments, systematic treatment variation, and so on. The results of the observational strategy should be highly persuasive under optimal conditions, but those may not be achieved easily.

The strategy of observing changes in cases from before to after treatment is employed widely; it has the advantage of simplicity and directness. What could be more straightforward than measuring some characteristic of a person before treatment, administering the treatment, and then measuring the characteristic of interest after treatment? Problems arise from the vulnerability of such simplistic approaches to a wide range of threats to validity of any causal interpretation of observed differences. Changes from pre- to postmeasures may be observed, because cases are changing anyway, because instruments change, because cases are expected to change (e.g., patient expectancies), because of secular historical events, and so on (Cook & Campbell, 1979). Therefore, such studies usually require design refinements, such as double pretesting (Boruch, 1974), quantification of treatment to reveal dose–response relationships, and monitoring for secular events and trends.

The best single step to strengthen interpretation of pre- and postdata is likely to be the addition of a comparison group that did not undergo the treatment of interest. Comparison groups can add greatly to the persuasiveness of conclusions. In fact, comparison groups are often essential. The critical issue in employing them has to do with the likelihood that comparison groups differ from experimental groups in no relevant way other than in not having had the treatment of interest. Comparability is reasonably well assured when sample sizes are not truly small and when cases are assigned randomly to treatments (i.e., when the design is a true or randomized experiment). Problems arise when treatment decisions are not made randomly, because then the experimental and comparison groups may be different in some other relevant way, causing the research to be referred to as a "nonequivalent comparison (control) group design" (Cook & Campbell, 1979), which often poses formidable analytic challenges (Reichardt, 1979). When the assumption of equivalence cannot be defended, and that is usually difficult to do when the design is not randomized, comparison group designs are subject to various threats to internal validity. On the other hand, not all threats to validity are especially plausible, and sometimes a combination of good theory, large differences, and the implausibility of some nonequivalencies may make comparison group designs quite persuasive. Often, it must be recognized, no other design choice that would be better is at the same time possible or feasible.

Data From Ongoing Medical Record Systems. Many different medical records are kept that might be exploited usefully for study of medical outcomes. Pharmacies keep records that might be examined to determine drug usage by patients treated under different regimens. For example, one might determine the number of refills for prescribed medications in groups of patients being treated in different behavioral therapies. Hospital records could provide information on a wide range of services delivered, charges levied, complications, lengths of stay, and so on. Medical insurance plans can be especially useful sources of information.

Ongoing medical records, including claims data, have several important advantages, as Wennberg, Roos, Sola, Schori, and Jaffe (1987) noted. If records are well kept and computerized, as most are likely to be these days, they can provide nearly immediate information, often at low cost. They also can make it possible to follow patients over long periods of time. Moreover, ongoing records are not likely to be biased with respect to the aims of researchers (e.g., pharmacies do not selectively record prescription refills), and second surgeries are not more likely to result in claims for some kinds of patients than for others. It is also possible, by relying on ongoing records, to assemble data on far larger numbers of cases than could be acquired on any other basis, thus providing for great statistical power and the opportunity to study relatively rare events. In their prostatectomy study, Wennberg et al. (1987) obtained data on 4,570 patients, ages 65 and older, who had undergone prostate surgery in a period of roughly 4 years in 1 of 16 hospitals.

However, the problems with ongoing record systems are important and result in often severe limitations on the conclusions they justify. To begin with, no one record system may contain all the information desirable for a given study, and matching records across systems may be difficult at best, or impossible altogether. For example, pharmacy records are unlikely to contain any information at all on patient diagnosis, and few record systems will provide more than crude information on outcomes. For instance, almost none will contain information on functional status, except in rehabilitation units, for which functional status is the outcome measure.

Sources of Bias. Upon undertaking any investigation, one should try to discern possible sources of bias in any existing data or to anticipate those sources in data to be collected. If one knows that data may be biased, one can either derive conclusions cautiously in light of that bias or, perhaps, take action to reduce or avoid the bias. Obviously, if one knows that bias exists and can estimate its extent, the data can be corrected for it statistically.

Bias often arises from reactivity of measures (Webb et al., 1981). Reactivity occurs when the act of measuring something changes the value of the measure. For example, patients who know that their pain is being assessed in relation to disability determination may respond differently from patients who know that their pain is being assessed to determine effectiveness of an analgesic. A physician who believes that he or she is being observed from behind a one-way mirror may behave differently from one who believes he or she is not being watched. Webb et al. (1981) offered many suggestions about how reactivity may be dealt with, but a strong, general recommendation is to use multiple sources of information that do not all share the same sources of reactivity (i.e., method variance).

When one wishes to make substantive generalizations across studies that apply different methods to measure related outcomes, the multitrait–multimethod approach (Campbell & Fiske, 1959) is often useful. This approach uses the evidence of converging results across different methods to identify common characteristics that are not limited to any single method of measurement, as well as of converging results across different traits to identify the systematic biases that may be introduced by any given measurement operation, regardless of what characteristic is being measured. It also uses the evidence of diverging results across different traits, regardless of the measurement operations used to assess them, to discriminate between discrepant characteristics that may otherwise be confounded by shared method bias. Recent advances in confirmatory factor modeling have aided greatly in the multivariate analysis of complex multitrait–multimethod data (Ferketich et al., 1991; Figueredo et al., 1991).

Other sources of bias include systematic error (e.g., as might arise from always giving one's institution the benefit of any doubt about a value), deliberate error, poorly calibrated instruments, and insufficiently trained staff. Any source of bias, reactivity or error, is a research hazard when the bias is more likely in one group or at one point than another. An instrument that systematically reads "too high" will not lead necessarily to erroneous conclusions if it is consistent throughout a project, but if an instrument drifts from a pretest to a posttest period, or if an instrument used in one office is less well calibrated than a similar instrument in another office, errors might be made that would affect conclusions about relative effectiveness of treatments.

Choice of Outcomes. The choice of outcome measures, or endpoints, is not always obvious and is often difficult or even arbitrary. For example, survival often is taken as the ultimate outcome in treatment of serious illnesses, but current medical knowledge often permits sustaining of life for long periods of time, but with minimal apparent additional gratifications. Adjustments to survival time to represent quality of life have been suggested in the form of the Index of Well-Being (see Kaplan, 1985) and Quality Adjusted Life Years (Weinstein & Stason, 1977). When outcomes are very different, as might be the case for survival time and for Quality Adjusted Life Years, aggregating outcomes across studies, as is required for a meta-analysis, may result in a nearly meaningless metric. On the other hand, confining outcome measurement to physiological parameters to achieve uniformity of meaning may be equally meaningless (Kaplan, 1990). Particularly troublesome is the indication of opportunistic selection of outcome measures to capitalize on observed differences (e.g., choosing patient satisfaction for one treatment or one study and a physiological parameter, e.g., reduction in seizure severity, in another).

Multivariate Independent Variables

Research of any complexity at all requires the use of multiple independent variables. In experimental work, only infrequently are more than two variables manipulated in the same study. Moreover, in multiple variable experimental studies, independent variables almost always are rendered orthogonal by the procedures of the experiment. By contrast, outside the laboratory and in problem areas as complex as treatment studies, independent variables, those from which expectations of differential outcomes are derived, may range from a few to numerous, and are rarely orthogonal. For example, in a study of treatment of seizure disorder, one might begin with two groups randomly assigned to receive either Drug X or Drug Y. That would constitute a very simple experiment, and, by randomization, the treatment variable would be expected to be orthogonal to all other variables. However, the investigators would likely be interested in the possibility of differential response to treatment related to gender, age, education, prior seizure status of patients, and so on. These variables would not be orthogonal to each other. Then, during the course of the experiment, some patients would be likely to drop out (attrition) of the study for one reason or another. Even if attrition were reasonably equal between groups, which it usually is not, the net result of attrition is almost always that the treatment variable is no longer orthogonal to other variables of interest. Sometimes even worse are the results of differential levels of compliance by subjects within and between conditions. Alternatively, patients may receive differing amounts of treatment, because the delivery system is faulty. Even the best planned experiment can end up disappointing when only a fraction of patients actually gets the treatment as originally planned. Treatment variations are also unlikely to be orthogonal to other variables. The net result, then, is that even well-conceived and properly designed experiments often end up requiring the same sorts of analytic approaches as required for quasiexperimental and observational studies. The vicissitudes of research outside the laboratory are inescapable.

Parenthetically, we would like to comment here that the difficulties in carrying out randomized experiments in real life should not be taken as a warrant for not trying. The very demands involved in planning and doing one's best to carry off a high-quality experiment are quite likely to result in better, more interpretable data than would otherwise result. In our experience, once a study has been planned and is underway, nothing ever happens to improve things. Quasiexperiments do not end up as well as they were planned either.

Several general strategies exist for analyzing multiple independent variables: univariate analyses, stepwise multiple regression, rationally prioritized analysis, hierarchical regression, and common-factor analysis. These strategies are not equally desirable or useful. What limits, or should limit, the choice of analyses are that mindless analyses permit capitalizing on chance, and multiple statistical tests, when done properly, use up degrees of freedom, thus decreasing statistical power. Whether used properly or not, multiple analyses result in alpha slippage (i.e., the probability of a Type I error is larger, perhaps much larger, than .05).

Stepwise regression, which one has labeled *unwise regression,* or some variant of it, consists of simply dumping all the data into a computer and seeing what happens. Stepwise regression first selects the variable with the highest zero-order correlation with the dependent variable. It then picks as the second variable the one with the largest partial correlation with the dependent variable (i.e., with the variance attributable to the first variable removed from both variables). A major problem is that stepwise regression permits capitalizing on chance in ways that can be completely misleading. Most data sets, and especially those involving background variables, are characterized by multicollinearity (i.e., substantial correlations between variables). Thus, for example, if education and income are highly correlated, but both are related to a dependent variable, stepwise regression first will pick the one that happens in the sample to have the highest correlation with the dependent measure. Then, because the other variable is highly correlated with the first, it may not enter into the regression at all. One can then unwisely reach the conclusion that education is an important predictor of perceived quality of life and that income is of no importance at all. On the other hand, because stepwise regression searches relentlessly for the predictors with the largest unique contribution, one can end up with a set of predictors and regression weights that bear little resemblance to the zero-order correlation matrix. A data set for which stepwise regression is the optimal analysis probably does not exist, at least not in the kinds of studies done in the social and behavioral sciences.

Rationally prioritizing variables for analysis may lack precision, because one person's rationality will not be the same as another's. Even so, it is preferable to trusting to the rationality of a set of computer software designed to look mindlessly through the data for the highest relationships. Rational prioritizing means simply that one analyzes data according to the best theory available, looking first for the relationships that are most critical or revealing. The theoretical judgments may be one's own if theory is reasonably explicit and well developed. Alternatively, one may use the aggregated judgments of a series of persons familiar with the problem.

For example, suppose one has available 20 background variables on a sample of persons who have undergone one of two behavioral interventions designed to avert minor seizures. One might suppose that response to the interventions might vary between different types of persons. One could look at 20 univariate analyses, or one could put all 20 variables into a stepwise regression analyses. Neither idea would be a very good one; both permit capitalizing on chance and both expend 20 degrees of freedom in one step. A preferable approach would be to have persons knowledgeable about the problem look through the prioritizing of variables, but one that depends on the same rational processes, is hierarchical regression. Hierarchical regression requires that an order for entering variables into an analysis be specified. Unlike stepwise regression, the order is not dependent on observed values of statistical parameters; the order should reflect the best theory available. Unlike univariate tests, hierarchal multiple regression conserves degrees of freedom and minimizes alpha slippage. Also, unlike univariate analyses, hierarchical regression yields an estimate of the strength of the overall model for explaining the dependent variable. If one has theory that will support the thinking necessary, hierarchical regression also permits testing of interactions between variables. One can construct new variables consisting of the products of two or more other variables, so that the regression coefficient associated with the product term will reflect the value of the interaction variable.

The final strategy for dealing with multiple dependent variables, and one we think should be used more often, is data reduction by way of common-factor analysis. For example, it is unlikely that one would have 20 orthogonal independent variables. Multicollinearity is almost certain to obtain within such a data set, and the collinearity points to the desirability of reducing the data set by combining variables that reflect the influence of a common factor. If income and education are highly correlated, that probably means that they both reflect some common factor of social advantage or the like. Factor analysis is the usual and generally most useful method of data reduction, but, again, rational methods can be used. That is, one can use theory or expert judgments to combine variables to produce indexes of more basic variables (factors). Common-factor index construction preserves degrees of freedom and reduces alpha slippage. Subsequent to the derivation of a small number of variables representing common factors, one then may analyze the derived variables by univariate analyses, making allowances for alpha slippage by a Bonferroni procedure (Kirk, 1982) or some equivalent, or one can enter the derived variables into hierarchical regression analyses.

Multiple Dependent Variables

The number of dependent variables in research is ordinarily smaller than the number of independent variables, usually much smaller, and often limited to only a single variable. If one is testing a treatment meant to reduce frequency of seizures, then the frequency of seizures is a single, critical outcome variable. Things are rarely that simple, however. For example, even if one were interested in reduction of frequency of seizures, one might also want to assess severity of seizures and overall quality of life. Turning six mild seizures per day into two severe seizures would not be much of a gain, nor would prevention of those seizures at the cost of eliminating most pleasures in a patient's life.

The most common way to deal with multiple dependent variables (outcomes) is to treat each one as a separate outcome (or endpoint) and do separate analyses of each. Integration of findings, then, is done subsequently in a more or less common sense way. If both frequency and severity of seizures are reduced by the intervention, then no problem arises. If one is reduced but not the other, then one discusses the implications of that finding. If two findings end up with opposite valences, the discussion usually includes mention of trade-offs or some similar quasieconomic concept.

Analysis of dependent variables can be facilitated by reducing their number if several such variables reflect a common factor. For example, reduction in seizure frequency, increased optimism, and decrease in absence from work might all reflect a common factor of improvement. Because those variables are assessed in entirely different metrics, one cannot simply add them together to produce a single variable. However, if one supposes that they are of approximately equal importance, one can standardize each variable separately and then add them to produce a common variable. That variable would then be the focus of interest in assessing an intervention.

An objection might be raised that the three variables might still possess unique variance of interest. That is dealt with easily by residualizing each variable on the common factor. Three new variables result, each reflecting the variance not associated with the common factor. An immediate following objection would be that one now has four outcome variables, where there were previously only three. What one actually has, however, is a common factor of improvement and three residuals. One can determine whether the intervention affects any or all of the specific variables over and above its effects on the common factor. For instance, one might find that the intervention had an effect on the common factor, but also an effect on the optimism residual but not on the other two. That finding would mean that the intervention had the effect of improving patients' situations generally, but that it also had an effect on optimism over and above its specific effects on seizures and absences from work. That kind of detailed insight into outcomes is well beyond knowing that an intervention affects all three variables considered separately. If the intervention had no effect on any residual variable, that also would be a critical insight, because it would suggest that whatever improvement is produced is quite general in nature.

RESEARCH DESIGNS

The concept of *research design* would be better thought of as part of a set of research tactics aimed at dealing with various of the issues described previously. For example, references to a "wait-list control" design often are found in the literature. In fact, no one wait-list control design should be considered as a separate entity. Wait-listing is a way of getting around what are seen as ethical problems with no-treatment conditions, but research subjects may be assigned randomly to wait-lists, they may get on such lists on a first-come, first-served basis, or may be assigned to them in any other way. Wait-list procedures may be associated with cross-sectional, longitudinal, or time-series data. They may result in data to be analyzed by any statistical procedure in the analyst's range of competencies. Similarly, most other research designs may be seen as flexible parts of larger strategies, and their nature cannot be understood fully outside the context of strategic considerations.

Randomized experiments, often called clinical trials in biomedical literature, generally are regarded as the method of choice for research, because they are thought to provide the strongest basis for causal inferences. The essential feature of randomized, or true, experiments is that treatments are assigned randomly to cases (or vice versa). Hence, if they are reasonably large, groups can be regarded as initially equivalent with respect to unobserved variables that might affect, or be correlated with, outcomes. In a true experimental design, the independent variable (e.g., a drug or surgery) is usually under the direct control of the investigator. But it only may be that exposure to the independent variable is controlled (e.g., patients might be assigned to different clinics without any direct involvement of investigators in those clinics). However, control over treatment is not a distinguishing feature of randomized experiments, because that control may be exercised equally in nonexperimental designs (e.g., nonequivalent control groups, pretest–posttest designs without control groups, etc.).

Randomized experiments often provide a strong basis for causal conclusions, but they do not resolve all research issues. In fact, randomized experiments may not always be the method of choice even if they are feasible. One reason is that randomized experiments are easier to plan than to carry out in most cases. Very often, randomized experiments require such intricate and precarious arrangements that they cannot be implemented successfully. For example, if experimental treatment conditions are too different and seemingly disadvantageous to one group or another, subjects may drop out of that condition more readily, rendering the randomization process irrelevant at the point of analysis. Randomized experiments may require such special arrangements that sample sizes are necessarily small, thus limiting their statistical power. Moreover, randomized experiments are likely to be carried out in the context of such special arrangements, such as inclusion–exclusion criteria for patients, intrusiveness of measurement, and so on, that the external validity of findings is limited exceptionally. In biomedical research, a distinction is made between efficacy and effectiveness studies. Efficacy studies are those carried out under more or less ideal conditions; effectiveness studies are carried out under real-life conditions. Treatments that are found efficacious very often are found limited in effectiveness when clinicians cannot carry out the treatments, patients will not comply, and the like. Randomization and the consequent strength in local molar validity may not always represent a good trade-off when critical issues have to do with generalizability, and that will be particularly the case if the strength of the randomized experiment cannot be maintained anyway.

If a randomized experiment seems like the best choice, the researcher must recognize that any such experiment has a point of randomization (i.e., a particular point in the total experimental procedure at which randomization must take place). The point chosen for randomization can have important consequences for interpretation of ultimate research findings and for their generalizability. For example, suppose the effects of phenytoin versus carbamazepine on the lipid levels of patients suffering from tonic–clonic seizures is to be evaluated. Patients who are prospective research subjects must be approached to determine whether they are willing to participate in an experiment, and they must be assigned to one of the two experimental conditions. Prospective patients could be assigned randomly to one of the groups and then asked whether they will participate. In that way, all eligible patients are in one group or another, but some may refuse to participate in the experiment and others may refuse to participate once they find out what the experimental conditions are. Unfortunately, the assumptions involved in randomization require that all patients randomly assigned be regarded as having been in the experiment, even if they do not participate further. With randomization at the early point, one runs the risk that any experimental effects would wash out because of nonparticipation. Alternatively, one might first ascertain that patients are willing to participate in the experiment and then assign them randomly to experimental conditions. However, in that case, the results would be generalizable only to persons willing to volunteer for experiments. That might not be so much of a limitation in a study comparing two similar drugs, but suppose the drugs had serious side effects or suppose one of the conditions were surgery. The limitation of generalizability to volunteers might be troublesome.

The *Nonequivalent Comparison Group Design* (NCGD) is not really a research design in the way that, for example, a "two-way factorical ANOVA with randomized blocks" is a design. Rather, the NCGD is a generalized set of tactics for implementing a comparison group strategy. The only thing one can say for certain about the NCGD is that at least one group not getting the treatment of interest is available for comparison with the (experimental) group getting the treatment, and that subjects have not been assigned randomly to the groups. (Strictly speaking, any randomized experiment in which *any* subjects are lost or dropped from the study for any reason has become a NCGD.) How the comparison group will have been selected, how similar it will be to the treatment group, and whether more than one comparison group will be available are all unspecified. Almost certainly, however, the NCGD is the most common quasiexperimental research approach.

The major problem with the NCGD is that if groups were not really comparable prior to the treatment, one cannot be certain that any subsequent differences between them are attributable to the treatment (i.e., the causal inference is jeopardized). Various approaches exist for trying to discern and deal with initial inequalities between groups (e.g., analysis of selection bias by "selection modeling") (Heckman & Hotz, 1989), correction of scores on the dependent variable for initial differences (Reichardt, 1979), and so on. None of these approaches is completely satisfactory, because no way exists for knowing whether corrections made were exactly, or even nearly, right.

The value of the NCGD cannot solely depend on the sophistication of statistical analyses. Instead, its value depends on the crucial role it can play in an overall strategy of argument in showing that the hypothesis of a treatment effect is plausible. The NCGD can help greatly to rule in a cause. The remainder of the case for the causal effect generally must lie in the logic of the inquiry and the consistency of the findings. For example, the argument must be structured in such a way as to support the proposition that the outcomes found are not only plausible in relation to the nature of the treatment, but that they are not so readily explained by hypothesized biases (i.e., threats to validity). Thus, weak outcomes easily may be written off as reflections of bias in the study, but it may be much more difficult to dispose of strong, large effects in the same way.

That latter proposition suggests that an important part of the overall research strategy, especially when one knows that the research design will be weak and open to attack, is to implement the treatment in as strong a form and in as well controlled a way as possible. It also suggests that a good theory of the treatment will be relatively more important when a NCGD must be relied on. The parts of an overall strategy must be carefully conceived and they must fit together.

Time-series designs might not seem to be of much use in studying interventions related to seizure disorder, because of the large number of data points needed—usually 50 or more. Still, the interrupted time-series deserves mention, because it is reasonably robust against most threats to validity. An interrupted time-series is one for which a number of observations are available for a baseline period, which is then interrupted by an intervention, following which a number of additional observations are made. To be concrete about it, one might have observations of frequency of seizures for a patient over some period of time, then a surgical intervention a subsequent set of observations. Converting these data into a time-series would require disaggregating the data into seizures per some consistent unit of time and then testing a plausible model to account for any changes from the pre- to the postintervention period. Time-series analysis takes advantage of the series of observations to determine a trend and error around it; to do that, at least 25 observations are recommended for either side of the intervention. That seems like a lot of observations, but if one understands that the time periods might be days or weeks (i.e., in contrast to months or years), the time frame is not so objectionable. The number of observations depends on the stability of the data considerably, and if, to revert to the example, the number of seizures per day differed wildly, more observations would be necessary.

Analysis of time-series data depends on the ability to model the effects expected. A simple change at the intercept (e.g., a drop in number of seizures per day) is relatively easy to model, and time-series is best suited to instances in which the intervention is fairly abrupt and limited in time. Interventions that must be phased in, as might be the case for a drug that requires time to build up in body tissue, are more difficult to study by time-series, because their effects are more difficult to model. For such treatments, one would need to know when to expect to begin to observe some effects, what the rate of change (slope) would be, when asymptote might be achieved, and so on. Nonetheless, time-series is potentially a useful and underused addition to the armamentarium of research tactics available to the researcher.

Simple pretest–posttest comparisons are a tempting option to evaluate treatment, but they usually are not persuasively interpretable. However, it is useful to explicate the conditions under which they may be interpretable, both to show why they are not often dependable and the infrequent circumstances under which they might be considered for use. A simple pretest–posttest comparison would be exemplified by a case in which a patient had averaged four seizures per day for nearly 4 months and then was put on a drug, with an observed decrease in seizure frequency. The investigator might want to conclude that the drug was effective in reducing seizure frequency.

Under what circumstances might outsiders view findings from such a study with some degree of acceptance? At least some of the conditions are easy to specify:

1. The theoretical basis for the intervention should be strong.
2. The measurements should be done carefully.
3. The dependent variable should not be subject to much fluctuation or spontaneous recovery.
4. The change should be substantial, not easily explained except with reference to the intervention.
5. The investigator must be objective and disinterested.

Such conditions may only be attainable infrequently; but when they are, investigators should seize on the opportunities.

Multiplism and Patched-Up Designs

All of the designs mentioned can be strengthened greatly by multiple approaches, some of which may be regarded as replications and some as patching up of designs. For example, a time-series done on one patient may be of interest, but if it can be replicated across several patients, the results will, if they are consistent, be enhanced greatly in persuasiveness. That will be particularly true if some irrelevant features are heterogeneous (e.g., if the different patients are observed at different times of the year, in different places, etc.). Similarly, a simple pretest–posttest comparison will, if consistently replicated across cases but in the context of variable specific features, be more persuasive. Even a NCGD may be more persuasive if it involves multiple groups, both treatment and control, because with multiple instances collected under the right circumstances, it becomes less and less credible that any consistent bias should have operated across all observations.

To be fully interpretable, even randomized experiments may require multiple control groups. For example, a no treatment control group may be needed to demonstrate that the case for any treatment effect at all is credible, and another may be needed to show that the treatment effect is specific (e.g., that it is not a placebo effect). NCGDs can often benefit from multiple comparison groups, each of which addresses some subset of threats to the preferred causal interpretation of the experiment. The use of multiple comparisons in quasiexperimentation sometimes is called patched-up design. In some instances, the multiple comparisons may involve extra groups. One group might be observed because it would help to rule out the threat of maturation, and another group might help to rule out regression artifacts. A time-series may be strengthened by an additional time-series lacking the critical interruption. In some instances, however, multiple comparisons may be in the form of multiple measures. A time-series may be enhanced by a parallel series of observations on a measure not thought to be susceptible to the intervention, or a comparison of two groups in terms of treatment effects may be enhanced by showing that they do not differ in some other critical variables thought to be related to susceptibility to change.

Evident from the foregoing is the fact that planning of a satisfactory research strategy is not a matter of following some set of formulae; a great deal of judgment, some verging on artistry, is involved. Goethe supposedly once said: "Science is an art—it isn't a science" (Howard, 1986, p. 131). We could not agree more.

REFERENCES

Bentler, P. M. (1989). *EQS: Structural equations program manual.* Los Angeles: BMDP Statistical Software, Inc.

Boruch, R. (1974). Double pretesting as a strategy for dealing with regression artifacts in quasi-experimental designs. Unpublished manuscript, Northwestern University, Evanston, IL.

Campbell, D. T. (1986). Relabeling internal and external validity for applied social scientists. In W. Trochim (Ed.), *Advances in quasi-experimental design and analysis* (pp. 67–77). San Francisco: Jossey-Bass.

Campbell, D. T., & Fiske, D. W. (1959). Convergent and discriminant validation by the multitrait–multimethod matrix. *Psychological Bulletin, 56,* 81–105.

Campbell, D. T., & Stanley, J. C. (1966). *Experimental and quasi-experimental designs for research on teaching.* Chicago: Rand McNally.

Canivet, J., Deuil, R., Eschwege, E., Hazard, J., Lubetzki, J., Tchobroutsky, G., & Valleron, A. (1971). Do oral antidiabetics play a part in the cardiovascular mortality of diabetics? Apropos of the University Group Diabetes Program report and the controversies it has raised. *Presse Medicale, 79,* 2437–2444.

Chamberlain, T. (1965). The method of multiple working hypotheses. *Science, 148,* 754–759. (Original work published 1895)

Cook, T. D. (1985). Postpositivist critical multiplism. In L. Shotland & M. M. Mark (Eds.), *Social science and social policy* (pp. 21–62). Beverly Hills, CA: Sage.

Cook, T. D. (1990). The generalization of causal connections: Multiple theories in search of clear practice. In L. Secrest, E. Perrin, & J. Bunker (Eds.), *Research methodology: Strengthening causal interpretations of non-experimental data.* U. S. Department of Health & Human Services.

Cook, T. D., & Campbell, D. T. (1979). *Quasi-experimentation: Design and analysis for field settings.* Boston: Houghton-Mifflin.

Cordray, D. S. (1986). Quasi-experimental analysis: A mixture of methods and judgment. In W. M. K. Trochim (Ed.), *Advances in quasi-experimental design and analysis. New Directions in Program Evaluation* (No. 31, pp. 9–28). San Francisco: Jossey-Bass.

Craik, K. H. (1986). Personality research methods: A historical perspective. *Journal of Personality, 54,* 18–51.

Cronbach, L. J., Gleser, G. C., Nanda, H., & Rajaratnam, N. (1972). *The dependability of behavioral measurements: Theory of generalizability of scores and profiles.* New York: Wiley.

Devine, E. G., & Cook, T. D. (1983). The meta-analytic analysis of effects of psychoeducational: Interventions on length of post-surgical hospital stay. *Nursing Research, 32,* 267–274.

Einhorn, H. J., & Hogarth, R. M. (1986). Judging probable cause. *Psychological Bulletin, 99,* 3–19.

Ferketich, S. L., Figueredo, A. J., & Knapp, T. R. (1991). The multitrait–multimethod approach to construct validity. *Research in Nursing and Health, 14,* 315–320.

Figueredo, A. J., Ferketich, S. L., & Knapp, T. R. (1991). More on MTMM: The role of confirmatory factor analysis. *Research in Nursing and Health, 14,* 387–391.

Heckman, J. J., & Hotz, J. (1989). Choosing among alternative nonexperimental methods for estimating the impact of social programs: The case of manpower training. *Journal of the American Statistical Association, 84,* 862–877.

Howard, G. S. (1986). *Dare we develop a human science?* Notre Dame, IN: Academic Publications.

Kaplan, R. M. (1985). Quantification of health outcomes for policy studies in behavioral epidemiology. In R. M. Kaplan & M. H. Criqui (Eds.), *Behavioral epidemiology and disease prevention* (pp. 31–54). New York: Plenum.

Kaplan, R. M. (1990). Behavior as the central outcome in health care. *American Psychologist, 45,* 1211–1220.

Kirk, R. E. (1982). *Experimental design: Procedures for the behavioral sciences* (2nd ed.). Belmont, CA: Brooks, Cole.

Lipsey, M. W. (1990). Theory as method: Small theories of treatments. In L. Sechrest, E. Perrin, & J. Bunker (Eds.), *Research methodology: Strengthening causal interpretations of nonexperimental data* (pp. 33–51). Rockville, MD: DHHS, Agency for Health Care Policy and Research.

Lord, F. M. (1963). Elementary models for measuring change. In C. W. Harris (Ed.), *Problems in measuring change* (pp. 21–38). Madison: University of Wisconsin Press.

Lord, F. M., & Novick, M. R. (1968). *Statistical theories of mental test scores.* Reading, MA: Addison-Wesley.

Meehl, P. E. (1967). Theory testing in psychology and physics: A methodological paradox. *Philosophy of Science, 34,* 103–115. [Reprinted in D. E. Morrison & R. E. Henkel (Eds.). (1970). *The significance test controversy.* Chicago: Aldine.]

Meehl, P. E. (1990). Why summaries of research on psychological theories are often uninterpretable. *Psychological Reports, 66,* 195–244.

Reichardt, C. S. (1979). The statistical analysis of data from nonequivalent group designs. In T. D. Cook & D. T. Campbell (Eds.), *Quasi-experimentation: Design and analysis issues for field settings* (pp. 147–206). Boston: Houghton-Mifflin.

Reichardt, C. S., & Gollub, H. F. (1986). Satisfying the constraints of causal modeling. In W. M. K. Trochim (Ed.), *Advances in quasi-experimental design and analysis. New directions in program evaluation* (No. 31, pp. 91–107). San Francisco: Jossey-Bass.

Schwartz, R. D., & Orleans, S. (1967). On legal sanctions. *University of Chicago Law Review, 34,* 274–300.

Sechrest, L., & Cohen, R. Y. (1979). Evaluating outcomes in health care. In G. C. Stone, F. Cohen, & N. E. Adler (Eds.), *Health psychology handbook* (pp. 369–394). San Francisco: Jossey-Bass.

Sechrest, L., & Figueredo, A. J. (in press). Approaches used in conducting outcomes and effectiveness research. In P. Budetti (Ed.), *A health research agenda for outcomes and effectiveness research.* Alexandria, VA: Health Administration Press.

Sechrest, L., Maller, S., & Hu, J. (1992). *Approaches to the analysis of small data sets.* Manuscript in preparation, based on papers given at Southwestern and Rocky Mountain Regional Meeting of the American Association for the Advancement of Science, Tucson, AZ.

Sechrest, L., West, S. G., Phillips, M. A., Redner, R., & Yeaton, W. (1979). Some neglected problems in evaluation research: Strength and integrity of treatments. In L. Sechrest, S. G. West, M. A. Phillips, R. Redner, & W. Yeaton (Eds.), *Evaluation studies review annual* (Vol. 4, pp. 15–36). Beverly Hills, CA: Sage.

Sechrest, L., White, S., & Brown, E. (1979). *Rehabilitation of criminal offenders: Problems and prospects*. Washington, DC: National Research Council.

Sechrest, L., & Yeaton, W. H. (1981). Empirical bases for estimating effect size. In R. F. Boruch, P. M. Wortman, D. S. Cordray, & Associates (Eds.), *Reanalyzing program valuations: Policies and practices for secondary analysis of social and educational programs*. (pp. 212–224). San Francisco: Jossey-Bass.

Shadish, W. (1989). Critical multiplism: A research strategy and its attendant tactics. In L. Sechrest, H. Freeman, & A. Mulley (Eds.), *Health services research methodology: A focus on AIDS* (pp. 5–28). Rockville, MD: National Center for Health Services Research and Health Care Technology Assessment.

Shadish, W. (1991, October). *Programming and implementation implications from a family therapy meta-analysis*. Paper presented at the meeting of American Evaluation Association, Chicago.

Smith, M. L., Glass, G. V., & Miller, T. I. (1980). *The benefits of psychotherapy*. Baltimore, MD: Johns Hopkins University Press.

Sutcliffe, J. P. (1980). On the relationship of reliability to statistical power. *Psychological Bulletin, 88,* 509–515.

Webb, E., Campbell, D. T., Schwartz, R. D., & Sechrest, L. (1966). *Unobtrusive measures: Nonreactive measures in the social sciences*. Chicago: Rand McNally.

Webb, E., Campbell, D. T., Schwartz, R. D., Sechrest, L., & Grove, J. (1981). *Nonreactive measures in the social sciences*. Boston: Houghton-Mifflin.

Weinstein, M. C., & Stason, W. B. (1977). Foundations of cost-effectiveness analysis for health and medical practice. *New England Journal of Medicine, 296,* 716.

Wennberg, J. E., Roos, N., Sola, L., Schori, A., & Jaffe, R. (1987). Use of claims data systems to evaluate health care outcomes: Mortality and reoperation following prostatectomy. *Journal of the American Medical Association, 257,* 933–936.

Wood, J., & Sechrest, L. (1992, March). *Natural experiments in the social sciences*. Paper presented at the meeting of Southwestern and Rocky Mountain Region of American Association for the Advancement of Science, Tucson, AZ.

Author Index

Note: Italicized page numbers refer to bibliography pages.

Z

Subject Index

T

UV

WZ